Obstetrics and
Gynecology
at a Glance

Obstetrics and Gynecology at a Glance

Errol R. Norwitz

MD, PhD(Oxon), FACOG
Louis E Phaneuf Professor of Obstetrics & Gynecology
Tufts University School of Medicine
Chairman, Department of Obstetrics & Gynecology
Tufts Medical Center
Boston, MA, USA

John O. Schorge

MD, FACOG, FACS
Associate Professor of Obstetrics, Gynecology and Reproductive Biology
Harvard Medical School
Chief, Gynecologic Oncology Service
Department of Obstetrics and Gynecology
Massachusetts General Hospital,
Boston, MA, USA

Fourth Edition

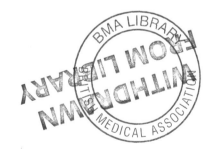
WILEY-BLACKWELL

A John Wiley & Sons, Ltd., Publication

Library of Congress Cataloging-in-Publication Data

Norwitz, Errol R., author.
  Obstetrics and gynecology at a glance / Errol R. Norwitz, John O. Schorge. – Fourth edition.
      p. ; cm. – (At a glance)
  Includes bibliographical references and index.
  ISBN 978-1-118-34173-5 (pbk. : alk. paper) – ISBN 978-1-118-34478-1 (Mobi) –
ISBN 978-1-118-34479-8 (ePub) – ISBN 978-1-118-34480-4 (ePdf) – ISBN 978-1-118-73234-2 –
ISBN 978-1-118-73241-0
  I. Schorge, John O., author.   II. Title.   III. Series: At a glance series (Oxford, England)
  [DNLM: 1. Genital Diseases, Female–Handbooks.   2. Pregnancy Complications–Handbooks.
WP 39]
  RG110
  618–dc23
                           2013017944

A catalogue record for this book is available from the British Library.

Contents

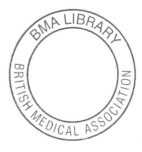

List of contributors

Laura Baecher-Lind, MD, MPH
Assistant Professor of Obstetrics and Gynecology
Tufts University School of Medicine
Boston, MA, USA

Lori R. Berkowitz, MD
Assistant Professor of Obstetrics, Gynecology and Reproductive
Biology
Massachusetts General Hospital, Harvard Medical School
Boston, MA, USA

Brian K. Bond, PharmD, MD
Assistant Professor of Obstetrics and Gynecology
Associate Director, Obstetrics and Gynecology Residency Program
Tufts University School of Medicine
Boston, MA, USA

Kelley E. Conroy, MD
Clinical Fellow in Maternal-Fetal Medicine
Tufts University School of Medicine
Boston, MA, USA

Alissa R. Dangel, MD
Assistant Professor of Obstetrics and Gynecology
Tufts University School of Medicine
Boston, MA USA

Kristen P. Eckler, MD
Assistant Professor of Obstetrics, Gynecology and Reproductive
Biology
Massachusetts General Hospital, Harvard Medical School
Boston, MA, USA

Trevin C. Lau, MD
Instructor of Obstetrics, Gynecology and Reproductive Biology
Massachusetts General Hospital, Harvard Medical School
Boston, MA, USA

Samantha J. Pulliam, MD
Assistant Professor of Obstetrics, Gynecology and Reproductive
Biology
Division of Urogynecology and Pelvic Reconstructive Surgery
Massachusetts General Hospital, Harvard Medical School
Boston, MA, USA

Aaron K. Styer, MD
Assistant Professor of Obstetrics, Gynecology, and Reproductive
Biology
Vincent Reproductive Medicine and IVF
Vincent Center for Reproductive Biology
Massachusetts General Hospital, Harvard Medical School,
Boston, MA, USA

Hong-Thao N. Thieu, MD
Assistant Professor of Obstetrics and Gynecology
Director, Obstetrics and Gynecology Residency Program
Tufts University School of Medicine
Boston, MA, USA

Carey M. York-Best, MD
Assistant Professor of Obstetrics, Gynecology and Reproductive
Biology
Chief, Division of General Obstetrics and Gynecology
Massachusetts General Hospital, Harvard Medical School
Boston, MA, USA

Preface

The medical and scientific problems of this world cannot be solved by skeptics whose horizons are limited by practical realities. We need women and men who dream of things that cannot be and ask why not.

Professor Egon Diczfalusy, Karolinska Institute,
Stockholm, Sweden, 1992

Medicine continues to attract the brightest and most dedicated students to its ranks. The opportunity to nurture the talented young minds that will one day rise up to lead the medical community remains the single greatest privilege for the academic clinician. Nowhere is this privilege – and challenge – more apparent than in obstetrics and gynecology, a discipline that remains more art than science. Although clinicians in all disciplines aspire to practice rational evidence-based medicine, many basic questions in the field of obstetrics and gynecology remain unanswered. While cardiologists measure changes in calcium flux within a single myocardial cell and nephrologists estimate changes in osmotic gradient along a single nephron, obstetrician–gynecologists continue to debate such questions as: How is the LH surge regulated? What causes endometriosis? Why is there still no effective screening test for ovarian cancer? What triggers labor?

This text is written primarily for medical students starting their clinical rotations. It is designed to give the reader a succinct yet comprehensive review of obstetrics and gynecology. Each chapter consists of two pages: a page of text and an accompanying set of images or algorithms that serve to complement the text. It is the sincere hope of the authors that the readers will find this book interesting, easy to read, and informative. Not all questions can be answered in a formal text format. Students should be encouraged to question and challenge their clinical teachers. Only then can the field move forward. Remember: "We need women and men who dream of things that cannot be and ask why not."

Errol R. Norwitz, MD, DPhil, FACOG
John O. Schorge, MD, FACOG, FACS

Acknowledgments

To my wife, Ann; my parents, Rollo and Marionne; and my children, Nicholas, Gabriella, and Sam.

E.R.N.

I would like to thank my wife, Sharon; and my children, Dante, Lena, and Rocco for their support during the completion of this book. In addition, I would like to express my deep appreciation for the mentors who inspired me during my obstetrics and gynecology training – most notably Isaac Schiff, Fred Frigoletto, John Repke, Ross Berkowitz, and Sam Mok.

J.O.S

About the companion website

Visit the companion website at:

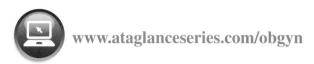 www.ataglanceseries.com/obgyn

The website includes:

• Multiple-choice questions
• Case studies from the book
• Flashcards with label on/off functionality

All of these are interactive so that you can easily test yourself on the topics in each chapter.

1 History taking and physical examination

Figure 1.1 LEOPOLD MANEUVERS

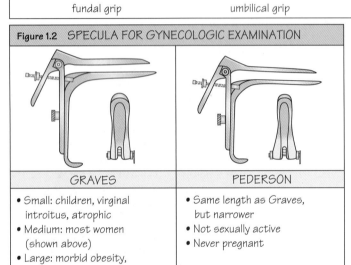

First maneuvre:
fundal grip

Second maneuvre:
umbilical grip

Third maneuvre:
Pawlick's grip

Fourth maneuvre:
pelvic grip

Figure 1.2 SPECULA FOR GYNECOLOGIC EXAMINATION

GRAVES	PEDERSON
• Small: children, virginal introitus, atrophic • Medium: most women (shown above) • Large: morbid obesity, grand multiparas	• Same length as Graves, but narrower • Not sexually active • Never pregnant

Figure 1.3 PERFORMING A PAP SMEAR

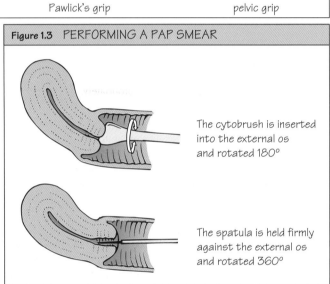

The cytobrush is inserted into the external os and rotated 180°

The spatula is held firmly against the external os and rotated 360°

Figure 1.4 PELVIC EXAMINATION

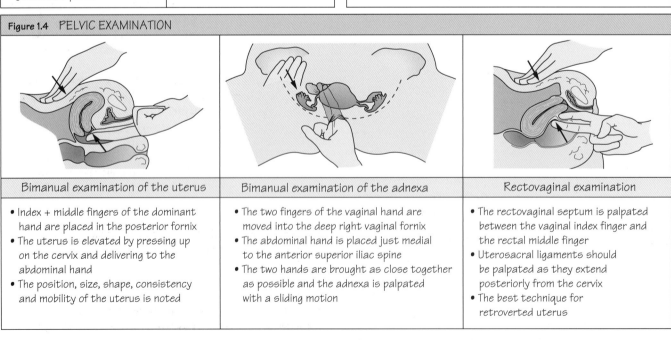

Bimanual examination of the uterus	Bimanual examination of the adnexa	Rectovaginal examination
• Index + middle fingers of the dominant hand are placed in the posterior fornix • The uterus is elevated by pressing up on the cervix and delivering to the abdominal hand • The position, size, shape, consistency and mobility of the uterus is noted	• The two fingers of the vaginal hand are moved into the deep right vaginal fornix • The abdominal hand is placed just medial to the anterior superior iliac spine • The two hands are brought as close together as possible and the adnexa is palpated with a sliding motion	• The rectovaginal septum is palpated between the vaginal index finger and the rectal middle finger • Uterosacral ligaments should be palpated as they extend posteriorly from the cervix • The best technique for retroverted uterus

Obstetrics and Gynecology at a Glance, Fourth Edition. Errol R. Norwitz and John O. Schorge.

General comments

- Dress appropriately and conduct yourself in a professional manner. Smile whenever appropriate and try to focus on putting the patient at ease.
- Introduce yourself by name and explain your role. Be welcoming to anyone else who may be with the patient. If you have other members of your team, introduce them as well.
- Begin by taking a brief history and trying to establish rapport before asking the patient to undress for her physical examination. Sit facing her and make direct eye contact.
- Listen carefully and invite questions to foster a trusting relationship. Try to understand the problem from her point of view in order to develop the most effective management plan. Acknowledge important points in the history by verbal or non-verbal cues (nodding).
- Occasionally, sensitivity to cultural expectations will require a change in approach. For example, some cultures discourage shaking hands whereas in others the husband or male family members will answer questions directed at the woman.

History

Taking an effective history involves a complicated interplay of multiple conflicting issues. The physician must create a comfortable environment, not appear rushed, and listen to all concerns, but at the same time stay focused and put limits on his or her time. The interview should be comprehensive, but tailored appropriately.

- *Chief complaint.* Patients should be encouraged to express, in their own words, the main purpose of the visit.
- *Present illness.* Pertinent open-ended questions can help clarify the details of the chief complaint and provide additional perspective.
- *Past medical and surgical history.* All significant health problems should be noted and any recent changes explored in more detail if indicated. Patients should be asked for an updated list of current medications and allergies. Prior surgical procedures, especially any involving the abdomen, pelvis, or reproductive organs, should be documented.
- *Gynecologic history.* Age-appropriate questions may include a detailed menstrual history (age of menarche or menopause, cycle length and duration, last menstrual period), contraceptive usage, prior vaginal or pelvic infections, and sexual history.
- *Obstetric history.* The number of pregnancies and their outcome should be detailed, including gestational ages, pregnancy-related complications, and other information if applicable to the visit.
- *Family history.* Serious illnesses (diabetes, cardiovascular disease, hypertension) of affected family members, particularly first-degree relatives, may have implications for the patient.
- *Social history.* To provide some context, questions should be asked about her occupation and where and with whom she lives. Patients should also routinely be asked about cigarette smoking, illicit drug use, and alcohol use.
- *Review of systems.* Consistently inquiring about the presence of physical symptoms is invaluable to uncover seemingly (to the patient) innocuous aspects of her health. Areas of importance include: constitutional (weight loss or gain, hot flushes), cardiovascular (chest pain, shortness of breath), gastrointestinal ("irritable bowel syndrome," constipation), genitourinary (incontinence, hematuria), neurologic (numbness, decreased sensation), psychiatric (depression, suicidal ideations), and other body systems.

Physical examination

1 General examination

- The patient should be asked to disrobe for a complete physical examination. Before discreetly stepping out of the room, it is the physician's responsibility to provide an appropriate gown and to assuage any anxiety by explaining what the examination will involve.
- A female chaperone should be present during the examination, regardless of physician gender.
- A comprehensive, but reasonably focused, examination should be conducted to assess her general health and provide insights that may have direct relevance to the chief complaint.

2 Abdominal examination

- The abdomen should be carefully: *inspected* for symmetry, scars, distension, and hair pattern; *palpated* for organomegaly or masses; and *auscultated* for bowel sounds.
- If a woman is pregnant, the four Leopold maneuvers should be performed (Figure 1.1): (1) palpate the woman's upper abdomen to identify either the fetal head or buttocks; (2) determine location of the fetal back; (3) identify whether fetal head or buttocks is lying above the inlet within the lower abdomen; and (4) locate the fetal brow.

3 Pelvic examination

- The patient should be asked to lie supine on the examining table and place her feet in stirrups.
- *Inspection* of the perineum involves assessment of the hair pattern, skin, presence of lesions (vesicles, warts), evidence of trauma, hemorrhoids, and abnormalities of the perineal body. Genital prolapse can be assessed by gently separating the labia and inspecting the vagina while the patient bears down (Valsalva maneuver).
- *Speculum examination* begins by choosing the appropriate type and size of speculum (Figure 1.2), inserting the blades through the introitus and guiding the tip in a downward motion toward the rectum. The blades are opened to reveal the cervix. The vaginal canal should be examined for erythema, lesions, or discharge. The cervix should be pink, shiny, and clear.
- The *Papanicolaou (Pap) smear* (Figure 1.3) samples the transformation zone of the cervix (the junction of the squamous cells lining the vagina and the columnar cells lining the endocervical canal).
- *Bimanual examination* (Figure 1.4) allows the physician to palpate the uterus and adnexae. In the normal and non-pregnant state, the uterus is approximately $6 \times 4\,cm$ (the size of a pear). A normal ovary is approximately $3 \times 2\,cm$ in size, but is often not palpable in obese or postmenopausal women.
- *Rectovaginal examination* (Figure 1.4) is especially valuable when pelvic organs are positioned in the posterior cul-de-sac, in preoperative planning, and in assessment of gynecologic cancers.
- *Rectal examination* performed separately and circumferentially with the examining finger can rule out distally located colorectal cancers. The physician may also note the tone of the anal sphincter and any other abnormalities (hemorrhoids, fissures, masses), and test a stool sample for occult blood.

Screening tests and preventive health

- Patients should routinely be counseled about the importance of screening tests, including:
  1 breast self-examinations
  2 mammograms
  3 Pap smears
- A discussion should also routinely be held about healthy lifestyle changes (diet, exercise), safe sexual practices, and contraception.

2 Anatomy of the female reproductive tract

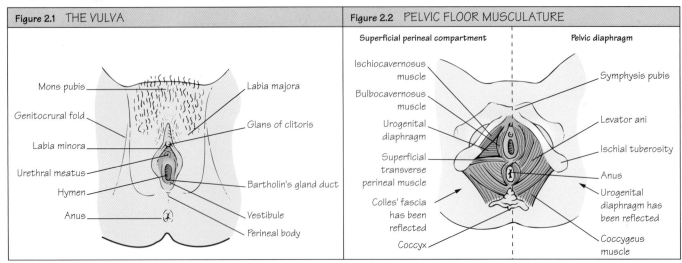

Figure 2.1 THE VULVA

- Mons pubis
- Genitocrural fold
- Labia minora
- Urethral meatus
- Hymen
- Anus
- Labia majora
- Glans of clitoris
- Bartholin's gland duct
- Vestibule
- Perineal body

Figure 2.2 PELVIC FLOOR MUSCULATURE

Superficial perineal compartment | Pelvic diaphragm

- Ischiocavernosus muscle
- Bulbocavernosus muscle
- Urogenital diaphragm
- Superficial transverse perineal muscle
- Colles' fascia has been reflected
- Coccyx
- Symphysis pubis
- Levator ani
- Ischial tuberosity
- Anus
- Urogenital diaphragm has been reflected
- Coccygeus muscle

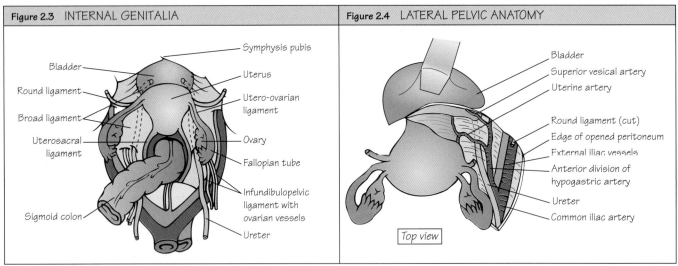

Figure 2.3 INTERNAL GENITALIA

- Bladder
- Round ligament
- Broad ligament
- Uterosacral ligament
- Sigmoid colon
- Symphysis pubis
- Uterus
- Utero-ovarian ligament
- Ovary
- Fallopian tube
- Infundibulopelvic ligament with ovarian vessels
- Ureter

Figure 2.4 LATERAL PELVIC ANATOMY

- Bladder
- Superior vesical artery
- Uterine artery
- Round ligament (cut)
- Edge of opened peritoneum
- External iliac vessels
- Anterior division of hypogastric artery
- Ureter
- Common iliac artery

Top view

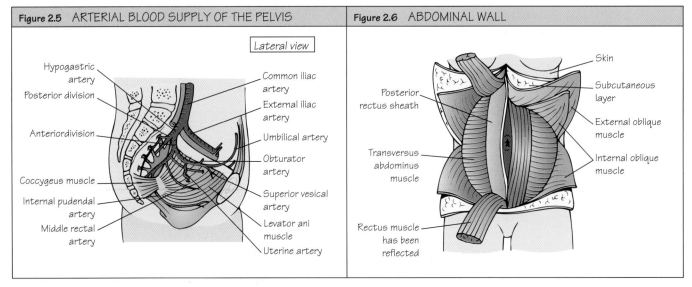

Figure 2.5 ARTERIAL BLOOD SUPPLY OF THE PELVIS

Lateral view

- Hypogastric artery
- Posterior division
- Anteriordivision
- Coccygeus muscle
- Internal pudendal artery
- Middle rectal artery
- Common iliac artery
- External iliac artery
- Umbilical artery
- Obturator artery
- Superior vesical artery
- Levator ani muscle
- Uterine artery

Figure 2.6 ABDOMINAL WALL

- Posterior rectus sheath
- Transversus abdominus muscle
- Rectus muscle has been reflected
- Skin
- Subcutaneous layer
- External oblique muscle
- Internal oblique muscle

Obstetrics and Gynecology at a Glance, Fourth Edition. Errol R. Norwitz and John O. Schorge.

The vulva and pelvic floor musculature

(Figures 2.1 and 2.2)

- The *vulva* is the visible external female genitalia bounded by the mons pubis anteriorly, the anus posteriorly, and the genitocrural folds laterally.
- The *perineum* is located between the urethral meatus and the anus, including both the skin and the underlying muscle.
- The *mons pubis* consists of hair-bearing skin over a cushion of adipose tissue that lies on the symphysis pubis.
- *Labia majora* are large, hair-bearing, bilateral, cutaneous folds of adipose and fibrous tissue extending from the mons pubis to the perineal body.
- The *clitoris* is a short, erectile organ with a visible glans. It is the female homolog of the male penis.
- *Labia minora* are thin, hairless, bilateral skinfolds medial to the labia majora, which originate at the clitoris.
- The *vestibule* is the cleft of tissue between the labia minora which is visualized when they are held apart.
- *Bartholin glands* are situated at each side of the vaginal orifice with duct openings at 5 and 7 o'clock.
- The *superficial perineal compartment* contains the ischiocavernosus, bulbocavernosus, and superficial transverse perineal muscles. It begins at the deep layer of superficial (Colles) fascia and extends up to the urogenital diaphragm.
- The *urogenital diaphragm (perineal membrane)* is a triangular sheet of dense, fibromuscular tissue stretched between the symphysis pubis and ischial tuberosities in the anterior half of the pelvic outlet. Its primary function is to support the vagina and perineal body.
- The *pelvic diaphragm* is found above the urogenital diaphragm and forms the inferior border of the abdominopelvic cavity. It is composed of a funnel-shaped sling of fascia and muscle (levator ani, coccygeus).

Internal genitalia and lateral pelvic anatomy (Figures 1.3 and 1.4)

- The *uterus* is a fibromuscular organ, the shape, weight, and dimensions of which vary considerably. The dome-shaped top is termed the "fundus."
- The *cervix* is connected to the uterus at the internal os. It is made up primarily of dense fibrous connective tissue. The cervical canal opens into the vagina at the external os.
- The *vagina* is a thin-walled, distensible, fibromuscular tube that extends from the vestibule of the vulva to the uterine cervix.
- The *fallopian tubes* (oviducts) are paired tubular structures that arise from the upper lateral portion of the uterus, widening in their distal third (ampulla) and ending at the fimbria.
- The *ovaries* are whitish-gray, almond-sized organs attached to the uterus medially by the utero-ovarian ligaments and to the pelvic side wall laterally by a vascular pedicle – the infundibulopelvic (IP) ligament.
- The *ureters* are bilateral, whitish, muscular tubes which serve as a conduit for urine from the kidney to the bladder trigone. They course over the common iliac bifurcation from lateral to medial at the level of the pelvic brim before passing under the uterine vessels just lateral to the cervix ("water under the bridge").
- The *bladder* is a hollow muscular organ that lies between the symphysis pubis and the uterus. The size and shape vary with the volume of urine.
- The *sigmoid colon* enters the pelvis on the left, forming the rectum at the level of the second and third sacral vertebrae and ending at the anal canal.
- The *round ligaments* are paired fibrous bands that originate at the uterine fundus and exit the pelvis through the internal inguinal ring. They provide little structural support.

- The *broad ligaments* are thin reflections of the peritoneum stretching from the pelvic side walls to the uterus. They provide virtually no suspensory support, but are draped over the fallopian tubes, ovaries, round ligaments, ureters, and other pelvic structures.
- The *cardinal (Mackenrodt) ligaments* provide the major support of the uterus and cervix. They extend from the lateral aspects of the cervix and vagina to the pelvic side walls.
- The *uterosacral ligaments* serve a minor role in the anatomic support of the cervix. They extend from the upper cervix posteriorly to the third sacral vertebra.

Arterial blood supply of the pelvis

(Figure 2.5)

- The *aorta* bifurcates at the fourth lumbar vertebra to form the two common iliac arteries which, in turn, bifurcate to form the external iliac and hypogastric (internal iliac) arteries.
- The *external iliac artery* passes under the inguinal ligament to become the femoral artery.
- The *hypogastric artery* branches into anterior and posterior divisions to supply the pelvis.
- The *ovarian arteries* originate from the infrarenal aorta and reach the ovaries via the IP ligament.
- The *inferior mesenteric artery* (IMA) arises from the lower aorta, about 3 cm above the bifurcation, to supply the descending colon. The IMA has significant collateral flow to the pelvis via branches of the hypogastric artery.
- The *internal pudendal artery* supplies the rectum, labia, clitoris, and perineum.

Innervation of the genital tract

- The *superior hypogastric plexus* is the main component of the autonomic nervous system providing innervation to the internal genital organs.
- The *iliohypogastric nerve* passes medial to the anterosuperior iliac spine in the abdominal wall to supply the skin of the suprapubic area. The slightly more medially located *ilioinguinal nerve* supplies the lower abdominal wall, upper portions of the labia majora, and the medial portions of the thigh. Either can be entrapped in the lateral closure of a transverse incision.
- The *pudendal nerve* arises from the sacral plexus and courses with the pudendal artery and vein through the pudendal (Alcock) canal to supply both motor and sensory fibers to the muscles and skin of the perineum.

Lymphatic drainage

- The vulva and distal third of the vagina are drained by an anastomotic series of coalescing channels which primarily lead to the *superficial* and *deep inguinal* lymph nodes.
- The upper two-thirds of the vagina and the cervix primarily drain to the *pelvic* (obturator, external iliac, hypogastric) lymph nodes.
- The uterus has a complex lymphatic system that variously drains to the *pelvic* and *para-aortic* (above and below the IMA) nodes.
- The ovaries and fallopian tubes' drainage systems follow the IP ligament to the *upper para-aortic* nodes near the origin of the ovarian arteries – above the IMA and below the renal vein.

Abdominal wall (Figure 2.6)

Layers of the abdominal wall include – from the outside to the inside – the *skin, subcutaneous layer* (Scarpa fascia), *musculoaponeurotic layer* (rectus sheath, external oblique muscle, internal oblique muscle, transversus abdominis), *transversalis fascia*, and *peritoneum*.

Figure 3.1 HORMONAL REGULATION OF OVULATION

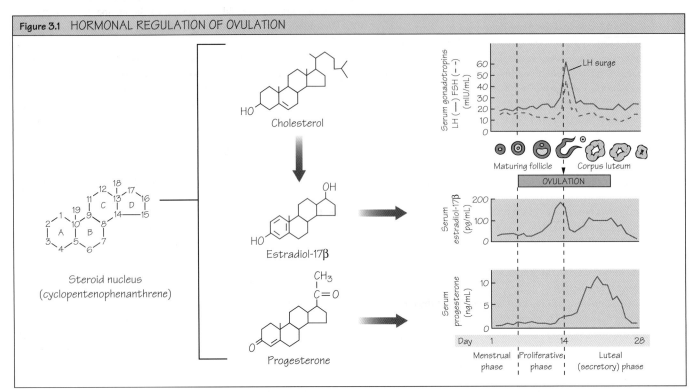

Figure 3.2 BIOLOGIC BASIS OF MENSTRUATION

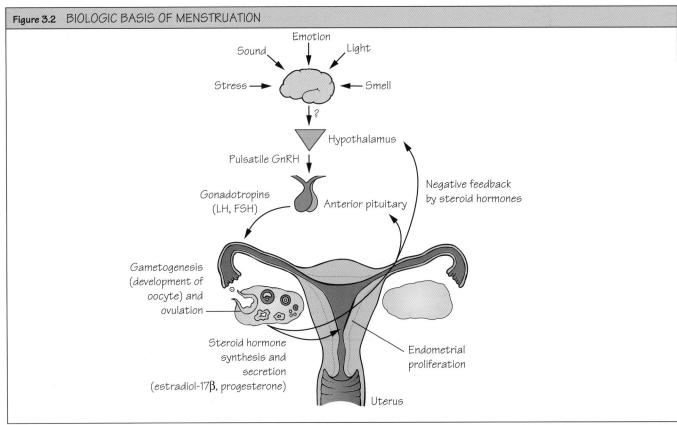

Obstetrics and Gynecology at a Glance, Fourth Edition. Errol R. Norwitz and John O. Schorge.

Definitions

• *Puberty* (see Chapter 21) is a general term encompassing the entire transition from childhood to sexual maturity.

• *Menarche* (the onset of menstruation) occurs at an average age of 12 years (normal range 8–16 years).

• *Menstrual cycles* or "periods" are often irregular through adolescence before settling into a more consistent ovulatory pattern ranging from 24 days to 35 days (average 28 days). The average duration of menstruation is 3–7 days and blood loss is typically about 80 mL.

• *Mittelschmerz* refers to periovulatory, unilateral, pelvic pain that some women consistently experience.

• *Menopause* (see Chapter 28) is defined as the cessation of menses and usually occurs around age 50. Women with continued bleeding beyond age 55 should be sampled to rule out malignancy.

Hormonal regulation of ovulation (Figure 3.1)

The cyclopentenophenanthrene ring structure is the basic carbon skeleton for all steroid hormones. Cholesterol is the parent steroid from which all the glucocorticoids, mineralocorticoids, and gonadal steroids are derived.

Phases of the menstrual cycle

• The *menstrual phase* begins on day 1 with the onset of bleeding and continues for several more days until the shedding of the endometrial lining stops (usually day 4–5).

• The *proliferative phase* begins at the end of the menstrual phase and ends at ovulation (usually day 13 or 14). This phase is characterized by endometrial thickening and ovarian follicular maturation.

• The *luteal (secretory) phase* starts at ovulation and lasts through day 28 before the entire process starts over again on day 1.

Biologic basis of menstruation (Figure 3.2)

Coordination of the menstrual cycle depends on a complex interaction of the brain, pituitary, ovaries, and endometrium.

Brain

• The hypothalamus is located at the base of the brain and essentially functions as the central processing unit of the reproductive system.

• Neuronal stimuli from the cerebral cortex are converted by the hypothalamus into pulses of neuropeptides (gonadotropin-releasing hormone, GnRH).

• Hypothalamic GnRH production is modulated by *negative feedback* of steroid hormones (estradiol-17β, progesterone).

Pituitary

• Located just below the hypothalamus, the pituitary gland consists of the neurohypophysis (posterior lobe) and the adenohypophysis (anterior lobe). It is the anterior pituitary that gives rise to gonadotropin (luteinizing hormone [LH] and follicle-stimulating hormone [FSH]) production.

• Pulsatile GnRH from the hypothalamus initiates the synthesis and secretion of LH and FSH. Similar to the hypothalamus, the anterior pituitary is subject to negative feedback regulation by the steroid hormones.

• In women of reproductive age, LH and FSH levels generally remain in the 10–20 mIU/mL range. After the menopause or surgical oophorectomy, estradiol-17β levels decline and LH and FSH are released from negative feedback, achieving circulating concentrations of more than 50 mIU/mL.

Ovaries

• Primitive germ cells (oogonia) divide by mitosis during fetal embryogenesis, peaking at around 7 million by 5 months of gestation.

• Meiotic division then begins, resulting in formation of primary oocytes. However, rapid atresia reduces the number of available follicles to 2 million at birth. At puberty, only around 300,000–400,000 follicles remain.

• Oocytes remain "resting" in *meiotic prophase* until puberty. Resting ovarian follicles are surrounded by thecal and granulosa cells: FSH stimulates the granulosa cells and LH stimulates the thecal cells.

• Only a single "dominant follicle" develops each menstrual cycle. When it produces enough estrogen to sustain a circulating estradiol-17β concentration of about 200 pg/mL for 48 hours, the hypothalamic–pituitary axis responds by secreting a surge of gonadotropins, primarily LH. This *LH surge* precedes ovulation by 24–36 hours.

• Following ovulation, the follicle collapses to form the *corpus luteum*. This endocrine organ mainly synthesizes progesterone to prepare the endometrium for pregnancy.

• If implantation does not occur, the corpus luteum will degenerate, resulting in a precipitous decline in circulating steroid hormone levels and the onset of menstruation. The decreasing steroid hormone levels release the negative feedback mechanism, inducing the pituitary to increase gonadotropin secretion. As a result, a new cycle of follicular recruitment is initiated.

• If implantation does occur, the embryo will rescue the corpus luteum by producing human chorionic gonadotropin (hCG) to prevent menstruation. At 7–9 weeks of gestation, the placenta takes over the production of progesterone from the corpus luteum.

Endometrium

• Dramatic monthly cyclic changes occur in the endometrium under the control of steroid hormones produced by the ovaries.

• Estradiol-17β production by the ovarian follicles induces endometrial proliferation. Progesterone synthesis by the corpus luteum then acts to mature the estrogen-primed endometrium in preparation for blastocyst implantation.

• Lowered steroid hormone levels in the late secretory phase cause a collapse of the endometrial vasculature, resulting in menstruation.

Premenstrual syndrome (PMS)

• *Definition.* Cyclic appearance of a constellation of myriad symptoms which affect lifestyle or work.

• Common manifestations include abdominal bloating, weight gain, constipation, anxiety, breast tenderness, depression, cravings for sugar or salt, and irritability.

• The diagnosis relies on a patient self-reporting symptoms that are predictably cyclic in nature and of sufficient severity to interfere with a day's normal events.

• PMS is quite common and typically mild; 5–10% of women report severe symptomatology at some point in their lives and 1% have such severe PMS that it threatens their work and interpersonal relationships.

• Multiple etiologic factors have been proposed, but there is no unifying theory to explain the pathophysiology of PMS.

• *Treatment.* Supportive therapy, aerobic exercise, and diet modification. *Fluoxetine* or *sertraline* has been shown to reduce symptoms of depression, anger, and anxiety.

4 Abnormal vaginal bleeding

Figure 4.1 ORGANIC CAUSES OF ABNORMAL VAGINAL BLEEDING

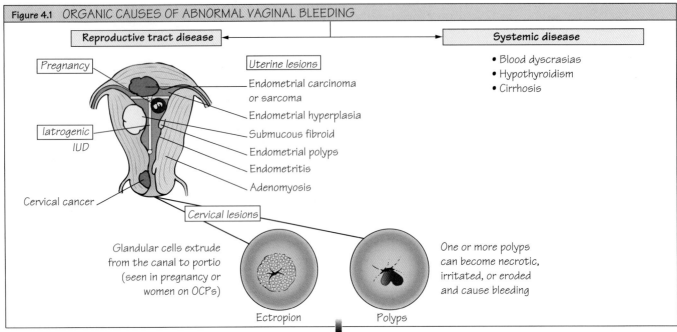

Reproductive tract disease

Pregnancy

Iatrogenic
IUD

Cervical cancer

Uterine lesions
- Endometrial carcinoma or sarcoma
- Endometrial hyperplasia
- Submucous fibroid
- Endometrial polyps
- Endometritis
- Adenomyosis

Cervical lesions

Glandular cells extrude from the canal to portio (seen in pregnancy or women on OCPs)

Ectropion

One or more polyps can become necrotic, irritated, or eroded and cause bleeding

Polyps

Systemic disease
- Blood dyscrasias
- Hypothyroidism
- Cirrhosis

Figure 4.2 FURTHER EVALUATION OF THE UTERUS

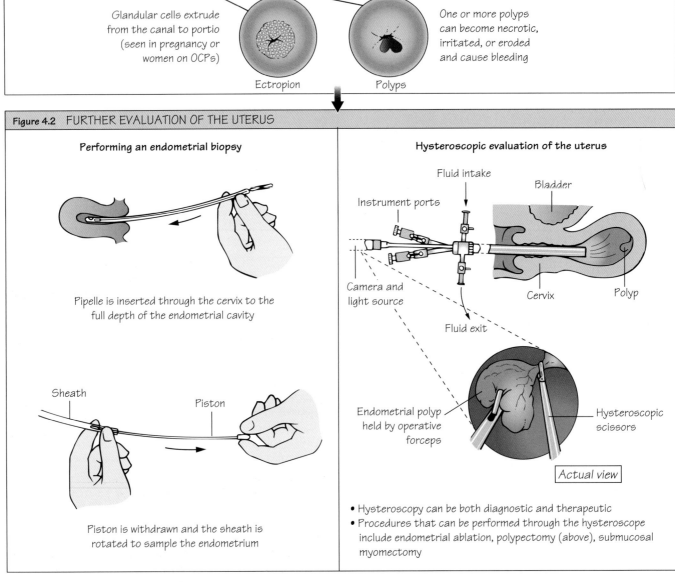

Performing an endometrial biopsy

Pipelle is inserted through the cervix to the full depth of the endometrial cavity

Sheath
Piston

Piston is withdrawn and the sheath is rotated to sample the endometrium

Hysteroscopic evaluation of the uterus

Fluid intake
Bladder
Instrument ports
Camera and light source
Fluid exit
Cervix
Polyp

Endometrial polyp held by operative forceps

Hysteroscopic scissors

Actual view

- Hysteroscopy can be both diagnostic and therapeutic
- Procedures that can be performed through the hysteroscope include endometrial ablation, polypectomy (above), submucosal myomectomy

Obstetrics and Gynecology at a Glance, Fourth Edition. Errol R. Norwitz and John O. Schorge.

Definitions

- *Menorrhagia.* Prolonged (>7 days) and/or heavy (>80 mL) uterine bleeding occurring at regular intervals.
- *Metrorrhagia.* Variable amounts of intermenstrual bleeding occurring at irregular but frequent intervals.
- *Polymenorrhea.* An abnormally short interval (<21 days) between regular menses.
- *Oligomenorrhea.* An abnormally long interval (>35 days) between regular menses.

Causes of abnormal vaginal bleeding

Organic causes (Figure 4.1)

1 Reproductive tract disease

- *Pregnancy-related conditions* are the most common causes of abnormal vaginal bleeding in women of reproductive age (threatened, incomplete, and missed abortion [see Chapter 15]; ectopic pregnancy [see Chapter 5]; and gestational trophoblastic disease [see Chapter 34]). Implantation bleeding is also quite common at about the time of the first missed menstrual period.
- *Uterine lesions* commonly produce menorrhagia or metrorrhagia by increasing endometrial surface area, distorting the endometrial vasculature, or having a friable/inflamed surface.
- *Cervical lesions* usually result in metrorrhagia (especially postcoital bleeding) due to erosion or direct trauma.
- *Iatrogenic causes* include the intrauterine device (IUD), oral/injectable steroids for contraception or hormone replacement, and tranquilizers or other psychotropic drugs. Oral contraceptives are often associated with irregular bleeding during the first 3 months of use, if doses are missed or the patient is a smoker. Long-acting progesterone-only contraceptives (Depo-Provera, Nexplanon) frequently cause irregular bleeding. Some patients may be unknowingly taking herbal medications (St John's wort, ginseng) that have an impact on the endometrium.

2 Systemic disease

- Blood dyscrasias such as von Willebrand disease and prothrombin deficiency may present with profuse vaginal bleeding during adolescence. Other disorders that produce platelet deficiency (leukemia, severe sepsis) may also present as irregular bleeding.
- Hypothyroidism is frequently associated with menorrhagia and/or metrorrhagia. Hyperthyroidism is usually not associated with menstrual abnormalities, but oligomenorrhea and amenorrhea are possible.
- Cirrhosis is associated with excessive bleeding secondary to the reduced capacity of the liver to metabolize estrogens.

Dysfunctional (endocrinologic) causes

The diagnosis of dysfunctional uterine bleeding (DUB) can be made after organic, systemic, and iatrogenic causes for abnormal vaginal bleeding have been ruled out (diagnosis of exclusion).

1 Anovulatory DUB

- The predominant type in the postmenarchal and premenopausal years due to alterations in neuroendocrinologic function.
- Characterized by continuous production of estradiol-17β without corpus luteum formation and progesterone release.
- Unopposed estrogen leads to continuous proliferation of the endometrium which eventually outgrows its blood supply and is sloughed in an irregular, unpredictable pattern.

2 Ovulatory DUB

- Incidence: up to 10% of ovulatory women.
- Mid-cycle spotting following the LH surge is usually physiologic. Polymenorrhea is most often due to shortening of the follicular phase of menstruation. Alternatively, the luteal phase may be prolonged by a persistent corpus luteum.

Diagnosis

- Patient age is the most important factor in the evaluation.
- Ruling out pregnancy-related complications should be the *first priority* in all women of reproductive age.
- A complete list of medications is essential to rule out their interference with normal menstruation.
- Non-gynecologic physical findings (thyromegaly, hepatomegaly) may suggest the presence of an underlying systemic disorder. Genitourinary (urinary infection) or gastrointestinal (hemorrhoids) bleeding may also be mistakenly interpreted by the patient as vaginal bleeding.
- Pelvic examination may reveal an obvious structural abnormality (cervical polyp), but frequently additional evaluation is necessary.
- Measurement of serum hemoglobin concentration, iron levels, and ferritin levels is an objective measure of the quantity and duration of menstrual blood loss. Additional laboratory tests (thyroid-stimulating hormone, coagulation profile) may be indicated.
- A *menstrual calendar* may be helpful in accurately determining the amount, frequency, and duration of the bleeding.
- Ovulation can be assessed by careful history taking and, if necessary, *ovulation prediction kits* (see Chapter 25).
- Further evaluation of the uterus (Figure 4.2) can be achieved in non-pregnant women by performing an *endometrial biopsy* or hysteroscopy. Pelvic ultrasound may also be indicated if the cause of bleeding cannot be confirmed.

Medical management

The majority of women with abnormal vaginal bleeding can be treated medically, particularly in the absence of a structural lesion.

- *Oral contraceptives* effectively correct the vast majority of common menstrual irregularities (anovulatory and ovulatory DUB). However, DUB can occasionally present as an acute hemorrhage requiring short-term, high-dose oral or intravenous estrogen therapy to transiently support the endometrium.
- *Non-steroidal anti-inflammatory drugs* (mefenamic acid) have been shown to reduce menstrual blood loss, particularly in ovulatory patients.

Surgical management

Structural abnormalities frequently require surgical intervention to alleviate symptoms.

- *Dilation and curettage (D&C)* can be both diagnostic and therapeutic, especially in women with acute vaginal bleeding due to endometrial overgrowth.
- *Hysteroscopy* is an office or day-surgery procedure that can be used to diagnose and treat abnormal uterine lesions. The uterine cavity is distended with fluid, allowing direct visualization of the abnormality and use of hysteroscopic instruments.
- *Endometrial ablation* (such as NovaSure) can dramatically reduce the amount of cyclic blood loss.
- *Hysterectomy* (see Chapter 17) is usually reserved for women with structural lesions not amenable to more conservative surgery (multiple large leiomyomas, uterine prolapse). It may also be indicated in women with persistent DUB, but only if medical therapy has failed.

5 Ectopic pregnancy

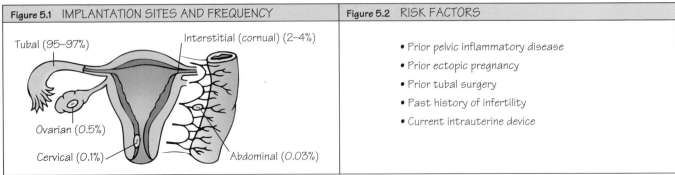

Figure 5.1 IMPLANTATION SITES AND FREQUENCY

Tubal (95–97%)
Interstitial (cornual) (2–4%)
Ovarian (0.5%)
Cervical (0.1%)
Abdominal (0.03%)

Figure 5.2 RISK FACTORS

- Prior pelvic inflammatory disease
- Prior ectopic pregnancy
- Prior tubal surgery
- Past history of infertility
- Current intrauterine device

Figure 5.3 DIAGNOSIS

- History
- Examination
- Serial β-hCG measurements
- Ultrasound
- Endometrial sampling to determine if intrauterine products of conception (e.g., chorionic villi) are present unless desired pregnancy

Figure 5.4 MEDICAL THERAPY

Criteria for receiving methotrexate	Contraindications to medical therapy

Absolute indications
  Hemodynamically stable without active
   bleeding or signs of hemoperitoneum
  Patient desires future fertility
  General anesthesia poses
   significant risk
  Patient is able to return for follow-up care
Relative indications
  Unruptured mass <3.5 cm at its
   greatest dimension
  No fetal cardiac motion detected
  Patient whose β-hCG level does not
   exceed a predetermined level
   (6000 – 15,000 mIU/mL)
	Absolute contraindications
	  Breastfeeding
	  Immunodeficiency
	  Alcoholism or other chronic liver disease
	  Blood dyscrasias,
	  Leukopenia, thrombocytopenia,
	   or significant anemia
	  Known sensitivity to methotrexate
	  Active pulmonary disease
	  Peptic ulcer disease
	  Hepatic, renal or hematologic dysfunction
	  B-hCG > 15,000 mIU/mL
	Relative contraindications
	  Gestational sac > 3.5 cm
	  Embryonic cardiac motion

Medical therapy

Surgical therapy

Definitive surgery (salpingectomy)

Conservative surgery

Figure 5.5 LAPAROSCOPIC LINEAR SALPINGOSTOMY FOR TUBAL ECTOPIC PREGNANCY

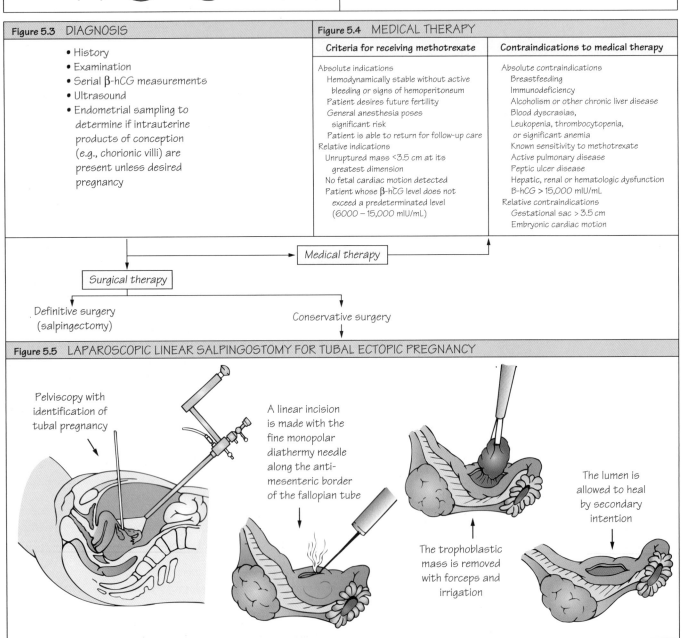

Pelviscopy with identification of tubal pregnancy

A linear incision is made with the fine monopolar diathermy needle along the anti-mesenteric border of the fallopian tube

The trophoblastic mass is removed with forceps and irrigation

The lumen is allowed to heal by secondary intention

Obstetrics and Gynecology at a Glance, Fourth Edition. Errol R. Norwitz and John O. Schorge.

Definition

Any gestation in which implantation occurs at a location other than the endometrial lining (Figure 5.1).

Epidemiology and risk factors

- *Incidence* in the UK and USA is roughly 20/1000 conceptions.
- *Mortality.* Ten percent of pregnancy-related maternal deaths (most common cause of death in the first half of pregnancy).
- *Risk factors* (Figure 5.2). Past history of *pelvic inflammatory disease* (see Chapter 8), especially that caused by *Chlamydia trachomatis*, is most important. However, >50% of patients have no risk factors.
- *Etiology.* The major cause of ectopic pregnancy is *acute salpingitis*: permanent agglutination of the folds of the endosalpinx can allow passage of the smaller sperm while the fertilized ovum (morula) gets trapped in blind pockets formed by adhesions. Contraception failure, hormonal alterations, and previous termination also contribute to an increased risk of ectopic pregnancy.

Symptoms and signs

Frequently the diagnosis is established before symptoms or signs develop due to the use of early serum testing and vaginal sonography.

- *Abdominal pain, absence of menses, and irregular vaginal bleeding* (usually spotting) are the main symptoms.
- Ruptured ectopic pregnancies cause shoulder pain in 10–20% of cases as a result of diaphragmatic irritation from the hemoperitoneum. Syncope also may occur due to intense, sudden pain. Other symptoms may include dizziness and an urge to defecate.
- The most common presenting sign in a woman with symptomatic ectopic pregnancy is *abdominal tenderness*. Half of women will have a palpable adnexal mass. Profound intraperitoneal hemorrhage will lead to tachycardia and hypotension.

Diagnosis (Figure 5.3)

A thorough history and physical examination are essential. The extent should be dictated by the severity of symptoms at presentation.

- Serial quantitative levels of the *β-subunit of human chorionic gonadotropin (βhCG)* are important. In normal early pregnancy, serum βhCG levels should double every 48 hours in early pregnancy.
- *Transvaginal sonography* can detect an intrauterine gestational sac at a serum βhCG level of 1,500–2,000 mIU/mL (approximately 5 weeks from last monthly period [LMP]); ≥6,000 mIU/mL are required to see an intrauterine gestational sac by transabdominal sonography.
- *Culdocentesis* may be performed in the office or emergency room and can quickly confirm the presence of free blood in the peritoneal cavity. When non-clotting blood is aspirated, the test is positive. This procedure is seldom performed in current practice.
- *Uterine curettage* (or biopsy) can effectively exclude an ectopic pregnancy by demonstrating histologic evidence of products of conception. This procedure may disrupt an intrauterine pregnancy, however; the patient should be informed of this risk, and the procedure should be performed when the probably of viable intrauterine pregnancy is low or if the pregnancy is undesired.
- *Laparoscopy* (see Chapter 17) may ultimately be indicated in some circumstances to make the diagnosis and initiate treatment.

Management

Due to earlier diagnosis, the goal of treatment has shifted from preventing mortality to reducing morbidity and preserving fertility. Once the diagnosis is confirmed, expectant management is rarely justified. However, if left untreated, about half of ectopic pregnancies will abort via the fallopian tube.

Medical therapy (Figure 5.4)

- *Methotrexate (MTX)* (50 mg/m^2 intramuscular injection) is effective treatment for select patients who meet the criteria. The dose is administered on day 1, but serum βhCG levels may continue to rise for several days. An acceptable response is defined as a ≥15% decrease in serum βhCG levels from day 4 to day 7. The levels of βhCG should thereafter be followed weekly.
- Most cases will be successfully treated with one dose of MTX, but up to 25% will require two or more doses if the βhCG level eventually plateaus or rises. Patients with a gestational sac >3.5 cm, starting βhCG >15,000 mIU/mL, or fetal cardiac motion are at higher risk for MTX "failure" and should be managed surgically.
- MTX side effects (nausea, vomiting, bloating, transient transaminitis) are generally mild.
- Increased abdominal pain will occur in up to 75% of patients due to tubal abortion or serosal irritation caused by hematoma stretching. Sonography can be used to rule out significant hemoperitoneum. However, all MTX patients should be closely monitored during follow-up due to the risk of rupture and hemorrhage.

Surgical therapy

- Definitive surgery (salpingectomy) is the treatment of choice for women who present as *hemodynamically unstable*.
- Conservative surgery can be considered for the *hemodynamically stable* patient:

  1 *Laparoscopic linear salpingostomy* (Figure 5.5). The injection of vasopressin before the linear incision can be used to markedly decrease bleeding. Serum βhCG levels must be followed until undetectable in conservatively managed patients because 5–10% will develop a *persistent ectopic pregnancy* and may require further treatment with MTX.

  2 Partial salpingectomy involves removal of the damaged portion of the fallopian tube and is indicated when there is extensive damage or continued bleeding after salpingostomy. This procedure should not be performed unless reanastomosis is planned.
- The only indication for oophorectomy is to achieve hemostasis.

Interstitial (cornual) pregnancy

- Implantation of the embryo into the fallopian tube where it passes through the myometrium.
- Frequently associated with severe morbidity because patients become symptomatic later in gestation and are difficult to diagnose, and lesions often produce massive hemorrhage when they rupture.
- Laparotomy with *cornual resection* or *hysterectomy* is often required.
- Maternal mortality rate is 2%.

Ovarian pregnancy

- Patients are usually thought to clinically have a ruptured corpus luteum cyst.
- Usually associated with profuse hemorrhage.

Cervical pregnancy

- Most occur after a previous sharp uterine curettage.
- May be successfully treated by MTX, but more advanced cases require hysterectomy.

Abdominal pregnancy

- Most occur secondary to tubal abortion with secondary implantation in the peritoneal cavity.
- Laparotomy with removal of the fetus is necessary. The placenta may be ligated and left *in situ* because it often derives its blood supply from the gastrointestinal tract and can be difficult to remove.

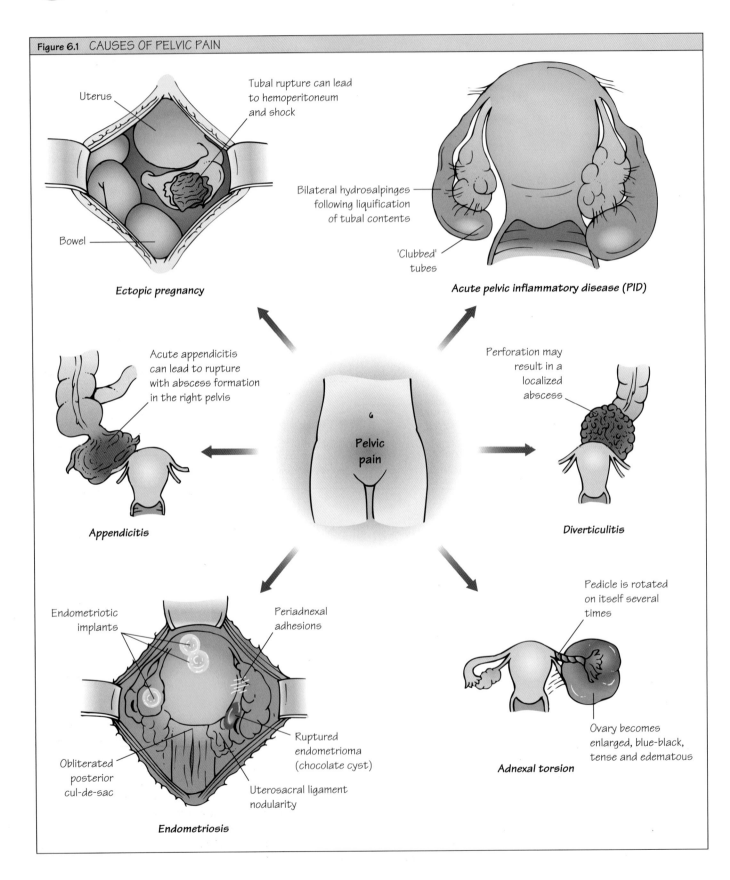

Figure 6.1 CAUSES OF PELVIC PAIN

Uterus

Tubal rupture can lead to hemoperitoneum and shock

Bowel

Ectopic pregnancy

Bilateral hydrosalpinges following liquification of tubal contents

'Clubbed' tubes

Acute pelvic inflammatory disease (PID)

Acute appendicitis can lead to rupture with abscess formation in the right pelvis

Appendicitis

Pelvic pain

Perforation may result in a localized abscess

Diverticulitis

Endometriotic implants

Periadnexal adhesions

Ruptured endometrioma (chocolate cyst)

Uterosacral ligament nodularity

Obliterated posterior cul-de-sac

Endometriosis

Pedicle is rotated on itself several times

Ovary becomes enlarged, blue-black, tense and edematous

Adnexal torsion

Obstetrics and Gynecology at a Glance, Fourth Edition. Errol R. Norwitz and John O. Schorge.

20 © 2013 John Wiley & Sons, Ltd. Published 2013 by John Wiley & Sons, Ltd.

- As pain arising from the pelvis is a subjective perception rather than an objective sensation, accurately determining the etiology is often difficult.
- Dysmenorrhea (uterine pain associated with menses) is the most common gynecologic pain complaint.

Evaluation strategies

- The history provides a description of the nature, intensity, and distribution of the pain. However, imprecise localization is typical with intra-abdominal processes.
- Physical examination includes a comprehensive gynecologic examination. Specific attention should be paid to trying to reproduce the pain symptoms.
- Chlamydia/gonorrhea cervical cultures and urinalysis with culture are frequently helpful.
- Ultrasonography and other imaging studies may be indicated.
- Specialized diagnostic studies based on the presumptive diagnosis may require consultation with other specialists in anesthesiology, orthopedics, neurology, or gastroenterology.

Acute pelvic pain

Potentially catastrophic causes (ruptured appendix) require timely intervention to quickly diagnose and treat.

Gynecologic causes

Three main categories: rupture, infection, and torsion.
- *Ectopic pregnancy* (Figure 6.1; see Chapter 5). In all women of reproductive age, the first priority in evaluating acute pelvic pain is to rule out the possibility of a ruptured ectopic pregnancy.
- *Acute pelvic inflammatory disease* (PID) (Figure 6.1; see Chapter 8) is an ascending bacterial infection that often presents with high fever, severe pelvic pain, nausea, and evidence of cervical motion tenderness in sexually active women.
- *Rupture of an ovarian cyst.* Intra-abdominal rupture of a follicular cyst, corpus luteum, or endometrioma is a common cause of acute pelvic pain. The pain may be severe enough to cause syncope. The condition is usually self-limiting with limited intraperitoneal bleeding.
- *Adnexal torsion* (Figure 6.1) is seen most commonly in adolescent or reproductive age women. By twisting on its vascular pedicle, any adnexal mass (ovarian dermoid, hydatid of Morgagni) can cause severe pain by suddenly compromising its blood supply. The pain will frequently wax and wane with associated nausea and vomiting.
- *Threatened, inevitable,* or *incomplete miscarriages* are generally accompanied by midline pelvic pain, usually of a crampy, intermittent nature (see Chapter 15).
- *Degenerating fibroids* or *ovarian tumors* may cause localized sharp or aching pain.

Non-gynecologic causes

- *Appendicitis* (Figure 6.1) is the most common acute surgical condition of the abdomen, occurring in all age groups. Classically, the pain is initially diffuse and centered in the umbilical area but, after several hours, localizes to the right lower quadrant (McBurney point). It is often accompanied by low-grade fever, anorexia, and leukocytosis.
- *Diverticulitis* (Figure 6.1) occurs most frequently in older women. It is characterized by left-sided pelvic pain, bloody diarrhea, fever, and leukocytosis.
- *Urinary tract disorders* (cystitis, pyelonephritis, renal calculi) can cause acute or referred suprapubic pain, pressure, and/or dysuria.

- *Mesenteric lymphadenitis* most often follows an upper respiratory infection in young girls. The pain is usually more diffuse and less severe than in appendicitis.

Chronic pelvic pain

Most women, at some time in their lives, experience pelvic pain. When the condition persists for longer than 3–6 months, it is considered chronic.
- Accounts for 10% of all visits to gynecologists and 20–30% of laparoscopies.
- Frequently there is little correlation between the objective severity of abdominal disease and the amount of perceived pain: a third of women who undergo laparoscopy for chronic pelvic pain will have no identifiable cause.
- Ten to twenty percent of hysterectomies are performed for chronic pelvic pain. Postoperatively, 75% of women will experience significant improvement in their symptoms.
- Patients and physicians may both become frustrated because the condition is difficult to cure or manage adequately.

Gynecologic causes

- *Dysmenorrhea* is the most common etiology. Primary dysmenorrhea is not associated with pelvic pathology, and is thought to be due to excessive prostaglandin production by the uterus. Secondary dysmenorrhea is usually due to acquired conditions (such as endometriosis). Oral contraceptives and non-steroidal anti-inflammatory drugs are helpful.
- *Endometriosis* (Figure 6.1; see Chapter 11) has a spectrum of pain that ranges from dysmenorrhea to severe, intractable, continuous pain which may be disabling. The severity of pain often does not correlate with the degree of pelvic pathology.
- *Adenomyosis* (see Chapter 11) is a common condition that is usually only confirmed by hysterectomy. Most frequently, women are asymptomatic and this is an incidental pathology finding. An enlarged, boggy uterus that is mildly tender to bimanual palpation is suggestive of the diagnosis.
- *Fibroids* (see Chapter 10) are the most frequent (benign) tumors found in the female pelvis. They may cause pain by either putting pressure on adjacent organs or undergoing degeneration.
- *Ovarian remnant syndrome* is characterized by persistent pelvic pain after removal of both adnexa. In such cases, a cystic portion of the ovary is usually identified as the source.
- *Genital prolapse* (see Chapter 20) may lead to complaints of heaviness, pressure, a dropping sensation, or pelvic aching.
- *Chronic PID* is usually as a result of persistent hydrosalpinx, tubo-ovarian cyst, or pelvic adhesions.

Treatment depends on the suspected etiology, but non-surgical options may include a discussion of nutritional supplementation, physical therapy modalities, acupuncture/acupressure, or antidepressants.

Non-gynecologic causes

- *Gastrointestinal disturbances* such as inflammatory bowel disease.
- *Musculoskeletal problems* such as muscle strain or disc herniation.
- *Interstitial cystitis* (chronic inflammatory condition of the bladder).
- *Somatoform disorders* are characterized by physical pain and symptoms that mimic disease, but are related to psychological factors (domestic discord, sexual abuse). Patients do not have conscious control over their symptoms and are not intentionally trying to confuse the doctor or complicate the process of diagnosis. Women often have long histories of unsuccessful medical or surgical treatments with multiple different physicians.

Figure 7.1 VAGINITIS

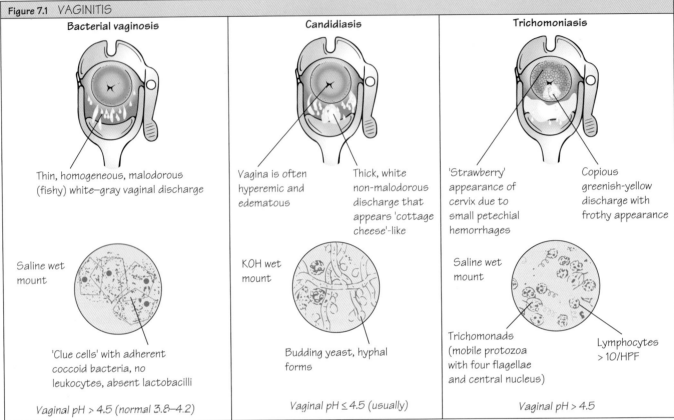

Bacterial vaginosis

Thin, homogeneous, malodorous (fishy) white–gray vaginal discharge

Saline wet mount

'Clue cells' with adherent coccoid bacteria, no leukocytes, absent lactobacilli

Vaginal pH > 4.5 (normal 3.8–4.2)

Candidiasis

Vagina is often hyperemic and edematous

Thick, white non-malodorous discharge that appears 'cottage cheese'-like

KOH wet mount

Budding yeast, hyphal forms

Vaginal pH ≤ 4.5 (usually)

Trichomoniasis

'Strawberry' appearance of cervix due to small petechial hemorrhages

Copious greenish-yellow discharge with frothy appearance

Saline wet mount

Trichomonads (mobile protozoa with four flagellae and central nucleus)

Lymphocytes >10/HPF

Vaginal pH > 4.5

Figure 7.2 INFECTIONS OF THE VULVA

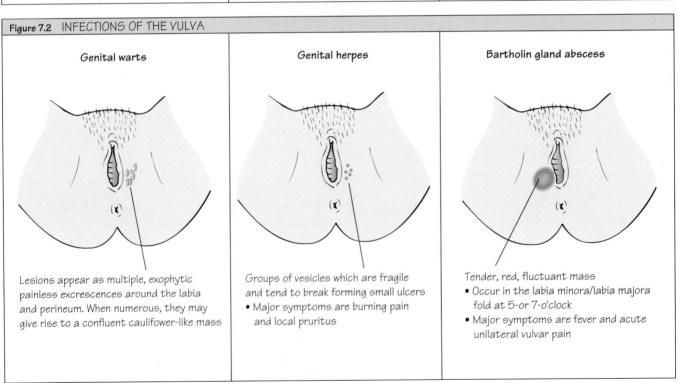

Genital warts

Lesions appear as multiple, exophytic painless excrescences around the labia and perineum. When numerous, they may give rise to a confluent cauliflower-like mass

Genital herpes

Groups of vesicles which are fragile and tend to break forming small ulcers
• Major symptoms are burning pain and local pruritus

Bartholin gland abscess

Tender, red, fluctuant mass
• Occur in the labia minora/labia majora fold at 5-or 7-o'clock
• Major symptoms are fever and acute unilateral vulvar pain

Obstetrics and Gynecology at a Glance, Fourth Edition. Errol R. Norwitz and John O. Schorge.

22 © 2013 John Wiley & Sons, Ltd. Published 2013 by John Wiley & Sons, Ltd.

Vulvovaginitis is the most common gynecologic problem for which women seek treatment. Symptoms may include vaginal discharge, vulvar pruritis and vaginal odor. The etiological agents responsible can commonly be identified in the office by obtaining an appropriate sample of the vaginal discharge for microscopic examination.

Bacterial vaginosis (BV) (Figure 7.1)
• *Etiology.* Overgrowth of several bacterial species in the vagina – specifically a decrease in lactobacilli and an increase in anaerobic organisms.
• *Incidence.* The most common cause of vaginitis in young women.
• *Symptoms.* Non-pruritic vaginal discharge with a "fishy" odor, but 50% of women are asymptomatic.
• *Diagnosis.* Positive KOH "whiff" test, pH >4.5, >20% clue cells on saline wet-mount, gray, homogeneous discharge (need three of four clinical criteria).
• *Treatment.* Oral/intravaginal metronidazole or clindamycin.

Candidiasis (Figure 7.1)
• *Etiology.* Over 200 strains of *Candida albicans* can colonize and cause vaginitis. It is unknown why *Candida* species is pathogenic in some women, but not in others.
• *Incidence.* The second most common cause of symptomatic vaginitis.
• *Symptoms.* Intense pruritus and vulvovaginal erythema.
• *Diagnosis.* KOH wet-mount to see the presence of branched and budding hyphae. Culture in Sabouraud medium may be indicated for selected cases.
• *Treatment.* topical clotrimazole (Canestin) or oral fluconazole (Diflucan).

Trichomoniasis (Figure 7.1)
• *Etiology. Trichomonas vaginalis* is an anaerobic protozoan and humans are the only known host.
• *Incidence.* This common sexually transmitted infection (STI) affects 180 million women worldwide.
• *Symptoms.* Profuse malodorous vaginal discharge, postcoital bleeding, vulvovaginal erythema.
• *Diagnosis.* Trichomonads seen on saline wet-mount are pathognomonic. Other features include an abundance of leukocytes and pH > 4.5. Organisms may be evident on a Pap smear in asymptomatic women.
• *Treatment.* Oral (not vaginal) metronidazole.

Chlamydial cervicitis
• *Etiology. Chlamydia trachomatis* is an obligate intracellular bacterial parasite of columnar epithelial cells.
• *Incidence.* The most prevalent STI in the UK and the USA; 30% of infections are associated with gonorrhea.
• *Symptoms.* Purulent or mucoid discharge, postcoital bleeding and vaginitis, but many asymptomatic women are identified through screening or contact tracing.
• *Diagnosis.* DNA probe test obtained vaginally (preferred) or by urine sample, or enzyme-linked immunosorbent assay.
• *Treatment.* Oral azithromycin or doxycycline.

Gonococcal cervicitis/vaginitis
• *Etiology. Neisseria gonorrhoeae* is a Gram-negative aerobic diplococcus.
• *Incidence.* Common but less prevalent STI than *Chlamydia* sp.
• *Symptoms.* Profuse, odorless, non-irritating, creamy white or yellow vaginal discharge, but may also be asymptomatic. Ten to twenty percent of women develop acute salpingitis with fever and pelvic pain; 5% exhibit disseminated gonorrhea infection with chills, fever, malaise, asymmetric polyarthralgias, and painful skin lesions.
• *Diagnosis.* A positive culture on selective media such as modified Thayer–Martin agar; 20% of patients will have detectable infection at multiple sites (pharynx, rectum).
• *Treatment.* Oral ciprofloxacin (the USA practice favors intramuscular ceftriaxone or oral cefixime, with dual treatment with azithromycin or doxycycline).

Genital warts (condyloma acuminatum) (Figure 7.2)
• *Etiology. Human papillomavirus* (HPV) infection is transmitted by skin-to-skin contact.
• *Incidence.* The most common viral STI.
• *Symptoms.* Uncomplicated cases are asymptomatic.
• *Diagnosis.* Usually clinical inspection is sufficient, but colposcopy and/or biopsy may be required.
• *Treatment.* Office cryotherapy or self-administered medical therapy, or other less common options depending on the extent: local cytotoxic agents (trichloroacetic acid, podofilox). Outpatient excision or laser surgery, local cytotoxic agents (trichloroacetic acid, podofilox).

Genital herpes (Figure 7.2)
• *Etiology. Herpes simplex virus* (HSV) type 1 (15%) or type 2 (85%).
• *Incidence.* This STI is the most common cause of genital ulcers.
• *Symptoms.* First-episode primary HSV infection is characterized by systemic symptoms, including malaise and fever. However, genital herpes is a recurrent infection with periods of active infection separated by periods of latency.
• *Diagnosis.* Usually clinical inspection is sufficient, but viral isolation by tissue culture is also very reliable.
• *Treatment.* Oral aciclovir or valaciclovir (topicals are not effective).

Syphilis
• *Etiology.* The spirochete *Treponema pallidum.*
• *Incidence.* An endemic STI in Europe in the fifteenth century, but its prevalence has declined dramatically.
• *Symptoms.* A systemic disease with myriad clinical presentations. Primary infection is marked by a painless, solitary ulcer at the site of acquisition. Secondary symptoms include a facial-sparing rash with involvement of the palms and soles. The classic skin lesion of late syphilis is the solitary gumma nodule.
• *Diagnosis.* Dark-field examination of scrapings from a lesion and/or serologic screening (rapid plasma reagin test).
• *Treatment.* Intramuscular benzathine penicillin.

Other infections
• *Bartholin gland abscess* (Figure 7.2). *Treatment:* surgical incision and placement of a Word catheter for drainage.
• *Pediculosis pubis* (scabies) is an intensely pruritic STI caused by the crab louse. *Treatment:* lindane (Kwell).
• *Molluscum contagiosum* is an asymptomatic, papular STI of the vulva caused by the poxvirus. Most cases resolve without treatment.
• *Necrotizing fasciitis* is a rapidly progressive, frequently fatal infection. *Treatment:* immediate wide surgical debridement and parenteral antibiotics.
• *Hydradenitis suppurativa* is a staphylococcal or streptococcal infection of the vulvar apocrine glands. *Treatment:* excision.
• *Rare vulvar* STIs include: *lymphogranuloma venereum* (caused by *Chlamydia trachomatis*), *chancroid* (caused by *Haemophilus ducreyi*), *donovanosis/granuloma inguinale* (caused by *Calymmatobacterium granulomatis*).

8 Pelvic inflammatory disease (PID)

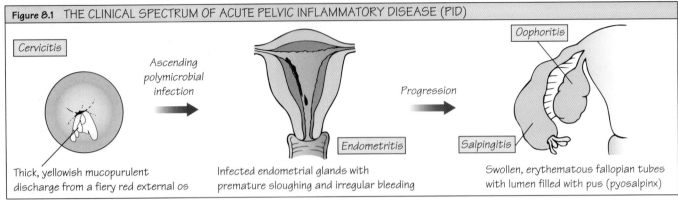

Figure 8.1 THE CLINICAL SPECTRUM OF ACUTE PELVIC INFLAMMATORY DISEASE (PID)

Cervicitis — Thick, yellowish mucopurulent discharge from a fiery red external os

Ascending polymicrobial infection

Endometritis — Infected endometrial glands with premature sloughing and irregular bleeding

Progression

Oophoritis / Salpingitis — Swollen, erythematous fallopian tubes with lumen filled with pus (pyosalpinx)

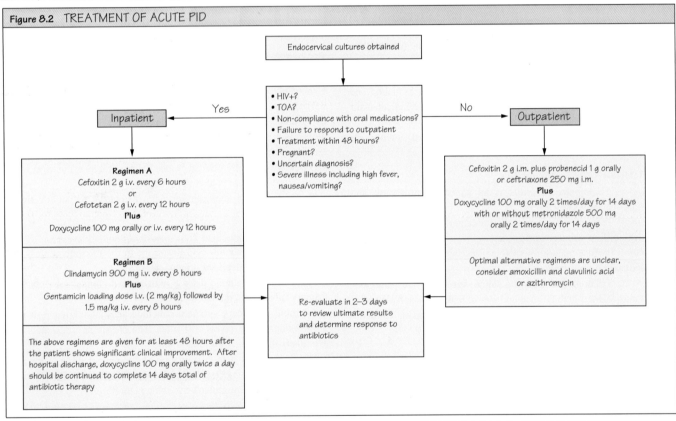

Figure 8.2 TREATMENT OF ACUTE PID

Endocervical cultures obtained

- HIV+?
- TOA?
- Non-compliance with oral medications?
- Failure to respond to outpatient
- Treatment within 48 hours?
- Pregnant?
- Uncertain diagnosis?
- Severe illness including high fever, nausea/vomiting?

Yes → Inpatient

Regimen A
Cefoxitin 2 g i.v. every 6 hours
or
Cefotetan 2 g i.v. every 12 hours
Plus
Doxycycline 100 mg orally or i.v. every 12 hours

Regimen B
Clindamycin 900 mg i.v. every 8 hours
Plus
Gentamicin loading dose i.v. (2 mg/kg) followed by 1.5 mg/kg i.v. every 8 hours

The above regimens are given for at least 48 hours after the patient shows significant clinical improvement. After hospital discharge, doxycycline 100 mg orally twice a day should be continued to complete 14 days total of antibiotic therapy

No → Outpatient

Cefoxitin 2 g i.m. plus probenecid 1 g orally or ceftriaxone 250 mg i.m.
Plus
Doxycycline 100 mg orally 2 times/day for 14 days with or without metronidazole 500 mg orally 2 times/day for 14 days

Optimal alternative regimens are unclear, consider amoxicillin and clavulinic acid or azithromycin

Re-evaluate in 2–3 days to review ultimate results and determine response to antibiotics

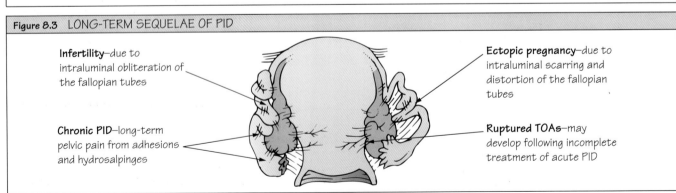

Figure 8.3 LONG-TERM SEQUELAE OF PID

Infertility—due to intraluminal obliteration of the fallopian tubes

Chronic PID—long-term pelvic pain from adhesions and hydrosalpinges

Ectopic pregnancy—due to intraluminal scarring and distortion of the fallopian tubes

Ruptured TOAs—may develop following incomplete treatment of acute PID

Obstetrics and Gynecology at a Glance, Fourth Edition. Errol R. Norwitz and John O. Schorge.

24 © 2013 John Wiley & Sons, Ltd. Published 2013 by John Wiley & Sons, Ltd.

Definition: a clinical spectrum of infection (Figure 8.1) that may involve the cervix, endometrium, fallopian tubes, ovaries, uterus, broad ligaments, intraperitoneal cavity, and perihepatic region.
• Infectious inflammation of the pelvic organs may lead to tissue necrosis and abscess formation. Eventually, the process evolves into scar formation with development of adhesions to nearby structures.
• Acute PID (salpingitis) is the typical clinical syndrome.
• Chronic PID is an outdated term that refers to the long-term sequelae.

Etiology
• The pathogenesis is incompletely understood but involves a polymicrobial infection ascending from the bacterial flora of the vagina and cervix.
• *Chlamydia trachomatis* and/or *Neisseria gonorrhoeae* is detectable in >50% of women. These pathogens are probably responsible for the initial invasion of the upper genital tract, with other organisms becoming involved secondarily.
• Fifteen percent of cases follow a surgical procedure (endometrial biopsy, intrauterine device [IUD] placement) which breaks the cervical mucous barrier and directly transmits bacteria to the upper genital tract.

Risk factors
• The classic example of a high-risk patient is a menstruating teenager who has multiple sexual partners, does not use contraception and lives in an area with a high prevalence of STIs.
• Seventy-five percent of women diagnosed are <25 years.
• Premenarchal, pregnant, or postmenopausal patients are rare.
• Having multiple partners increases the risk by fivefold.
• Frequent vaginal douching increases the risk by threefold.
• Barrier (condom, diaphragm) contraception decreases the risk.
• IUD insertion is a risk factor in the first 3 weeks after placement.
• Previous PID is a risk factor for future episodes: 25% of women will develop another infection.

Epidemiology
• 1 million women in the USA (200,000 in the UK) are diagnosed annually.

Symptoms and signs
• PID can occur and cause serious harm without causing any noticeable symptoms.
• Lower abdominal pain is the most common complaint.
• Patients may also have fever, painful intercourse, irregular menstrual bleeding, nausea, and vomiting.
• Seventy-five percent have a mucopurulent cervical discharge on examination.
• Five percent present with *Fitz–Hugh–Curtis syndrome* (perihepatic inflammation and adhesions), characterized by pleuritic right upper quadrant pain.

Diagnosis
• The Centers for Disease Control and Prevention (CDC) recommends diagnosis by *minimal* criteria of lower abdominal pain and uterine/adnexal tenderness or cervical motion tenderness on exam.
• *Supportive* criteria include temperature >101°F, mucopurulent cervical or vaginal discharge, abundant white blood cells (WBCs) on saline wet-mount, elevated C-reactive protein (CRP), elevated erythrocyte sedimentation rate (ESR), and positive gonorrhea or chlamydia testing.
• *Confirmatory* criteria traditionally include plasma cell endometritis on endometrial biopsy and visualization on laparoscopy. The sensitivity and specificity of these "gold standard" criteria are debated.
• Women meeting the criteria for PID may have a separate pathologic process (appendicitis, endometriosis, rupture of an adnexal mass) or a normal pelvis in up to 50% of cases.

Treatment of acute PID (Figure 8.2)
• Antibiotic treatment should be started as soon as possible.
• Patients may be managed as outpatients or inpatients, depending on their clinical picture.
• Tubo-ovarian abscesses (TOAs) should be drained percutaneously or surgically.
• Management should include treatment of sexual partners, screening for other sexually transmitted infections, and education on the prevention of re-infection.

Surgical management
• Ruptured TOAs are a surgical emergency. The mortality risk is 5–10% chiefly due to the development of septic shock and adult respiratory distress syndrome.
• Patients with a TOA that does not respond to antibiotics and percutaneous drainage also require surgery.
• Bilateral salpingo-oophorectomy with hysterectomy yields the highest chance of success. Leaving any of the reproductive organs *in situ* risks re-emergence of infection, but conservative surgery should be considered in young patients who desire future fertility.

Long-term sequelae of PID (Figure 8.3)
Although the acute infection may be treated successfully, subsequent effects are often permanent. This makes early identification very important in preventing damage to the reproductive system.
• *Infertility* occurs in 10–15% of women with a single episode of PID and depends on the severity of the infection.
• *Chronic PID* is a recurrent pain syndrome that develops in 20% of women as a result of inflammation.
• *Ectopic pregnancy* is increased six- to tenfold.

Rare causes
Actinomycosis
• *Actinomyces israelii* is an anaerobic, Gram-positive, non-acid-fast, pleomorphic bacterium.
• The diagnosis should be suspected if such organisms are identified on cervical Gram stain or if an endometrial biopsy shows "sulfur granules." However, definitive diagnosis requires a positive culture.
• *Treatment.* High-dose parenteral penicillin plus oral doxycycline for 6 weeks.

Pelvic tuberculosis
• A common cause of chronic PID and infertility in developing countries.
• *Mycobacterium tuberculosis* is the causative agent.
• Definitive diagnosis requires histologic evidence of granulomas, giant cells, and caseous necrosis.
• *Treatment.* Multiple antituberculosis drugs for 18–24 months.

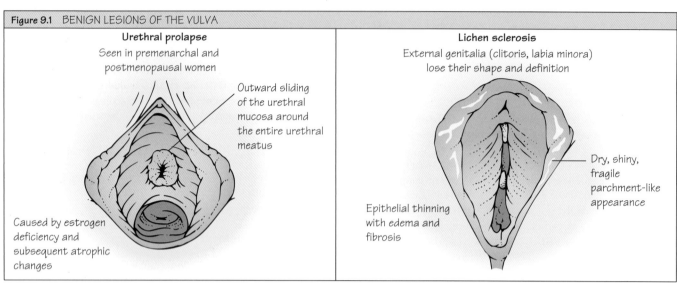

Figure 9.1 BENIGN LESIONS OF THE VULVA

Urethral prolapse

Seen in premenarchal and postmenopausal women

Outward sliding of the urethral mucosa around the entire urethral meatus

Caused by estrogen deficiency and subsequent atrophic changes

Lichen sclerosis

External genitalia (clitoris, labia minora) lose their shape and definition

Dry, shiny, fragile parchment-like appearance

Epithelial thinning with edema and fibrosis

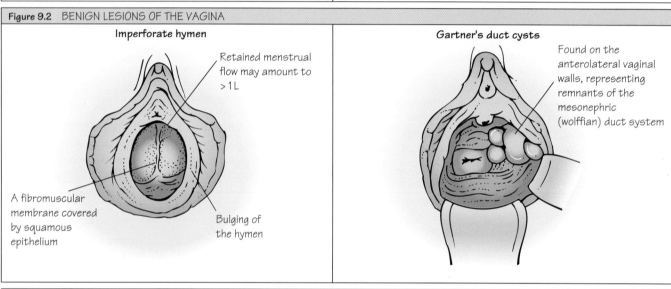

Figure 9.2 BENIGN LESIONS OF THE VAGINA

Imperforate hymen

Retained menstrual flow may amount to >1 L

A fibromuscular membrane covered by squamous epithelium

Bulging of the hymen

Gartner's duct cysts

Found on the anterolateral vaginal walls, representing remnants of the mesonephric (wolffian) duct system

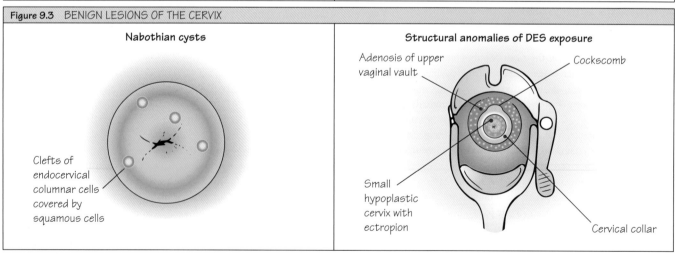

Figure 9.3 BENIGN LESIONS OF THE CERVIX

Nabothian cysts

Clefts of endocervical columnar cells covered by squamous cells

Structural anomalies of DES exposure

Adenosis of upper vaginal vault

Cockscomb

Small hypoplastic cervix with ectropion

Cervical collar

Obstetrics and Gynecology at a Glance, Fourth Edition. Errol R. Norwitz and John O. Schorge.

26 © 2013 John Wiley & Sons, Ltd. Published 2013 by John Wiley & Sons, Ltd.

Vulvar lesions
Urethral disorders
• *Urethral prolapse* (Figure 9.1) may cause dysuria, but often is asymptomatic. *Treatment*: topical estrogen cream, hot sitz baths, and antibiotics may reduce inflammation and infection; surgical excision is rarely needed.
• *Urethral diverticulum* is a sac or a pouch that connects with the urethra and may cause dysuria, dribbling incontinence urgency, or hematuria. *Treatment*: excision with layered closure or marsupialization.
• *Skenes*. Duct, cyst, or abscess is an obstruction of the periurethral glands. *Treatment*: abscess requires incision and drainage.

Vulvar cysts and benign tumors
• *Bartholin cysts* result from occlusion of the excretory duct. *Treatment*: most will resolve spontaneously with local care, but marsupialization is performed for large or recurrent lesions and abscess requires incision and drainage and often placement of a Word catheter.
• *Hernias (hydroceles, cysts) of the canal of Nuck* are abnormal dilations of the peritoneum that accompany the round ligament through the inguinal canal and into the labia majora. *Treatment*: excision of the hernia sac.
• *Epidermal inclusion cysts* are formed when a focus of epithelium is buried beneath the skin surface and becomes encysted. *Treatment*: *expectant management or* excision if symptomatic.

Non-neoplastic epithelial disorders
• Candida vulvitis is a symmetric bright red rash, causes itching and burning. *Treatment*: topical imidazole, oral fluconazole.
• *Lichen sclerosus* (Figure 9.1) is an atrophic change or thinning of the epidermis (onion skin, parchment like), more common in postmenopausal women. The main symptom, if any, is pruritus. Diagnosis can often be made by inspection alone, but biopsy is confirmatory. One percent annual risk of vulvar cancer. *Treatment*: topical testosterone or high-potency corticosteroids (clobetasol).
• *Squamous cell hyperplasia* is a diagnosis of exclusion that represents a thickening of the epidermis and lichenification, and is a chronic scratch–itch cycle reaction to fungus or other vulvitis, allergens, or unknown stimuli. Pruritus and excoriations are often evident. Pathologic findings are non-specific. *Treatment*: management of the inciting cause and/or topical corticosteroids.
• *Lichen planus* is a chronic inflammatory dermatitis of unknown etiology. It is characterized by multiple, small, shiny, purple, cutaneous papules. *Treatment*: vaginal corticosteroid suppositories.
• *Psoriasis* and *eczema of the vulva* are an incurable chronic inflammatory dermatitis that may involve the vulva. Diagnosis is made by inspection and asymmetric distribution, and biopsy is confirmatory. *Treatment*: ultraviolet light or topical corticosteroids.

Other benign vulvar lesions
• *Nevi* begin as pigmented nests of cells at the dermal–epidermal junction. *Treatment*: biopsy-proven diagnosis to rule out melanoma.
• *Hidradenitis suppurativa* is a chronic, progressive, inflammatory disorder characterized by apocrine gland plugging and superinfection. *Treatment*: antibiotics or surgical excision for refractory cases.
• *Provoked vulvodynia* is a chronic pain syndrome of unclear etiology that may be suggested on physical examination by reproducible exquisite pinpoint pressure tenderness to light touch with Q tip at vestibule. May interfere with sexual intercourse or tampon use. *Treatment*: topical estrogen cream, local topical anesthetic jelly, vaginal dilator therapy or pelvic floor, physical therapy agents or surgical excision, *or* tricyclic antidepressants.
• *Idiopathic vulvodynia* (vulvar pain) is a diagnosis of exclusion without specific physical findings. *Treatment*: tricyclic antidepressants.

Vaginal lesions
Congenital anomalies
• *Müllerian agenesis* (see Chapter 22) results from abnormal development of the distal müllerian ducts, and is usually associated with blind vaginal pouch and absence of the uterus and vagina. *Treatment*: progressive vaginal dilatation or surgical creation of a neovagina.
• *Imperforate hymen* (Figure 9.2) is a distal failure of vaginal vault canalization during embryogenesis. A *transverse vaginal septum* is a more proximal failure. Diagnosis is usually made at menarche when patients present with cyclic abdominal pain due to retained menstrual flow. *Treatment*: surgical hymenectomy.

Vaginal cysts and benign tumors
• *Epithelial inclusion cysts* are the most common cystic structures in the vagina, usually resulting from birth trauma or gynecologic surgery. *Treatment*: *expectant management, possible* surgical excision.
• *Gartner duct cysts* (Figure 9.2) or other embryonic epithelial remnants may be multiple and may occasionally be an incidental finding on routine physical examination. *Treatment*: expectant management, surgical excision if painful.

Other vaginal lesions
• *Vaginal lacerations* occur most commonly secondary to sexual intercourse. Other causes include blunt trauma (straddle) injuries and penetration injuries by foreign objects. *Treatment*: surgical repair.
• *Atrophic vaginitis* is a disorder of postmenopausal women. Lack of estrogen causes the vaginal mucosa to become thin, causing dryness and bleeding. *Treatment*: oral or topical estrogen.
• *Fistulae* from the bladder, ureter, and small or large bowel may occur in any part of the vaginal canal. *Treatment*: surgical repair.
• *Foreign bodies* (retained tampons, pessaries) can lead to ulceration and infection of the vagina. *Treatment*: removal and local care.

Cervical lesions
Cervical cysts and benign tumors
• *Nabothian cysts* (Figure 9.3) are so common that they are considered a normal feature of the adult cervix, with mucinous fluid within the cyst and often vascularity on the surface. *Treatment*: none.
• *Cervical polyps* are the most common benign neoplastic growths of the cervix. They usually originate from inflammation with focal hyperplasia and localized proliferation. *Treatment*: removal by twisting the stalk and gently pulling.

Cervical stenosis
• Acquired causes include cervical surgery, radiation, infection, neoplasia, and atrophic changes.
• Symptoms in premenopausal women may include dysmenorrhea, subfertility, abnormal vaginal bleeding, and amenorrhea. Postmenopausal women are usually asymptomatic.
• Complications may include development of a hydrometra (clear fluid in the uterus), hematometra (blood), or pyometra (pus). *Treatment* (if needed): cervical dilation to re-establish the patency of the canal.

Diethylstilbestrol exposure
• Diethylstilbestrol (DES) is a synthetic estrogen that was administered between the 1940s and 1970s to prevent miscarriage in some women with high-risk pregnancies.
• Women who were exposed to DES *in utero* frequently have extension of glandular epithelium on the ectocervix (ectropion) and upper vagina (vaginal adenosis), in addition to other structural anomalies. *Treatment*: none is needed. Associated with rare clear cell cancer of vagina or cervix.

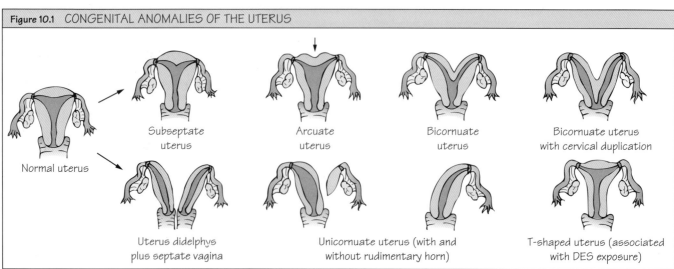

Figure 10.1 CONGENITAL ANOMALIES OF THE UTERUS

Normal uterus

Subseptate uterus

Arcuate uterus

Bicornuate uterus

Bicornuate uterus with cervical duplication

Uterus didelphys plus septate vagina

Unicornuate uterus (with and without rudimentary horn)

T-shaped uterus (associated with DES exposure)

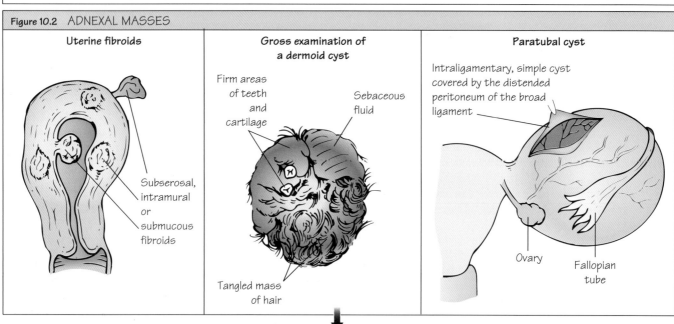

Figure 10.2 ADNEXAL MASSES

Uterine fibroids

Subserosal, intramural or submucous fibroids

Gross examination of a dermoid cyst

Firm areas of teeth and cartilage

Sebaceous fluid

Tangled mass of hair

Paratubal cyst

Intraligamentary, simple cyst covered by the distended peritoneum of the broad ligament

Ovary

Fallopian tube

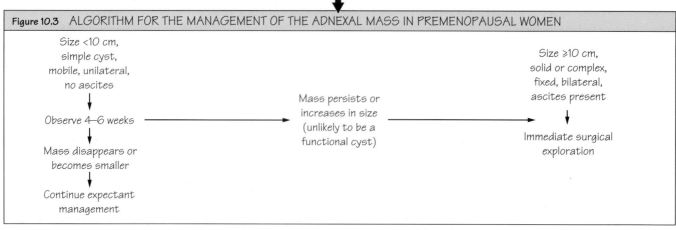

Figure 10.3 ALGORITHM FOR THE MANAGEMENT OF THE ADNEXAL MASS IN PREMENOPAUSAL WOMEN

Size <10 cm, simple cyst, mobile, unilateral, no ascites

Observe 4–6 weeks

Mass disappears or becomes smaller

Continue expectant management

Mass persists or increases in size (unlikely to be a functional cyst)

Size ≥10 cm, solid or complex, fixed, bilateral, ascites present

Immediate surgical exploration

Obstetrics and Gynecology at a Glance, Fourth Edition. Errol R. Norwitz and John O. Schorge.

Uterine lesions

Congenital anomalies (Figure 10.1)
• Normal müllerian duct fusion during embryogenesis results in a triangular-shaped uterine cavity and canalized upper vagina. Incomplete fusion results in a variety of congenital anomalies.

• *Uterine didelphys* is the most extreme form of incomplete fusion with two separate uteri and possibly two cervices, and a septate upper vagina. Partial fusion is more common, resulting in an *arcuate* septate, *bicornuate*, or *septate* uterus. A *unicornuate* uterus arises from one müllerian duct and its attached tube; the other müllerian duct may be rudimentary or absent.

Fibroids (leiomyomas, myomas) (Figure 10.2)
The most common neoplasm of the female pelvis present in about 50% of women and the leading indication for hysterectomy.

• *Etiology.* Uterine fibroids are benign proliferations of smooth muscle and fibrous connective tissue that originate from a single cell. They are usually multiple, range in diameter from 1 mm to >20 cm, and are surrounded by a pseudocapsule of compressed smooth muscle fibers. Fibroids may increase in size in response to estrogen therapy and most regress to some degree after menopause. Progestins, clomiphene, and pregnancy occasionally induce a rapid increase in size, with hemorrhagic degeneration and pain. Fibroids are more common in black women.

• *Classification.* All fibroids begin within the myometrium. Continued growth in one direction will ultimately determine how the fibroids are classified by location as subserosal, intramural, or submucosal. Occasional fibroids have more numerous mitotic figures (mitotically active leiomyoma) or densely cellular fascicles of smooth muscle (cellular leiomyoma). These subtypes do not meet diagnostic criteria for leiomyosarcoma and have no malignant risk.

• *Symptoms.* Most patients are asymptomatic. Women may seek treatment for abnormal uterine bleeding, pelvic pressure, or pain.

• *Diagnosis.* Palpation of an enlarged, irregular uterus on bimanual examination is suggestive. Ultrasound may be used to confirm the diagnosis. Grossly, fibroids can have a variety of appearances depending on the location and presence of degeneration.

• *Expectant management.* Most patients do not require any treatment. Fibroids may be monitored over time by examination or ultrasound. Intervention may be indicated if (1) the patient has bulky symptoms, (2) the patient has excessive bleeding, (3) there is a concern that the mass is a sarcoma – based on rapid growth, (4) the uterus is causing significant hydronephrosis, or (5) if there is distortion of the uterus cavity in women who are contemplating pregnancy or experiencing recurrent miscarriage.

• *Medical management. Oral contraceptive pills (OCPs), progestins, and the Mirena intrauterine system (IUS)* can all reduce excessive bleeding. Gonadotropin-releasing hormone (GnRH) agonists (ie, leuprolide acetate) induce a hypoestrogeniuc amenorrhea and can temporarily shrink fibroids, usually in anticipation of more definitive surgery.

• *Non-invasive surgical techniques.* Uterine artery embolization is an alternative to surgery that decreases blood flow to the fibroid uterus. Most patients have a significant decrease in bleeding symptoms and a reduction in uterine size; however, the benefit may be transient.

• *Minimally invasive surgery.* Hysteroscopic myomectomy for submucous fibroids up to 4 cm or endometrial ablation is primarily efficacious for control of bleeding. Laparoscopic or robotic myomectomy or hysterectomy can be performed safely if technically feasible, with intraoperative morcellation if needed. For very large, or more complex circumstances, a laparotomy may be required to safely perform the operation.

Endometrial polyps
Localized overgrowths of endometrial glands and stroma that usually arise at the uterine fundus. The majority are asymptomatic, but some present with abnormal vaginal bleeding. These may be removed hysteroscopically.

Adnexal masses
Five to ten percent of women will have surgery for an adnexal mass during their lifetime. Ultrasound is the imaging modality of choice. The sonographic appearance of irregular borders, ascites, papillations, or septations within an ovarian cyst should increase concern about malignancy.

Benign ovarian cystic masses
The sonographic appearance of irregular borders, ascites, papillations, or septations within an ovarian cyst should increase concern about malignancy (see Chapter 33).

• *Functional cysts* are the most common clinically detectable enlargements of the ovary occurring during the reproductive years. They may be large simple cysts or hemorrhagic corpus luteum cysts. The majority will resolve spontaneously within 4–6 weeks.

• *Dermoids (benign cystic teratomas;* Figure 10.2) represent 25% of all ovarian neoplasms. They vary in size from a few millimeters to 25 cm in diameter, and are bilateral in 10–15% of cases. They are usually complex cystic structures that contain elements from all three germ cell layers (endoderm, mesoderm, and ectoderm).

• *Serous cystadenomas* are common uni- or multilocular cysts; 10–20% are bilateral.

• *Mucinous cystadenomas* are multilocular, lobulated, and smooth surfaced. Bilateral lesions are rare. These lesions may become huge, occasionally weighing >50 kg.

• *Ovarian endometriomas* ("chocolate cysts") are cystic areas of endometriosis that are usually bilateral and may reach 15–20 cm in size. On bimanual examination, the adnexae are often tender and immobile due to associated inflammation and adhesions. Endometriomas are homogeneous complex masses that can be more clearly diagnosed with pelvic magnetic resonance imaging.

Benign ovarian solid neoplasms
• *Ovarian fibromas* are the most common variant. They are slow growing and vary widely in size. *Meigs syndrome* refers to the rare clinical triad of an ovarian fibroma, ascites, and hydrothorax.

• *Serous adenofibromas and cystadenofibromas* are partially solid tumors with a predominance of connective tissue; 25% are bilateral.

Fallopian tube lesions
• *Paratubal cysts* (Figure 10.2) are usually asymptomatic and discovered incidentally. The cysts are thin walled and filled with clear fluid. They are remnants of the embryonic wolffian (mesonephric) duct system.

• *Hydrosalpinges* are abnormally dilated fallopian tubes that represent sequelae of previous pelvic inflammatory disease (see Chapter 8).

Management of the adnexal mass
The overwhelming majority of adnexal masses are benign, regardless of patient age.

   Note: all women with a solid ovarian neoplasm should have excision.

   Note: the CA-125 tumor marker titer should not be used to determine the need for surgery.

• *Premenopausal women* (Figure 10.3).

• *Postmenopausal women.* Simple cysts often can be followed expectantly unless they are symptomatic. Many will resolve over time. All complex adnexal masses should be considered potentially malignant and surgically excised.

Figure 11.1 COMMON SITES OF ENDOMETRIOSIS

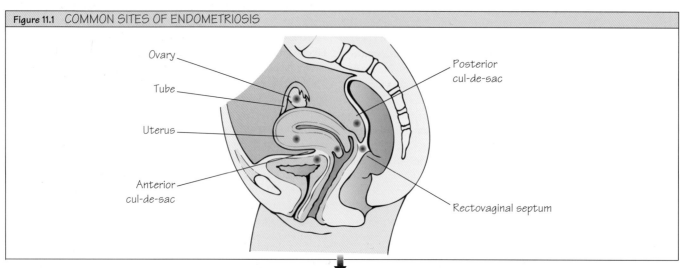

Figure 11.2 AMERICAN FERTILITY SOCIETY (AFS) CLASSIFICATION OF ENDOMETRIOSIS

		Points assigned for each lesion visualized at surgery		
	Endometriosis	<1 cm	1–3 cm	>3 cm
Peritoneum	Superficial	1	2	4
	Deep	2	4	6
Ovary	R Superficial	1	2	4
	Deep	4	16	20
	L Superficial	1	2	4
	Deep	4	16	20
	Posterior cul-de-sac obliteration	Partial		Complete
		4		40
	Adhesions	<1/3 enclosure	1/3–2/3 enclosure	>2/3 enclosure
Ovary	R Filmy	1	2	4
	Dense	4	8	16
	L Filmy	1	2	4
	Dense	4	8	16
Tube	R Filmy	1	2	4
	Dense	4	8	16
	L Filmy	1	2	4
	Dense	4	8	16

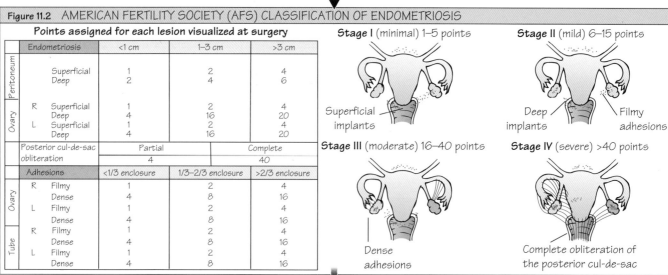

Stage I (minimal) 1–5 points

Superficial implants

Stage II (mild) 6–15 points

Deep implants — Filmy adhesions

Stage III (moderate) 16–40 points

Dense adhesions

Stage IV (severe) >40 points

Complete obliteration of the posterior cul-de-sac

Figure 11.3 LAPAROSCOPIC EXCISION OF OVARIAN ENDOMETRIOMA

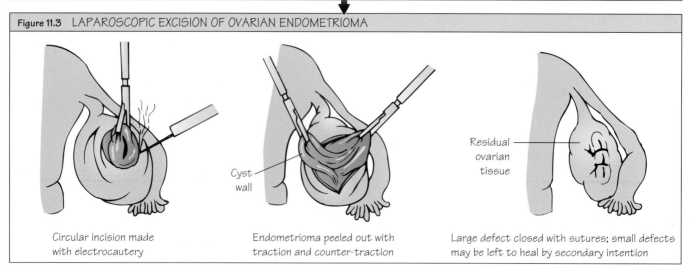

Circular incision made with electrocautery

Cyst wall

Endometrioma peeled out with traction and counter-traction

Residual ovarian tissue

Large defect closed with sutures; small defects may be left to heal by secondary intention

Endometriosis

• *Definition.* Functional endometrial glands and stroma outside the uterine cavity (Figure 11.1).
• *Prevalence.* Five to ten percent of women of reproductive age; 30–40% of infertile women; 80% of women with chronic pelvic pain (see Chapter 6).
• *Age.* Typically diagnosed in women during their 20s. Not found before menarche and characteristically regresses after the menopause.
• *Pathogenesis.* theories include (1) *retrograde menstruation* (viable endometrial cells reflux through the tubes during menstruation and implant in the pelvis), (2) *celomic metaplasia* (multipotential cells of the celomic epithelium are stimulated to transform into endometrium-like cells), (3) *hematogenous dissemination* (endometrial cells are transported to distant sites), and (4) *autoimmune disease* (a disorder of immune surveillance that allows ectopic endometrial implants to grow).

Symptoms and signs

• The most common symptoms are *pelvic pain* and *infertility*, but many patients are asymptomatic.
• *Cyclic pain* is the hallmark of endometriosis, including secondary dysmenorrhea (begins before or with menstruation and is maximal at the time of maximal flow), deep dyspareunia (pain with intercourse), pain with defecation, and sacral backache with menses.
• The severity of symptoms does not necessarily correlate with the degree of pelvic disease. Indeed, many women with minimal endometriosis complain of severe pelvic pain.
• Infertility may result from anatomic distortion of the pelvic architecture due to extensive endometriosis and adhesions, but also occurs in women with minimal disease for unknown reasons.
• Common physical findings include a fixed, retroverted uterus, nodularity of the uterosacral ligaments, and enlarged, tender adnexa.

Diagnosis

• History and physical examination may suggest the diagnosis because endometriotic lesions may occur anywhere in the body. The most common site is the ovary.
• Pelvic ultrasonography may demonstrate presence of one or more *endometriomas* (blood-filled ovarian cysts) which are commonly adherent to the surrounding pelvic structures.
• Laparoscopic surgery with direct visualization of endometriotic lesions and histologic examination of biopsy specimens is the standard for making the diagnosis. Early lesions on the peritoneal surface are small and vesicular. Later lesions have a typical "powder-burn" appearance, which refers to a puckered, black area surrounded by a stellate scar.

Classification

• The American Fertility Society classification system (Figure 11.2) is based on surgical findings with points subjectively assigned to each lesion depending on its size and depth. The presence and extent of adhesions are also scored.

Medical management

The primary goal of medical therapy is suppression of ovulation and induction of amenorrhea. Symptomatic relief of dysmenorrhea, dyspareunia, and/or pelvic pain is usually somewhat successful, but often short-lived. Medical therapy does not eradicate the lesions.
• *Non-steroidal anti-inflammatory drugs (NSAIDs)* not only reduce pain but also reduce menstrual flow. They are commonly used together with other therapy. For more severe cases, opiate prescription drugs may be required.

• *Progestins* counteract estrogen and inhibit the growth of the endometrium. Such therapy can reduce or eliminate menstruation in a controlled and reversible fashion.
• *Oral contraceptives (OCs)* reduce or eliminate menstrual flow and provide estrogen support. Typically, it is a long-term approach. Newer agents (Seasonale) were designed to reduce the number of cycles by inducing a menses every 3 months or even less. Alternatively, OCs can be taken continuously without the use of placebo pills, or, in the case of the use of NuvaRing or the contraceptive patch, without the break week. This eliminates monthly bleeding episodes.
• *Danazol* and *gestrinone* are suppressive steroids with some androgenic activity. Both agents inhibit the growth of endometriosis but their use remains limited because they may cause unsightly hirsutism.
• *Gonadotropin-releasing hormone (GnRH) agonists* induce a profound hypoestrogenic "medical menopause." Although quite effective, they induce unpleasant menopausal symptoms, and beyond 6 months may lead to osteoporosis. To counteract such side effects or to extend the treatment some estrogen may have to be given back (add-back therapy).
• "Empiric" therapy is used when signs and symptoms support the diagnosis of endometriosis, but definitive surgical diagnosis has not been achieved. A trial of OCs and NSAIDs is often attempted first, but a 3-month course of GnRH agonist (Lupron) may also be helpful in refractory patients.
• Patients who do not respond to empiric therapy generally warrant diagnostic laparoscopy to confirm the diagnosis before moving on to danazol, long-term GnRH agonist therapy with add-back, or opiates.

Surgical management (Figure 11.3)

• Young women desiring future fertility typically undergo laparoscopic surgery with a primary goal to excise or destroy as much of the endometriosis as possible while restoring normal anatomy and salvaging normal ovarian tissue. Multiple such operations over a period of years may occur in some cases.
• Laparoscopic surgery is generally advised when imaging suggests a larger ovarian endometrioma (>4 cm) or pelvic adhesions are clinically suspected. *Presacral neurectomy* and/or *uterosacral nerve ablation* has been reported to benefit selected patients.
• Pregnancy rates may be improved in women with moderate-to-severe endometriosis who undergo surgical treatment.
• Older women without concerns about future childbearing are usually the best candidates for more definitive surgery (hysterectomy with bilateral salpingo-oophorectomy).
• Patients should be counseled that pelvic pain may still be unrelieved and hormone replacement therapy (see Chapter 28) with estrogen is still an option. Alternatively, one or both ovaries may be retained, but the risk of reoperation for persistent pain is about 20%.
• Endometriosis often obliterates natural tissue planes and surgery can be very complex due to adhesions, generalized induration, and involvement of the rectum and bladder.

Adenomyosis

• *Definition.* Endometrial glands and stroma within the myometrium.
• *Prevalence.* Occurs to some degree in about 20% of women.
• *Symptoms and signs.* Dysmenorrhea, menorrhagia, dyspareunia, and a smoothly enlarged boggy uterus on pelvic examination.
• *Diagnosis* may be suggested by pelvic ultrasonography and/or magnetic resonance imaging, but adenomyosis is a histopathologic diagnosis.
• *Treatment.* May be treated with continuous OCPs, Depo-Provera or Mirena intrauterine system but in many there is no effective medical treatment – hysterectomy is curative for symptomatic women.

Figure 12.1 CONTRACEPTION OPTIONS

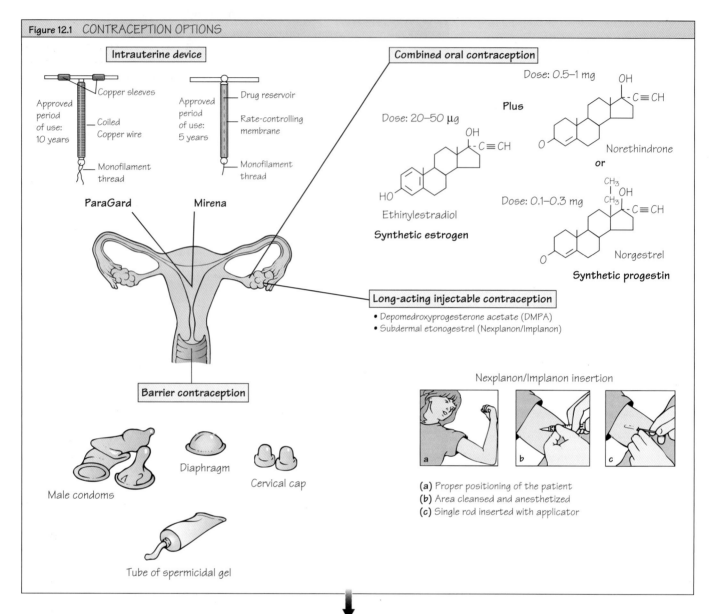

Intrauterine device

Copper sleeves
Approved period of use: 10 years
Coiled Copper wire
Monofilament thread

Drug reservoir
Approved period of use: 5 years
Rate-controlling membrane
Monofilament thread

ParaGard   Mirena

Combined oral contraception

Dose: 20–50 μg
Ethinylestradiol
Synthetic estrogen

Dose: 0.5–1 mg
Plus
Norethindrone
or
Dose: 0.1–0.3 mg
Norgestrel
Synthetic progestin

Long-acting injectable contraception
• Depomedroxyprogesterone acetate (DMPA)
• Subdermal etonogestrel (Nexplanon/Implanon)

Barrier contraception

Male condoms
Diaphragm
Cervical cap
Tube of spermicidal gel

Nexplanon/Implanon insertion

(a) Proper positioning of the patient
(b) Area cleansed and anesthetized
(c) Single rod inserted with applicator

Figure 12.2 FAILURE RATES FOR VARIOUS CONTRACEPTIVE METHODS

Method	Percentage of women becoming pregnant within 1 year	
	Perfect use	Typical use
OCs, OrthoEvra, NuvaRing, 'mini-pill'	0.3	8
Male condoms	2	15
Diaphragm with spermicide	6	16
Paraguard IUD	0.6	0.8
Mirena IUS	0.2	0.2
Depo-Provera	0.3	3
Nexplanon/Implanon	<0.1	<0.1

Obstetrics and Gynecology at a Glance, Fourth Edition. Errol R. Norwitz and John O. Schorge.

- *Definition.* The voluntary prevention of pregnancy ("birth control").
- *Contraceptive options* (Figure 12.1) depend primarily on the motivation of the user, but none is 100% effective, immediately available, and low cost. Of the methods, only male and female condoms reduce the risk of sexually transmitted infections.

Oral contraceptives (OCs)

The most popular method of reversible contraception in the USA and the UK.
- *Composition.* Most are combinations that contain both a synthetic estrogen and a progestin. The progestin-only pill ("minipill") is less popular since it is associated with a higher incidence of irregular bleeding.
- *Administration.* For simplicity, the first pill is often taken on the first day of the period, or on the first Sunday after the first day of the period. Thereafter, one tablet is taken every day for a total of 21 days, followed by 7 days of a placebo pill. An anovulatory (withdrawal) bleed will then occur. Most OC preparations contain 28 tablets to allow a woman to take a tablet every day, which reduces mistakes and missed pills. Alternative contraception (typically condoms) is generally advisable when starting OCs.
- *Formulations.* Recently, some OCs have been designed to induce menses quarterly instead of monthly (Seasonale). Other combined hormone alternatives include a weekly transdermal patch (OrthoEvra), a vaginal ring (NuvaRing) changed every 3 weeks, or a monthly injection (Lunelle; not available in the USA).
- *Mechanism of action.* All types prevent ovulation through central inhibition of the mid-cycle luteinizing hormone (LH) surge, act peripherally to decrease oviductal function, and thicken cervical mucus.
- *Health benefits.* OCs reduce menstrual cramps and decrease uterine bleeding. They protect against benign breast disease, prevent formation of ovarian cysts, and reduce the incidence and severity of pelvic inflammatory disease (PID). In addition, OCs reduce the risk of endometrial and ovarian cancer, and possibly endometriosis.
- *Side effects.* Irregular breakthrough bleeding (especially if doses are missed), nausea, headache, elevated blood pressure, weight gain, breast pain.
- *Absolute contraindications.* Thromboembolic disease, chronic liver disease, undiagnosed uterine bleeding, pregnancy, and estrogen-dependent neoplasia.
- *Relative contraindications.* Smoking in women >35 years, migraine headaches, cardiac disease, diabetic complications.

Long-acting injectable contraception

Depomedroxyprogesterone acetate (DMPA, Depo-Provera)
- *Dosing.* This is 150 mg intramuscularly every 12 weeks.
- *Mechanism.* Prevents ovulation by blocking the mid-cycle LH surge.
- *Side effects.* markedly irregular vaginal bleeding, amenorrhea, weight gain, alopecia, reduced libido, depression, and osteopenia.

Subdermal etonogestrel (Nexplanon/Implanon)
- *Dosing.* Single-rod subdermal implant inserted beneath the skin of the upper arm is effective for 3 years.
- *Mechanism.* Prevention of ovulation in addition to impaired oocyte maturation and thickened cervical mucus.
- *Side effects.* Similar to DMPA. Removal usually takes longer than placement and may be mildly uncomfortable due to fibrosis.

Barrier contraception

Works by blocking sperm from getting into the female reproductive tract.

Male condoms (prophylactics, rubbers)
- The most popular barrier method, a latex or polyurethane sheath placed over the penis, prevents deposition of semen in the vagina.
- Disposable, convenient to use, inexpensive, widely available, and prevents the spread of sexually transmitted infections (STIs).

Intravaginal devices
- The *diaphragm* is a circular patch of latex rubber held in place by a collapsible metal frame. It prevents passage of sperm into the cervical canal. It must be used with a spermicidal gel and left in place for 6 hours after intercourse.
- The *female condom* fits loosely inside the vagina and covers the perineum. It is used infrequently.

Spermicides
- Nonoxynol-9, a non-toxic detergent that destroys the cell membrane of sperm, is the main active ingredient.
- Available without prescription as foam, cream, or suppositories.
- Most commonly used with a diaphragm.

Intrauterine device (IUD), also known as LARC (long-acting reversible contraception)

The most commonly used reversible contraceptive worldwide and endorsed as a first-line product regardless of parity.
- *Terminology.* In the USA, all devices that are placed in the uterus to prevent pregnancy are referred to as IUDs. In the UK, only copper-containing devices are called IUDs and hormonal intrauterine contraceptives are referred to by the term intrauterine system (IUS).
- *Dosing.* May be inserted at any time in the menstrual cycle once a pre-existing pregnancy has been excluded. Uterine perforation may occur at the time of insertion, but is rare. The expulsion rate is 5% in the first year.
- *Mechanism.* Prevents fertilization and implantation by inducing a local, sterile, inflammatory reaction that is hostile to the oocyte, sperm, and zygote.
- *Side effects.* Menorrhagia and dysmenorrhea are the primary reasons for early removal of the copper T-380A (ParaGard) IUD. Conversely, the levonorgestrel (Mirena) IUS reduces menstrual blood flow and cramping. There is a very low risk of uterine infection for the first 3 days after insertion of the device.

Emergency contraception (morning-after pill)
- Not recommended as a first-line method. It is typically used after failure of another method or after unprotected sex.
- The risk of pregnancy can be reduced by 75% if taken within 72 hours of unprotected intercourse.
- *Dosing.* Single dose of 1.5 mg levonorgestrel (UK standard) or two pills (each: 0.05 mg ethinylestradiol, 0.25 mg levonorgestrel) followed by a second dose 12 hours later (USA standard). Alternatively, an IUD may be placed to prevent implantation.

Failure rates (Figure 12.2)

The *rhythm method* (periodic abstinence), *coitus interruptus* (withdrawal of the penis before ejaculation), *postcoital douching*, and *prolonged breastfeeding* are unreliable and not considered methods of contraception because of their high failure rates.

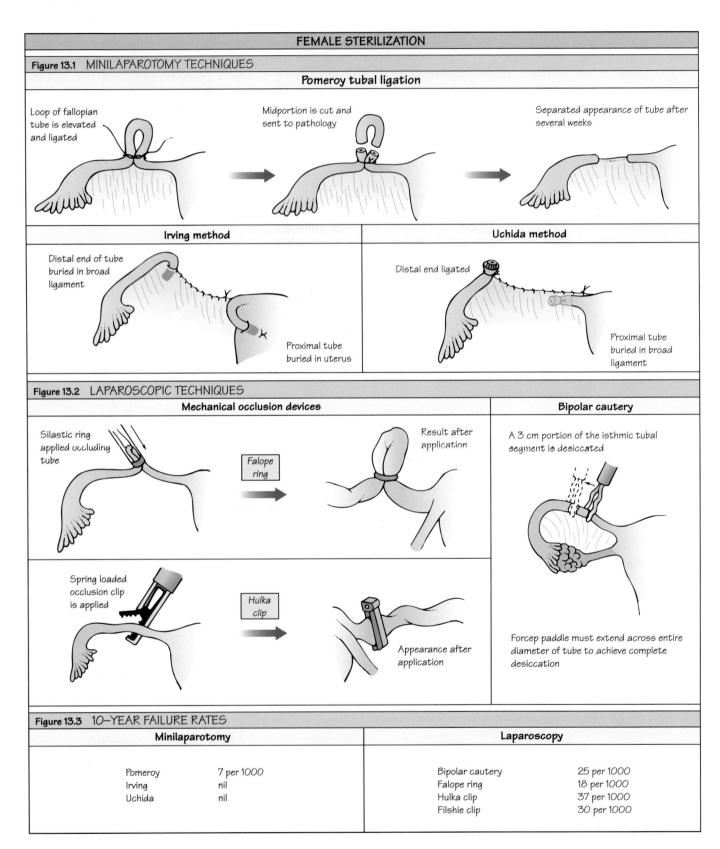

FEMALE STERILIZATION

Figure 13.1 MINILAPAROTOMY TECHNIQUES

Pomeroy tubal ligation

Loop of fallopian tube is elevated and ligated

Midportion is cut and sent to pathology

Separated appearance of tube after several weeks

Irving method

Distal end of tube buried in broad ligament

Proximal tube buried in uterus

Uchida method

Distal end ligated

Proximal tube buried in broad ligament

Figure 13.2 LAPAROSCOPIC TECHNIQUES

Mechanical occlusion devices

Silastic ring applied occluding tube

Falope ring

Result after application

Spring loaded occlusion clip is applied

Hulka clip

Appearance after application

Bipolar cautery

A 3 cm portion of the isthmic tubal segment is desiccated

Forcep paddle must extend across entire diameter of tube to achieve complete desiccation

Figure 13.3 10–YEAR FAILURE RATES

Minilaparotomy		Laparoscopy	
Pomeroy	7 per 1000	Bipolar cautery	25 per 1000
Irving	nil	Falope ring	18 per 1000
Uchida	nil	Hulka clip	37 per 1000
		Filshie clip	30 per 1000

Obstetrics and Gynecology at a Glance, Fourth Edition. Errol R. Norwitz and John O. Schorge.

- *Definition.* A surgical procedure that is aimed at permanently blocking or removing part of the female or male genital tracts to prevent fertilization.
- *Frequency.* The most common method of family planning worldwide. More than 220 million couples use surgical sterilization for contraception, 90% of whom live in developing countries.
- *Ratio* of female : male sterilization is 3 : 1.
- *Risks.* All patients undergoing surgical sterilization should be aware of the nature, efficacy, safety, and complications of the operation as well as alternative methods of contraception. Patients should be informed of the risk of regret. Many couples are under the false impression that sterilization procedures are easily reversed. It is the responsibility of the surgeon to make it clear that such procedures are intended to be permanent.

Female sterilization

- Can be performed at cesarean delivery, immediately postpartum, post-abortion, or as an interval procedure unrelated to pregnancy.
- In developing countries, tubal ligation is generally a popular form of birth control and is widely available, although some Muslim countries (e.g. Egypt and Indonesia) do not permit it.
- Faith-based medical institutions in developed countries will sometimes refuse to perform tubal ligations.
- *Advantages.* Tubal ligation is permanent, effective, and safe. Long term, it reduces a woman's risk of developing ovarian cancer by 50%.
- *Complications.* The mortality rate (4/100,000 procedures) mainly reflects anesthetic risks. Other potential complications include hemorrhage, infection, erroneous ligation of the round ligament, and injury to adjacent structures.
- *Regret.* The strongest indicator of future regret is young age (age <25) at the time of sterilization. Risk factors for regret also include parity, marital status, and health of children.
- *Reversal.* One in 500 sterilized women will undergo microsurgical tubal reanastomosis. This procedure has excellent results if a small segment of the tube has been damaged. Pregnancy rates after reanastomosis vary with age of the woman and the method of sterilization (electrocoagulation approximately 40%, clips or rings approximately 70–80%).

Techniques (Figures 13.1 and 13.2)
1 Laparotomy
Location of the incision depends on the size of the uterus:
- *Interval tubal ligation* is performed through a 2- to 3-cm midline *suprapubic* incision. The abdomen is entered, the uterus identified, and the fallopian tube elevated with a finger or Babcock clamp. After the tube has been identified by its fimbriated end, the tubal ligation is then performed.
- *Postpartum tubal ligation* is either performed at cesarean section or after vaginal delivery. The latter procedure is ideally performed while the uterine fundus is high in the abdomen (within 48 hours of delivery), using a 2- to 3-cm *subumbilical* incision. Maternal and neonatal wellbeing should be confirmed before sterilization.

2 Laparoscopic tubal ligation
The most popular method of interval tubal ligation in the developed world:

- Mechanical occlusion devices – such as the spring-loaded clip (Filshie clip, Hulka clip) or a Silastic rubber band (Falope ring) – are most commonly used. Special applicators are necessary and each requires skill for proper application. Adhesions or a thickened or dilated fallopian tube increase the risk of misapplication and subsequent failure. Clips (5 mm) and rings (2 cm) destroy less oviductal tissue, making reversal more likely to succeed.
- Bipolar electrocoagulation is the most commonly used laparoscopic occlusion method in the USA. To maximize effectiveness, at least 3 cm of the isthmic portion of the fallopian tube must be completely coagulated by using sufficient energy.

3 Essure (transcervical, hysteroscopic approach)
Available since 2002, but not widely used or universally offered.
- Microinserts are placed into the proximal fallopian tubes by a catheter passed through a hysteroscope.
- Once in place, the device is designed to elicit scarring in and around the microinsert to form a blockage.
- Unlike other forms of tubal ligation, no general anesthetic or incisions are required.
- Three months post-procedure, a hysterosalpingogram is performed to confirm blockage. Patients are instructed to use another form of contraception until confirmation of tubal blockage.

Failure rates of female sterilization (Figure 13.3)
- Varies by technique, the skill of the operator, and characteristics of the patient (age, pelvic adhesions, hydrosalpinx).
- Resultant pregnancies are more likely to be ectopic.

Male sterilization (vasectomy)
- *Method.* Vasectomy involves permanent surgical interruption of the vas deferens (the duct that transports sperm during ejaculation). It can be performed on an outpatient basis within 15 minutes under local anesthesia, but is not immediately effective. Spermatozoa normally mature in the vas deferens for around 70 days before ejaculation. For this reason, 3 months or 20 ejaculations are needed to completely deplete the vas deferens of viable sperm. Post-vasectomy semen analysis should be performed before unprotected intercourse.
- *Advantages.* When compared with female tubal ligation, vasectomy is safer, less expensive, and equally effective.
- *Complications.* The mortality rate is essentially zero. Wound hematomas are most common and self-limited. The primary long-term complication is a permanent feeling of testicular pain ("post-vasectomy pain syndrome").
- *Regret.* Some men experience depression or anger and go through a period of mourning over the loss of their reproductive ability. This emotion is similar to what some women experience after menopause. Half of vasectomized men prefer to keep their sterilization secret.
- *Reversal.* Fewer than 5% of men request vasectomy reversal. Vas deferens reanastomosis is a difficult and meticulous procedure that is costly and has only a 50% success rate.
- Failure rates are <0.5%.

14 Breast disease

Figure 14.1 ANATOMY OF THE BREAST

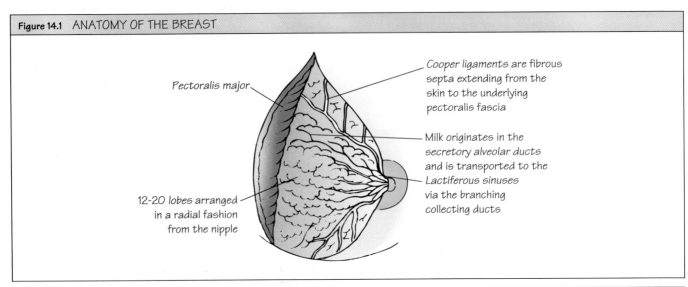

Pectoralis major

Cooper ligaments are fibrous septa extending from the skin to the underlying pectoralis fascia

Milk originates in the secretory alveolar ducts and is transported to the Lactiferous sinuses via the branching collecting ducts

12-20 lobes arranged in a radial fashion from the nipple

Figure 14.2 RISK FACTORS FOR BREAST CANCER

Age (risk increases in each decade)	
Previous cancer in the contralateral breast	
Family history of two close relatives	>4-fold
BRCA1 or BRCA2 mutation carrier	
Previous biopsy with premalignant histology	2.1-4 fold
Radiation exposure	
Nulliparity	
Residence in North America or northern Europe	
First birth age 35 or older	
Early menarche	
Late menopause	1.1-2 fold
Obesity	
Urban residence	
Upper socioeconomic status	
Other primary cancer in ovary or endometrium	

Figure 14.3 FINE NEEDLE ASPIRATION

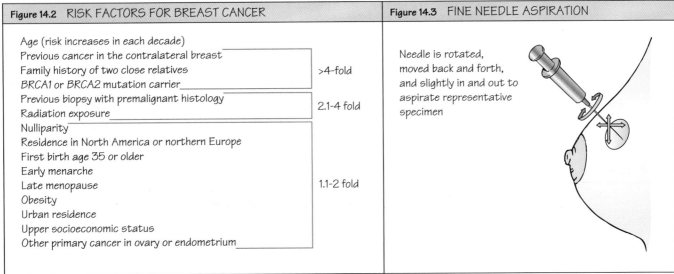

Needle is rotated, moved back and forth, and slightly in and out to aspirate representative specimen

---

Figure 14.4 MAMMOGRAM

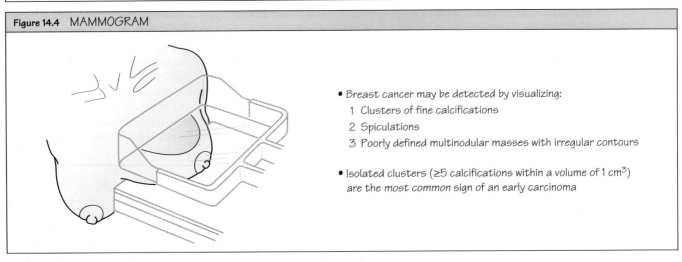

- Breast cancer may be detected by visualizing:
  1. Clusters of fine calcifications
  2. Spiculations
  3. Poorly defined multinodular masses with irregular contours

- Isolated clusters ($\geq$5 calcifications within a volume of 1 cm^3) are the *most common* sign of an early carcinoma

---

Obstetrics and Gynecology at a Glance, Fourth Edition. Errol R. Norwitz and John O. Schorge.

Anatomy and development (Figure 14.1)

• The breasts are large, modified sebaceous glands contained within the superficial fascia of the anterior chest wall.
• The average weight is 200–300 g during the menstruating years.
• Composed of 20% glands and 80% fat and connective tissue.
• Breast tissue is sensitive to the cyclic changes in hormonal levels – women often experience breast tenderness and fullness during the luteal phase of the cycle. Premenstrual symptoms are produced by an increase in blood flow, vascular engorgement, and water retention.
• Nearing the onset of puberty, the first change in the breast is the formation of the breast bud (see Chapter 21). The areola subsequently enlarges, and then the nipple begins to grow outwards.
• Estrogen is responsible for the initial stages of breast development, but further development requires adult levels of progesterone.

Physical examination

• Comprehensive breast examination is particularly important when symptoms are present.
• *Inspection* is the first step. This is usually done with the arms raised overhead, then with tension on the pectoralis muscles (by having the patient place her hands on her hips and press inward), and finally with the patient relaxed and leaning forward. These maneuvers accentuate skin and contour changes such as retraction, edema, or erythema, and nipple changes such as retraction, eczema, or erosion.
• *Palpation* is best performed with the patient in both sitting and supine positions. The examination is done in concentric circles, starting with the outermost breast tissue. The physician should attempt to elicit nipple discharge and examine the axilla carefully for adenopathy.

Benign breast disease

Fibrocystic changes

• *Definition.* Exaggeration of the normal physiologic response of breast tissue to the cyclic levels of ovarian hormones.
• *Frequency.* The most common of all benign breast conditions.
• *Symptoms and signs.* Cyclic bilateral breast pain, increased engorgement and density of the breasts, excessive nodularity, rapid change and fluctuation in the size of cystic areas, increased tenderness, and occasionally spontaneous clear nipple discharge.
• *Physical examination.* Marked tenderness of well-delineated, slightly mobile, cystic nodules or thickened areas.
• *Diagnosis.* A wide variety of histopathologic findings (cysts, adenosis, fibrosis, duct ectasia).
• *Treatment.* Well-fitting brassieres and light, loose clothing; decreased intake of coffee, chocolate, tea; smoking cessation. Oral contraceptives or progestins are helpful in up to 90% of patients. Danazol is effective for severe symptoms.

Fibroadenomas

• *Definition.* Firm, rubbery, freely mobile, solid, usually solitary masses.
• *Frequency.* The second most common type of benign breast disease.
• *Symptoms and signs.* Typically a young woman in her 20s discovers the painless mass accidentally while bathing. Growth of the mass is usually extremely slow, but occasionally can be quite rapid.
• *Physical examination.* Average size is 2.5 cm; multiple lesions are found in 15–20% of women.
• *Diagnosis.* Mammography is rarely indicated in a woman under age 30. Ultrasound may be helpful to distinguish a solid from a cystic mass.
• *Treatment.* If the etiology cannot be established by fine-needle aspiration (FNA), surgical removal is indicated. Any mass that rapidly increases in size should be removed, as should any solid mass in a woman over age 30.

Other benign conditions

• *Mastodynia* (breast pain) is a common symptom affecting women. Reduction of dietary fat can result in significant improvement.
• *Galactorrhea* (milky discharge) usually results from medication (hormones, phenothiazines) side effects, but may suggest a prolactin-secreting tumor.
• *Intraductal papilloma* is usually solitary and often causes a serous or bloody discharge.
• *Duct ectasia* results from subareolar dilation and periductal mastitis.
• *Fat necrosis* usually results from trauma and is the only benign lesion that causes skin dimpling.

Breast cancer

• More than 1 million new cases occur each year worldwide – making it the most common malignancy of women. One in eight women will be diagnosed with breast cancer by age 80.

Risk factors (Figure 14.2)

• *Inherited* cases (5–10%) are usually due to *BRCA-1* or *BRCA-2* germline mutations. Carriers have a 55–85% risk of developing cancer.
• *Prevention* by using tamoxifen or raloxifene in high-risk women is currently being evaluated. Prophylactic mastectomy is chiefly reserved for *BRCA-1* or *BRCA-2* mutation carriers.
• *Mammogram* (Figure 14.4) is the best technique for early detection, but the false-negative rate is 10%.

Screening recommendations

The UK. Mammogram every 3 years for women aged 50–70.
The USA. Mammogram every 2 years for women aged 50–74.
• High-risk patients, such as *BRCA-1* or *BRCA-2* carriers, may be screened earlier and more frequently with breast MRI.
• *Histopathology.* The most common type (70–80%) is infiltrating ductal carcinoma, followed by lobular carcinoma (5–8%). The incidence of ductal carcinoma *in situ* (DCIS) has increased dramatically with the advent of widespread mammography screening.
• *Staging* is based on the TNM system to determine the anatomic extent of malignant disease: primary tumor (T), lymph node involvement (N), and metastasis (M).

Diagnosis and treatment

1 *FNA* (Figure 14.3) *and core biopsy* are office procedures commonly used to diagnosis palpable breast masses. Excisional biopsy is a more agressive outpatient procedure to obtain complete histology. Needle-localised excisional biopsy or stereotactic mammography are indicated for non-palpable lesions.
2 *Excisional biopsy.* Outpatient procedure with complete histology.
3 *Needle-localized excisional biopsy or stereotactic mammography.* Performed for non-palpable lesions.
4 *Lumpectomy* is the most common form of breast-conserving surgery that yields superior cosmetic results. Infrequently, a type of mastectomy is required that necessitates reconstruction.
5 *Modified radical mastectomy.* Complete removal of the breast tissue, underlying fascia of the pectoralis major muscle, and the axillary lymph nodes.
6 *Reconstruction.* Tissue expanders with implant or myocutaneous flap:
• *Postoperative radiation* can benefit high-risk patients by preventing local recurrence.
• *Adjuvant chemotherapy* is a complex topic, but commonly depends on the patient age, estrogen and progesterone receptor status, and whether Her-2 expression is present. Doxorubicin, cyclophosphamide, and/or paclitaxel is a common cytotoxic drug. Tamoxifen and/or aromatase inhibitors are hormonal agents that are frequently used.

Figure 15.1 MISCARRIAGE

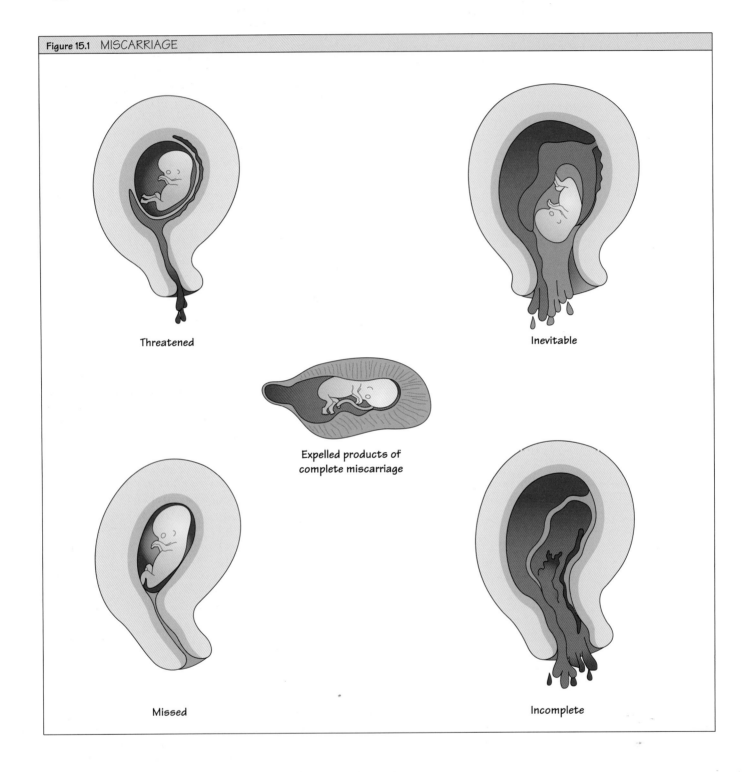

Threatened

Inevitable

Expelled products of
complete miscarriage

Missed

Incomplete

Obstetrics and Gynecology at a Glance, Fourth Edition. Errol R. Norwitz and John O. Schorge.

38 © 2013 John Wiley & Sons, Ltd. Published 2013 by John Wiley & Sons, Ltd.

- *Definition.* Expulsion or removal of an embryo or fetus from the uterus before it is capable of independent survival.
- Of all conceptions 50–75% abort spontaneously. Most are unrecognized because they occur before or at the time of the next expected menses.

Spontaneous miscarriage

- *Definition.* Loss of a clinically recognized pregnancy before 20 weeks' gestation or <500 g.
- Make up 15–20% of clinically diagnosed pregnancies.
- Risk factors include advanced maternal age, increasing gravidity, prior miscarriage, and smoking.
- *History.* Vaginal bleeding is the most common presenting complaint, followed by crampy abdominal pain.
- *Examination.* Initially, vital signs should be taken to rule out hemodynamic instability. Speculum examination allows visualization of the cervix and potentially the location of products of conception. Bimanual examination may help estimate gestational age.
- *Laboratory tests.* Serum human choronic gonadotropin (hCG), blood count, and rhesus (Rh) typing should be sent (virtually all Rh-negative patients should receive anti-D immunoglobulin prophylaxis [see Chapter 53]).

Etiology (see also Chapter 24)

- More than 80% of all miscarriages occur in the first trimester (<12 weeks' gestation). The exact mechanisms are not always apparent, but death of the embryo or fetus nearly always *precedes* spontaneous expulsion. As a result, finding the cause of early miscarriage involves ascertaining the cause of fetal death. At least half result from chromosomal abnormalities.
- Less than 20% of all miscarriages occur in the second trimester (12–20 weeks' gestation). The fetus frequently does not die before expulsion and anatomic factors are more likely to be causative.

Fetal factors

- *Chromosomal abnormalities.* Half of embryos and early fetuses that result in first-trimester miscarriages demonstrate aneuploidy. Autosomal trisomies (either chromosome 13, 16, 18, 21, or 22) are the most frequently identified anomalies. Monosomy X (45,X), the second most frequent chromosomal abnormality, usually results in miscarriage and much less frequently in live-born female infants (Turner syndrome, see Chapter 22). Triploidy is often associated with partial hydatidiform moles (see Chapter 34).
- *Abnormal development.* First-trimester miscarriages often display a developmental abnormality of the zygote, embryo, early fetus, or even placenta. A common example is having either a degenerated or absent embryo (ie, blighted ovum).

Maternal factors

The causes of miscarriages having normal (euploid) chromosomes are poorly understood, but a various medical disorders, environmental conditions, and developmental abnormalities have been implicated.
- *Uterine defects.* Even large and multiple uterine fibroids usually do not cause miscarriage. Asherman syndrome results from vigorous curettage that results in insufficient functional endometrium to support a pregnancy. It is controversial whether abnormal müllerian duct formation or fusion defects (see Chapter 24) cause miscarriage or whether surgical correction prevents it. Such corrective procedures should be done as a last resort, if at all. Incompetent cervix (see Chapter 58) is a potential fixable cause of miscarriage.
- *Infections, endocrine factors, environmental causes, and immunologic factors* (see Chapter 24).

- *Physical trauma.* Clearly, major abdominal trauma can precipitate miscarriage, but it is a minor contribution.

Classification and treatment

Threatened miscarriage (Figure 15.1)

- *Definition.* Uterine bleeding before 20 weeks with a closed cervical os and a confirmed viable intrauterine gestation.
- Vaginal spotting or heavier bleeding occurs in 20–25% of pregnant women and may persist for days or weeks. However, some bleeding near the time of expected menses may be physiologic.
- Half of these pregnancies will eventually miscarry, but the risk is substantially lower if fetal cardiac activity is demonstrated. Fetuses that do not miscarry remain at increased risk for preterm delivery, low birthweight, and perinatal death.
- *Treatment.* There are no effective therapies and patients are monitored expectantly unless the pregnancy is undesired or non-viable. Bed rest is often recommended, but does not alter the course.

Inevitable, incomplete, and complete miscarriage (Figure 15.1)

- *Definition.* Imminent, partial, or complete expulsion of products of conception before 20 weeks' gestation through a dilated cervix.
- When the placenta, in whole or in part, detaches from the uterus, bleeding ensues. Typically bleeding is profuse and associated with uterine cramping. During incomplete miscarriage, the internal os remains open and allows passage of blood. Following complete detachment and expulsion of the gestational products, the internal cervical os closes.
- Incomplete miscarriages usually occur between 6 and 14 weeks' gestation; complete miscarriages are most common <6 or >14 weeks.
- *Treatment.* Suction curettage is typically required for inevitable or incomplete miscarriage; complete miscarriages may be managed expectantly without evacuation.

Septic abortion

- *Definition.* Any threatened, inevitable, or incomplete miscarriage associated with a fever before 20 weeks' gestation.
- Retained products of conception after spontaneous miscarriage, legal termination of pregnancy, or illegal termination of pregnancy acts as a nidus for the development of a local infection that is potentially fatal if generalized sepsis ensues.
- Patients usually present with fever, chills, leukocytosis, uterine tenderness, and a foul-smelling cervicovaginal discharge.
- *Treatment.* Broad-spectrum intravenous antibiotics, prompt uterine evacuation, and supportive therapy in severe cases. However, a large, grossly infected uterus is at risk for perforation and may be allowed to evacuate with pitocin or prostaglandin stimulation.

Missed abortion (Figure 15.1)

- *Definition.* Fetal demise before 20 weeks' gestation without detachment of the placenta – resulting in retention of products of conception for days or weeks behind a closed cervical os.
- Typically, after the demise there is an episode of bleeding that subsides and is followed by a continuous brown vaginal discharge. Many women have no other symptoms. Very rarely, prolonged retention of a dead fetus after midpregnancy can result in coagulopathy.
- *Treatment.* Management is individualized, depending on the circumstances. Expectant management is often difficult for the patient to endure after being informed of the demise. Medical management is often the safest option.

16 Termination of pregnancy

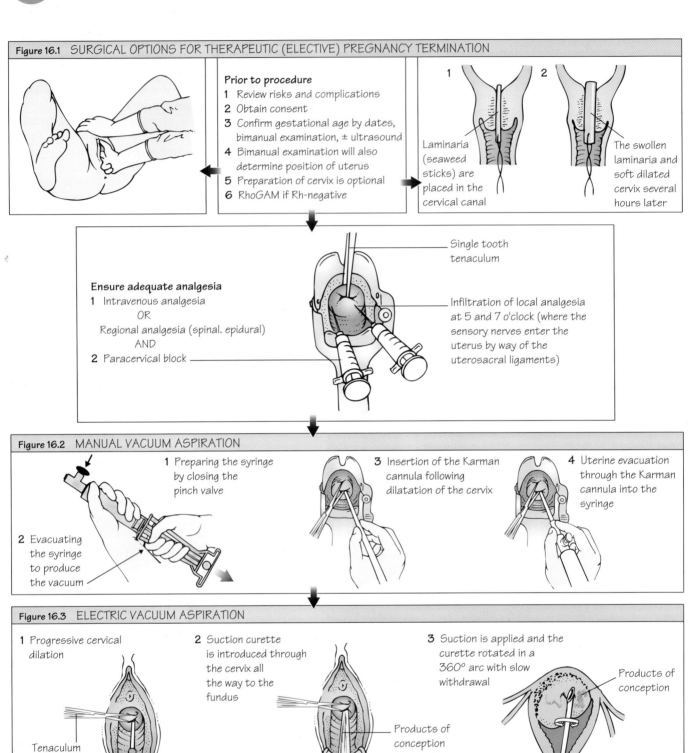

Figure 16.1 SURGICAL OPTIONS FOR THERAPEUTIC (ELECTIVE) PREGNANCY TERMINATION

Prior to procedure
1 Review risks and complications
2 Obtain consent
3 Confirm gestational age by dates, bimanual examination, ± ultrasound
4 Bimanual examination will also determine position of uterus
5 Preparation of cervix is optional
6 RhoGAM if Rh-negative

Laminaria (seaweed sticks) are placed in the cervical canal

The swollen laminaria and soft dilated cervix several hours later

Ensure adequate analgesia
1 Intravenous analgesia
   OR
   Regional analgesia (spinal. epidural)
   AND
2 Paracervical block

Single tooth tenaculum

Infiltration of local analgesia at 5 and 7 o'clock (where the sensory nerves enter the uterus by way of the uterosacral ligaments)

Figure 16.2 MANUAL VACUUM ASPIRATION

1 Preparing the syringe by closing the pinch valve

2 Evacuating the syringe to produce the vacuum

3 Insertion of the Karman cannula following dilatation of the cervix

4 Uterine evacuation through the Karman cannula into the syringe

Figure 16.3 ELECTRIC VACUUM ASPIRATION

1 Progressive cervical dilation

Tenaculum

Mechanical dilator

2 Suction curette is introduced through the cervix all the way to the fundus

Products of conception

Suction curette

3 Suction is applied and the curette rotated in a 360° arc with slow withdrawal

Products of conception

Suction curette

Obstetrics and Gynecology at a Glance, Fourth Edition. Errol R. Norwitz and John O. Schorge.

- *Definition.* Elective or voluntary "abortion" is the interruption of pregnancy before viability at the request of the woman.
- About 1.2 million terminations are performed annually in the USA. Half the women are younger than 25 years. About 88% are conducted up to 12 weeks, 10% from 13 weeks to 20 weeks, and 1–2% beyond 20 weeks.
- Worldwide, 44 million pregnancy terminations occur annually. Abortion rates (per 1,000 women aged 15–44) vary from 12 in western Europe to 32 in Latin America.
- Half the abortions worldwide are considered unsafe. Unsafe abortion accounts for an estimated 13% of all maternal deaths.

History

- Abortion has a long history and has been induced by various methods over the centuries, including herbal abortifacients, physical trauma, and insertion of non-surgical instruments (knitting needles, clothes hangers) into the uterus. These methods are rarely seen in developed countries where medical and surgical abortion is legal and available.
- Elective pregnancy termination in the UK has been legal since the Abortion Act was passed in 1967. Abortion was legalized in the USA with the Supreme Court's *Roe v. Wade* decision in 1973. Worldwide, abortion laws vary substantially by region. Some countries allow abortion by request (the USA, Canada, the UK, France, China, Russia). Some countries allow abortion only to save a woman's life (Ireland, Indonesia, Egypt). A few countries ban abortions without exception (Chile, Dominican Republic, Nicaragua).

Personal and social factors

- Women choose to undergo pregnancy termination for a variety of reasons, including a desire to delay or end childbearing, concern over the interruption of work or education, issues of financial or relationship stability, and perceived immaturity.
- In the USA and the UK, 1% of all abortions occur because of rape or incest, 6% because of potential health problems regarding either the mother or child, and 93% for social reasons (the pregnancy was unplanned).
- Societal pressures may also influence the decision to undergo termination. Examples include disapproval of single motherhood, insufficient economic support for families, lack of access to or rejection of contraceptive methods, or efforts toward population control (such as China's one-child policy).

Medical termination

- About 95% effective for pregnancies up to 9 weeks' gestation.
- Nearly 10% of all terminations in the USA and the UK.
- Becoming increasingly common due to safety and convenience.
- Two medications are given in sequence:
  1 *Mifepristone (RU486)* is a progesterone receptor antagonist that blocks the hormone needed to maintain the pregnancy. Within hours, the uterine lining begins to shed, the cervix begins to soften, and bleeding may occur.
  2 *Misoprostol* (Cytotec, USA) or *gemeprost* (UK) are both prostaglandin E_1 analogs. Side effects include profuse vaginal bleeding, uterine cramps, nausea, vomiting, diarrhea, headache, muscle weakness, and dizziness.
- US regimen: (1) mifepristone 600 mg orally followed 24–72 hours later by misoprostol 400 μg orally (Food and Drug Administration [FDA] approved for up to 7 weeks' gestation) or (2) mifepristone 200 mg orally followed 6–72 hours later by misoprostol 800 μg vaginally or buccally (evidence-based regimen).
- UK regimen: mifepristone 600 mg orally followed 48 hours later by gemeprost 1 mg vaginally.
- More than half the women will abort within a few hours of taking the gemeprost or misoprostol dose.
- In cases of failure of medical abortion, vacuum or manual aspiration is used to complete the abortion surgically.

Surgical techniques (Figures 16.1, 16.2 and 16.3)

- These are 99% effective.
- About 90% of all terminations in the USA and the UK.
- The cervix is first dilated, then the uterine cavity is mechanically evacuated.
- Surgical termination is a simple procedure and is safer than childbirth when performed before week 16.
  1 *Manual vacuum aspiration (MVA)* can be performed up to 6–7 weeks' gestation without regional anesthesia. A soft, flexible, plastic cannula is attached to a handheld self-locking syringe. Evacuation is accomplished by repetitive in-and-out, rotating movements.
  2 *Electric vacuum aspiration (EVA)* uses an electric pump, requires a paracervical block and cervical dilation, and is used for terminations between 6 and 15 weeks' gestation.
  3 *Dilation and evacuation (D&E)* is performed between 15 and 20 weeks' gestation. Due to the larger fetal size, the procedure is often done in the operating room under general anesthesia. Cervical preparation and dilation precedes mechanical destruction and evacuation of fetal parts using specialized (Sopher) forceps. The placenta and remaining tissue are then removed by suction curettage.
- Regardless of technique, identification of products of conception is mandatory before the procedure is considered complete.

Late pregnancy termination (20–24 weeks)

1 *Dilation and extraction (D&X)* is usually performed after intracardiac fetal injection (KCl or digoxin) to ensure cessation of fetal cardiac activity before the procedure. The technique is similar to a D&E. Cervical preparation is required and facilitates extraction of fetal parts while minimizing uterine or cervical injury. On a living fetus, this procedure has been termed "partial birth abortion" and is banned in the USA.
2 *Induction of labor* with systemic agents such as misoprostol, mifepristone, or high-dose oxytocin is used to induce contractions and promote expulsion of the fetus and placenta. The primary advantage compared with D&X is that the fetus delivers intact.
3 *Intra-amniotic infusion* of hypertonic saline and/or prostaglandin is used to induce contractions and promote expulsion of the fetus and placenta. This method is seldom used due to the availability and safety of the above methods.

Complications

- The frequency of complications depends on operator experience and gestational age (increased if <6 weeks or >16 weeks).
- *Immediate complications.* Hemorrhage, cervical injury, anesthesia complications. The use of osmotic dilators (laminaria) significantly reduces the risk of uterine perforation.
- *Late complications.* Retained products of conception, infection (endometritis), and Rh sensitization.
- *Mortality rate.* Fewer than 1/100,000 surgical procedures when a patient is under the care of an experienced clinician.

17 Gynecologic surgery

Figure 17.1 LAPAROSCOPIC SURGERY

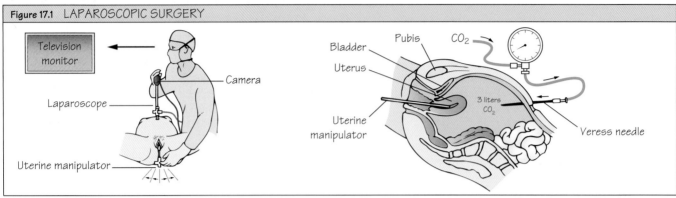

Television monitor

Camera

Laparoscope

Uterine manipulator

Bladder

Pubis

CO_2

Uterus

3 liters CO_2

Uterine manipulator

Veress needle

Figure 17.2 ABDOMINAL SURGERY

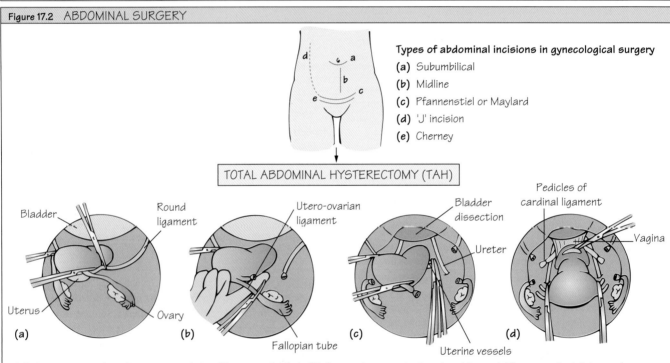

Types of abdominal incisions in gynecological surgery
- **(a)** Subumbilical
- **(b)** Midline
- **(c)** Pfannenstiel or Maylard
- **(d)** 'J' incision
- **(e)** Cherney

TOTAL ABDOMINAL HYSTERECTOMY (TAH)

Bladder
Round ligament
Uterus
Ovary
(a)

Utero-ovarian ligament
Fallopian tube
(b)

Bladder dissection
Ureter
Uterine vessels
(c)

Pedicles of cardinal ligament
Vagina
(d)

(a) Uterus grasped at the cornua and round ligament divided. **(b)** Ovarian ligament isolated and ligated (if ovary to be left in situ).
(c) After bladder dissection, uterine vessels are isolated and ligated. **(d)** Cardinal ligaments have been divided and the vagina is entered. The final step is cuff closure.

Figure 17.3 VAGINAL HYSTERECTOMY

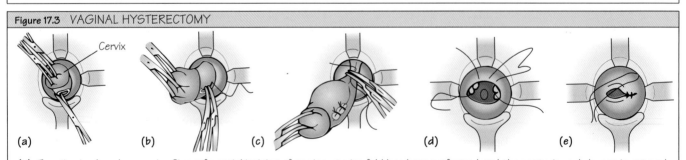

Cervix

(a) **(b)** **(c)** **(d)** **(e)**

(a) Traction is placed on cervix. Circumferential incision of cervico-uterine fold has been performed and the posterior cul-de-sac is entered.
(b) The cardinal and uterosacral ligaments are ligated. **(c)** Ovarian and round ligaments are ligated. **(d)** Purse-string closure of peritoneal cavity. **(e)** Reapproximation of the vaginal cuff.

Obstetrics and Gynecology at a Glance, Fourth Edition. Errol R. Norwitz and John O. Schorge.

Dilation and curettage (D&C)

• *Indications.* Diagnostic (postmenopausal bleeding) and therapeutic (dysfunctional uterine bleeding – DUB).
• *Technique.* The cervix is placed on traction and the cervical canal progressively dilated until the internal os is wide enough to admit the curette. The uterine cavity is then circumferentially scraped with a sharp curette.
• *Complications.* Creating a false tract for patients with cervical stenosis, bleeding, infection, uterine perforation.

Hysteroscopy (see also Chapter 4)

• *Indications.* Diagnosis of uterine anomalies, resection of submucous fibroids, endometrial ablation, numerous others.
• *Technique.* The hysteroscope is inserted after dilation of the cervical canal and the uterine cavity is distended with fluid (glycine, saline). A variety of instruments (rollerball coagulator, scissors, resectoscope) may be passed through the operative sheath to perform the procedure.
• *Complications.* Same as D&C, extravasation of hypotonic fluid into the circulation may cause acute hyponatremia and seizures.

Minimally invasive surgery

• There has been a revolution in the range of surgical procedures performed with laparoscopy due to advances in equipment and surgeon experience.
• Very recently, the daVinci robotic system has further expanded these options.
• Results in a shorter hospital stay, less postoperative discomfort, and a quicker return to work.

Laparoscopy (Figure 17.1)

• *Indications.* Tubal ligation, ectopic pregnancy, salpingo-oophorectomy, total laparoscopic hysterectomy, pelvic and para-aortic node dissection, sacrocolpopexy, tubal reanastomosis, myomectomy, and numerous others.
• *Technique.* A Veress needle is inserted at the umbilicus to achieve a pneumoperitoneum. The surgeon then punctures the abdominal wall with the trocar and inserts the laparoscope. Additional operating sites may then be inserted in the lower quadrants for ancillary instruments (probe, forceps, scissors, irrigator). Visualization of the pelvic organs is facilitated by transvaginal placement of an intrauterine manipulator.
• *Complications.* Injury to intra-abdominal organs, nerve injury (due to incorrect placement of the legs in surgical stirrups), laceration of large vessels, subcutaneous emphysema.

Robotic assisted

• *Indications.* All laparoscopic indications in addition to patients who might otherwise have limiting technical factors requiring an abdominal incision (obesity, adhesions).
• *Technique.* The initial steps are similar to laparoscopy. After trocar placement, the robot is "docked" to hold the camera and accessory sites. The surgeon breaks scrub and is seated at a separate "console" to control the instruments while an assistant remains by the patient to provide retraction or other functions. The visualization and range of motion are considered superior.
• *Complications.* Similar to regular laparoscopy.

Abdominal surgery (Figure 17.2)

Selecting an appropriate incision is critical to a successful operation:
• *Subumbilical.* Used for postpartum tubal ligation.
• *Midline.* Provides excellent exposure to the pelvis and may be extended to the upper abdomen.

• *Pfannenstiel* is most commonly used in gynecology; *Maylard* gives more exposure by dividing the rectus muscles.
• *"J."* The best option for extending a Pfannenstiel to the upper abdomen.
• *Cherney.* Similar to Maylard, but divides the tendon of the rectus at symphysis pubis.

Total abdominal hysterectomy (TAH) (Figure 17.2)

• The second most common major operation performed in the USA and the UK (after cesarean).
• *Indications.* Uterine fibroids (most common), endometrial cancer, pelvic pain, dysfunctional uterine bleeding, numerous others.
• *Technique.* Supracervical hysterectomy is a modification performed by amputating the cervix after ligation of the uterine vessels and suturing the distal stump.
• *Complications.* Bleeding, infection, distal ureteral injury, postoperative ileus.

Salpingo-oophorectomy

• *Indications.* Benign ovarian tumors, gynecologic malignancy, pelvic pain, numerous others.
• *Technique.* The retroperitoneal space is entered and the infundibulopelvic (IP) ligament is clamped above the ureter. The broad ligament attachments are dissected distally and the utero-ovarian ligament divided.
• *Complications.* Hematoma, ureteral injury at pelvic brim.

Myomectomy

• *Indications.* Symptomatic uterine fibroids, persistent menorrhagia, infertility.
• *Technique.* An incision is made through the uterine musculature overlying the fibroid. The myometrium is bluntly dissected from the fibroid pseudocapsule and the specimen removed. The uterine incisions are then closed to obliterate the dead space and provide hemostasis.
• *Complications.* Bleeding necessitating hysterectomy, postoperative adhesions.

Radical gynecologic surgery

• *Radical hysterectomy* is used to treat early cervical cancer (see Chapter 30) by removing additional soft tissue to achieve negative margins for cure.
• *Cytoreductive surgery* is performed for advanced ovarian cancer (see Chapter 33) and aims to remove all grossly visible disease within the abdomen.
• *Pelvic exenteration* is performed in selected patients with centrally recurrent cervical cancer. This operation involves removal of the bladder (anterior), rectum (posterior), or both organs (total), in addition to the uterus and adjacent soft tissues to achieve a negative margin.

Vaginal surgery

This results in quick recovery and short hospital stay compared with abdominal surgery.

Total vaginal hysterectomy (TVH) (Figure 17.3)

• *Indications.* Cervical dysplasia, symptomatic uterovaginal prolapse, numerous others.
• *Technique.* Surgical steps are almost in reverse order to TAH. Morcellation of uterine fibroids may allow resection of larger uteri.
• *Complications.* Bleeding, vaginal cuff cellulitis, bladder injury.
  Other vaginal operations are shown in Chapters 19 and 20.

Figure 18.1 FOUR TENETS OF PRINCIPLE-BASED ETHICS

1 *Respect for autonomy* acknowledges a patient's right to have their own views, to make choices, and to take actions based on their own personal values and beliefs.
2 *Beneficence* expresses the obligation of a physician to act in a way that is likely to benefit the patient.
3 *Nonmaleficence* requires the physician not to harm or cause injury ("First, do no harm.")
4 *Justice* is the obligation to treat equally those who are alike or similar according to whatever criteria are selected.

Figure 18.2 GUIDELINES FOR ETHICAL DECISION MAKING

- Identify the decision makers – "whose decision is it?"
- Collect data, establish facts
- Identify all medically appropriate options
- Evaluate options, according to the values and principles involved
- Identify ethical conflicts and set priorities
- Select the option that can be best justified
- Re-evaluate the decision after it is acted on

Figure 18.3 BASIC FUNDAMENTALS OF RISK MANAGEMENT

Office setting

- Telephone etiquette is vital to fostering an empathetic office environment.
- Misunderstanding can easily occur over the telephone by any of the office staff.
- Improper exchanges may result in an angry patient who subsequently considers filing a malpractice claim.
- The reception desk should be friendly and inviting.

- Patients should feel comfortable that all of their concerns have been addressed at each visit.
- Patients should be encouraged to call the office themselves for test results – so that inadvertent reports are not 'lost'.
- Pysicians should review any bill before it is turned over to a collection agency to avoid some instances of potential patient hostility.

Treatment and informed consent

- Patients must be comfortable with your impression of the diagnosis, what the treatment plan entails, what the alternatives might be and their prognosis if the treatment is refused.
- Patients have a right to receive an honest appraisal of the relevant risks that might reasonably occur and the anticipated outcome (e.g., possible sterility). *Physicians should work to master the ability to develop quick rapport with patients in the practice.

- The time sequence of the procedure and estimated recuperation time is vital to assuage concerns.
- Valid consent has four characteristics: voluntary, competent, informed and understanding.
- The use of a 'timeout' by the medical team has recently become commonplace to prevent errors (e.g., wrong-site surgery).

Medical records

- The written record can either save or hang the physician in a lawsuit. Legally, it is what matters.
- Progress notes not only document your evaluation and care of the patient, but the fact that you were present.
- Timeliness of completion of records, especially operative notes is imperative.
- Detrimental statements about the patient should be avoided, but it is prudent to document inappropriate patient behavior (e.g., noncompliance).

- If a record has been requested or a suit filed, the physician should NEVER alter the record – juries can interpret such changes as conclusive proof that negligent behavior was covered up.
- The proper way to correct a record is to draw a single line through the error, but never obliterate the error. Write the correction and the date, and initial it.
- Physicians are best served by refraining from criticizing colleagues in the record.

Communication

- Patients are least likely to sue a physician who is easy to talk to, answers questions, is accessible, is fair, shows respect, and provides good care.
- Good communication encourages questions and involvement of family members.

- More than half of what a patient perceives is obtained through nonverbal communication.
- Body language, posture and facial expressions all convey strong messages – positive or negative.

Ethics in obstetrics and gynecology

• The *Hippocratic oath* emphasizes the virtues that were historically expected to characterize and guide the behavior of physicians and other healthcare professionals who swore to practice medicine ethically and honestly.

• The vast expansion of medical technology over the past several decades has led to increasingly complex ethical questions for obstetrician–gynecologists.

• The availability of assisted reproductive technology, preimplantation genetics, selective abortion, and earlier gestational age viability is a sample of the dilemmas commonly encountered.

• Medical ethics is currently dominated by four tenets of principle-based ethics (Figure 18.1).

• These major principles may be used as guides to professional action. However, conflicts will still arise – requiring the physician to determine which principle(s) should have priority.

• Obstetric/gynecology (Ob/Gyn) physicians often face a conflict between principles of beneficence and nonmaleficence because a pregnant woman actually represents two patients.

• Frequently, more than one course of action may be morally justifiable, whereas in others no course of action seems acceptable because each may result in significant harms or else compromise important principles or values. Yet, the clinician must select one of the available options and be able to justify that decision with ethical reasons.

• The involvement of individuals with a variety of backgrounds and perspectives can be useful in addressing ethical questions. Consultation with a social worker or hospital ethics committee may be advantageous.

• Guidelines (Figure 18.2), consisting of several logical sequential steps, can aid the practitioner in analyzing and resolving an ethical problem.

• Ob/Gyn physicians who are familiar with the concepts of medical ethics will be better able to approach complex situations in an objective, structured way and minimize the likelihood of anger, injury, or litigation.

Professional liability

• Unfortunately, Ob/Gyn physicians are frequent targets for malpractice claims. In the USA, 75% of practitioners have been sued at least once in their careers.

• The impact is significant on many different levels, including: (1) fear of a future lawsuit making Ob/Gyn a less attractive career for prospective medical students, (2) exorbitant insurance fees resulting in sparse or no medical care in some areas, and (3) defensive medicine unnecessarily driving up healthcare costs.

• Most obstetrics lawsuits are birth related, typically due to an alleged failure to perform or to timely deliver a patient by cesarean section. Almost half the claims result from neurologically impaired infants or stillbirths.

• The stress of potential lawsuits leads many Ob/Gyn physicians to curtail or cease the obstetric portion of their practices.

• Most gynecology lawsuits involve sterilization, surgical complications, undiagnosed breast disease, or mismanagement of an ectopic pregnancy.

• *Medical malpractice* happens when a treatment is believed to be below the degree of care conducted by a typical physician under the same or similar sets of circumstances.

• Factors that have contributed to the current malpractice crisis include: (1) higher patient expectations, (2) an increasingly litigious

society, (3) excessive monetary awards, and (4) rising insurance premiums.

• Unfortunately, all of society suffers because the cost, quality, and availability of healthcare are adversely affected. Half the claims are eventually dropped by the plaintiff attorney or found to be without merit.

• The furor raised by the most outrageous payouts has given rise to a grassroots tort reform in the USA that has been successful in limiting non-economical damages (eg, pain and suffering) in some states.

• *Risk management* (Figure 18.3) refers to medical practices and procedures that reduce the risk of patient injury as well as the risk of being sued.

Disclosure of adverse events (AEs)

• Bad outcomes, especially preventable ones, are an uncomfortable reality of medical care.

• Disclosing such events is usually awkward, and physicians may know how it can best be facilitated.

• Whenever a complication is recognized, it should be treated quickly and appropriately. The patient and her family should be immediately informed. Frequent visits thereafter will convey compassionate concern for the problem. Avoidance will only escalate the distrust.

• Physicians should be quick to call a consultant to help and, if indicated, turn over most of the care to a specialist or other colleague.

• When the AE occurs from a physician's mistake, he or she is ethically required to inform the patient of the facts necessary to ensure understanding of what has occurred.

• Expressions of sympathy (acknowledgment of suffering) are always appropriate, but the appropriateness of an apology (accountability for suffering) will vary from case to case. Physicians may first wish to seek advice from the hospital's risk manager and his or her liability carrier.

• Disclosing information about unanticipated AEs should benefit both sides through a strengthened physician–patient relationship and a promotion of trust.

• Patients expect and want full disclosure of the AE, an acknowledgment of responsibility, an understanding of what happened, expressions of sympathy, and discussion of what is being done to prevent similar future outcomes.

• Disclosure of AEs can also be important for the physician's personal healing. Barriers are many, including shame, lack of training in how to disclose, and fear of lawsuits.

• Many patients who sue after an AE do so based on their suspicion of a cover-up or by desire for revenge.

The litigation process

• The underlying principle of law is the adversarial system, in which attorneys are bound to reveal only the evidence that benefits their clients, instead of the whole truth.

• To prevail in a case, the plaintiff's attorney must provide:

1 An established standard of care for the particular procedure or practice

2 Proof of a deviation from that standard

3 Proof of an identifiable injury

4 Proof that the specified deviation or negligence was the cause of the identified injury.

19 Urinary incontinence

Figure 19.1 DIAGNOSIS

Simple cystometry	Complex urodynamic testing

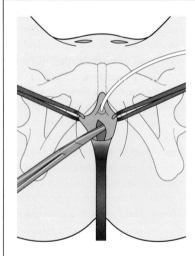

Allows determination of stress incontinence, detrusor overactivity, measurement of first sensation, desire to void, and bladder capacity

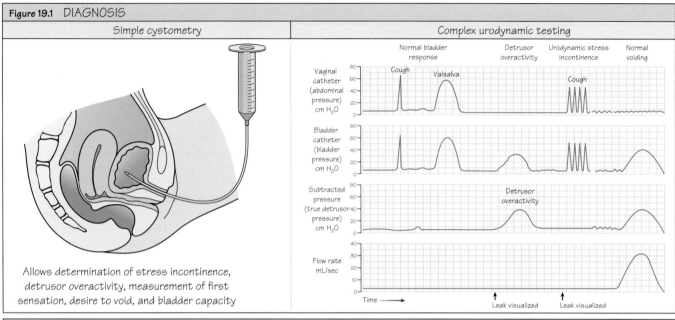

Figure 19.2 SURGICAL TREATMENT

Tension-free transvaginal tape (TVT) sling

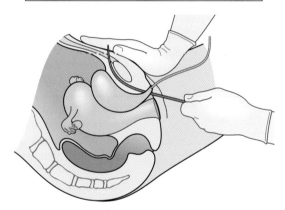

Note the small suprapubic abdominal incisions bilaterally

The needle tip is inserted into the paraurethral space, angulated laterally behind the surface of the pubic symphysis and a hand is used to guide it to the abdominal incision

The sling is adjusted to correct tension, the abdominal tape is cut at skin level, and incisions are closed

Burch colposuspension

- Often performed laparoscopically, but also accessible via a Pfannenstiel incision
- A plane is identified beneath the rectus abdominis and dissected to the pubis
- The space of Retzius is opened

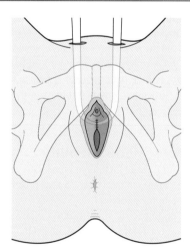

- A vaginal finger elevates the bladder neck
- 1-3 permanent sutures are placed lateral to the bladder neck and tied to Cooper ligaments

- *Definition.* Involuntary leakage of urine that is suffiecient enough in frequency and amount to cause physical and/or emotional distress.
- *Incidence.* Highly prevalent in women across their adult lifespan and severity increases linearly with age in women across their adult lifespan: 4–8% ultimately seek medical attention. One in three women aged >60 years has a bladder control problem.
- *Mechanism.* Continence and urination involve a balance between urethral closure and detrusor (bladder smooth muscle) activity. Urethral pressure normally exceeds bladder pressure, resulting in urine remaining in the bladder. Intra-abdominal pressure increases (coughing, sneezing) are normally transmitted to both urethra and bladder equally, maintaining continence. Disruption of this balance leads to various types of incontinence.

Diagnosis (six basic components)

1 *History.* A detailed history is important to determine the severity of symptoms and rule out medication causes. Emotional distress often does not correlate well with the amount of urine loss that can be demonstrated.

2 Physical examination (three areas):
- *General examination* to rule out delirium and, atrophic urethritis, restricted mobility, or stool impaction.
- *Urogynecologic examination* may reveal severe vulvar excoriation from continual dampness. The vaginal tissue should be inspected for signs of atrophy, stenosis, bladder neck mobility (*Q-tip test*), and atrophic urethritis. The patient is asked to cough repeatedly or undergo a Valsalva maneuver with a full bladder in the lithotomy or standing position to induce urine leakage. Rectal examination can evaluate rectal sphincter tone or the presence of fecal impaction.

3 *Urinalysis and urine culture.* Many relevant metabolic and urinary tract disorders can be screened by a simple urinalysis. A culture is essential to rule out infection before proceeding with further evaluation.

4 *Residual urine volume after voiding.* A catheterized post-void residual (PVR) urine specimen should be obtained to exclude urinary retention (normal PVR ≤100 mL) or infection.

5 *Frequency–volume bladder chart.* More than seven voids per day suggest a problem with frequency, but this is highly dependent on habit and fluid intake. Patients can be notoriously inaccurate in estimating urinary frequency and should be encouraged to keep a "urinary diary" for several days as part of their initial evaluation.

6 *Urodynamics* is a group of tests designed to aid in determining the etiology of lower urinary tract dysfunction.
- *Simple cystometry* (Figure 19.1) involves placing a catheter and gradually filling the bladder with sterile water. Involuntary "detrusor" contractions are demonstrated by a rise in water level during filling due to back-pressure. Normally, the first sensation to void occurs at 150 mL and bladder capacity is typically 400–600 mL.
- *Uroflowmetry* is used to determine the urinary flow rate and flow time to screen for the presence of outflow obstruction and abnormal detrusor contractility. Normally, women achieve a peak flow rate of 15–20 mL/s with a voided volume of 150–200 mL.
- *Complex urodynamic testing* (Figure 19.1) requires placement of an intravesical catheter to measure detrusor pressures and a vaginal or rectal catheter to indirectly measure intra-abdominal pressures.

Stress urinary incontinence (SUI)

Patients have loss of small amounts of urine with coughing, laughing, sneezing, exercising, or other movements that increase intra-abdominal pressure and thus increase pressure on the bladder.
- *Etiology.* Physical changes resulting from pregnancy, childbirth, and menopause often result in weaknesses in the pelvic floor, and urethral support structures and nerve damage.

- *Mechanism.* If the fascial support is weakened, the urethra can move downward at times of increased abdominal pressure, causing bladder pressure to exceed urethral sphincter closure pressure (hypermobile urethra). Incomplete urethral closure may be due to scarring or neuromuscular damage, and cause a more severe form of stress urinary incontinence – intrinsic sphincter deficiency.
- *Diagnosis.* SUI is suggested by history, physical examination, and a positive stress test (demonstrable loss of urine while the patient is being examined).
- *Non-surgical treatment.* pelvic muscle (Kegel) exercises, biofeedback (pressure measurement device notifies the patient when correct muscle contraction is performed and reinforces correct technique), pessaries (see Chapter 20).
- *Surgical treatment* (Figure 19.2):
  1 *Tension-free transvaginal tape* (TVT) or transobturator tape (TOT) are minimally invasive suburethral sling procedures that are rapidly becoming the "gold standard."
  2 *Burch colposuspension* involves suture placement at the Cooper ligament. The Marshall–Marchetti–Krantz (MMK) variation has sutures going through the periosteum of the pubic symphysis.
  3 *Anterior colporrhaphy* (see Chapter 20) has a poor long-term success rate.
  4 *Collagen periurethral injections (Coaptite, Macroplastique)* are designed as a treatment for SUI resulting from intrinsic sphincter deficiency.

Urge incontinence

Patients experience involuntary leakage for no apparent reason while suddenly feeling an urgent need to urinate. This may be accompanied by urinary frequency and nocturia, and patients often describe their bladder as "spastic" or "overactive."
- *Etiology.* Involuntary detrusor muscle contractions. Detrusor hyperactivity can be due to loss of central nervous system (CNS) inhibitory pathways, local irritants, or bladder outlet obstruction.
- *Mechanism.* Frequently idiopathic, but results from damage to the nerves of the bladder, the nervous system (spinal cord and brain), or the muscles themselves.
- *Treatment.* Behavior modification (bladder drills, biofeedback) and/or pharmacologic therapy (oxybutynin chloride, imipramine, mirabegron), injection of the detrusor muscle with botulinum toxin A, neuromodulation.

Overflow incontinence

Patients experience continuous, unstoppable dribbling of urine, or continuing to dribble for some time after they have passed urine.
- *Etiology.* The bladder is always full and overflows, resulting in frequent or continuous urine leakage.
- *Mechanism.* Weak bladder detrusor muscles, resulting in incomplete emptying, or a blocked urethra (outflow obstruction) due to advanced vaginal prolapse, or after an anti-incontinence procedure that has overcorrected the problem.
- *Treatment.* Catheter drainage, followed by treatment of the underlying condition.

Other types of incontinence

- *Mixed incontinence* usually refers to the common combination of stress and urge incontinence occurring together.
- *Transient incontinence* is often triggered by medications, urinary tract infections, mental impairment, restricted mobility, or stool impaction (severe constipation), which can push against the urinary tract and obstruct outflow.
- *Functional incontinence* occurs when a person does not recognize the need to go to the toilet, recognize where the toilet is, or get to the toilet in time due to confusion, dementia, poor eyesight, or poor mobility.

Figure 20.1 PELVIC ORGAN PROLAPSE

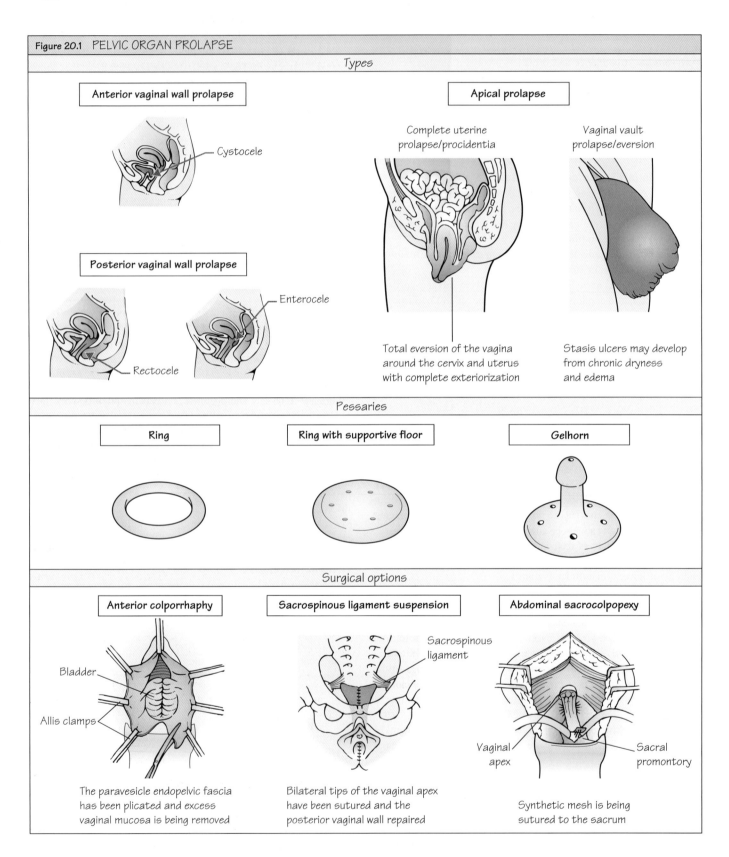

Types

Anterior vaginal wall prolapse

Cystocele

Posterior vaginal wall prolapse

Enterocele

Rectocele

Apical prolapse

Complete uterine prolapse/procidentia

Vaginal vault prolapse/eversion

Total eversion of the vagina around the cervix and uterus with complete exteriorization

Stasis ulcers may develop from chronic dryness and edema

Pessaries

Ring

Ring with supportive floor

Gelhorn

Surgical options

Anterior colporrhaphy

Bladder

Allis clamps

The paravesicle endopelvic fascia has been plicated and excess vaginal mucosa is being removed

Sacrospinous ligament suspension

Sacrospinous ligament

Bilateral tips of the vaginal apex have been sutured and the posterior vaginal wall repaired

Abdominal sacrocolpopexy

Vaginal apex

Sacral promontory

Synthetic mesh is being sutured to the sacrum

Obstetrics and Gynecology at a Glance, Fourth Edition. Errol R. Norwitz and John O. Schorge.

- *Definition.* Descent of one or more pelvic organs (uterine cervix, vaginal apex [after hysterectomy], anterior vagina, posterior vagina, or cul-de-sac peritoneum) through the pelvic floor into the vagina.
- *Incidence.* Half of parous women have prolapse on examination; 10% of women will undergo surgery for prolapse or urinary incontinence in their lifetime. Prolapse is the most common indication for hysterectomy in women after age 55.
- *Pelvic support.* The vagina and uterus have three levels of support in the pelvis: (1) the uterus, cervix, and upper vagina are supported by cardinal and uterosacral ligaments; (2) the arcus tendinus fascia (white line) and the levator ani fascia support the midvagina; and (3) the perineal muscles and membrane support the distal vagina. The levator ani complex of muscles (see Chapter 2) provides the major support for the pelvic organs.
- *Etiology*:
  1 *Vaginal parity.* Pregnancy, labor, and vaginal delivery may result in various degrees of damage to pelvic support structures, including the ligaments, fascia, muscles, and their nerve supply.
  2 *Race.* Prolapse occurs more frequently among white women than Asian and black ones. Inherited differences in pelvic architecture and the quality of supporting muscles/connective tissue are thought to be responsible.
  3 *Estrogen deficiency.* Pelvic tissues are estrogen sensitive. Prolapse often becomes symptomatic during the menopausal years as collagen fibers deteriorate.
  4 *Chronic conditions* that cause repeated increases in intra-abdominal pressure (obesity, "smokers' cough," heavy lifting, constipation) can contribute to significant pelvic relaxation.
  5 *Connective tissue disease.* Chronic steroid use, Ehlers–Danlos syndrome, and other related conditions can disrupt normal, collagen-based, pelvic tissue support.

Diagnosis

- *History.* Each woman's condition should be assessed to ascertain the nature, severity, and progression of her symptoms in addition to coexisting medical conditions, prior obstetric events and past/present medications.
- *Symptoms.* Mild degrees of genital prolapse are often asymptomatic, but the most common complaint is an annoying bulge at the vaginal introitus. Due to the effects of gravity, some women experience minimal symptoms in the morning with progressively more bulging as the day goes on. Patients may note incomplete bladder or rectal emptying.
- *Pelvic examination.* Uterine procidentia is obvious, but most patients have less pronounced prolapse:
  1 *Lithotomy.* The labia are spread and the protrusion identified. The patient is then asked to strain as though attempting defecation and also to cough. What appears first at the introitus may suggest the location of the major defect. Rectovaginal examination may indicate an enterocele that bulges into the space between the rectum and upper posterior vaginal wall, or a distal defect near the perineum.
  2 *Standing.* If the patient suggests that her prolapse is not being seen at its worst extent, she can be asked to strain while in the standing position.

Classification and management

Several systems (Baden-Walker, POP-Q) have been developed to classify pelvic organ prolapse:
- Women with mildly symptomatic prolapse can be counseled that treatment is appropriate only when symptoms warrant it. Non-specific pelvic pressure or back pain may not be alleviated with treatment anyway.

- *Pessaries* can be used to avoid surgery or improve symptoms while awaiting surgical correction. The goal of fitting is to provide satisfactory reduction of the protrusion, without causing discomfort or adversely affecting bladder function.
- *Pelvic floor muscle training* (Kegel exercises) is a simple, non-invasive intervention that is commonly recommended as adjunct therapy for women with prolapse and related symptoms.
- *Total vaginal hysterectomy* (TVH, see Chapter 17) alone is not a treatment for prolapse, but is commonly performed to provide vaginal access to the uterosacral ligaments for suspension of the vaginal apex.

Cystocele (Figure 20.1)
Surgical options
1 *Anterior colporrhaphy* involves vaginally plicating the endopelvic fascia in the midline to provide support and raise the bladder to correct its anatomic position.
2 *Paravaginal repair* replaces the anterolateral vaginal wall to its anatomic position.
3 The *McCall culdoplasty* shortens the uterosacral ligaments and reattaches them to the vaginal apex.

Rectocele (Figure 20.1)
Surgical options
Posterior colporrhaphy mimics the anterior procedure with a midline plication of endopelvic fascia. *Perineorrhaphy* is commonly required due to an attenuated perineal body or widened genital hiatus.

Enterocele (Figure 20.1)
Surgical options
As an enterocele is a true herniation of the peritoneal cavity at the pouch of Douglas which bulges into the rectovaginal septum, repair is usually performed at the same time as posterior colporrhaphy. The hernia sac is visualized as the vagina is separated from the rectum and it must be dissected free of underlying tissue. The neck of the hernia is then isolated and sutured. Fixing the uterosacral ligaments to the sac will help prevent recurrence.

Uterine procidentia (Figure 20.1)
Surgical options
TVH is common, but anterior and posterior colporrhaphy generally do not provide sufficient long-term apical support:
1 *Sacrospinous ligament suspension* (SSLS) may be concomitantly performed vaginally by suspending the fascia of the apex to one or both ligaments.
2 *Abdominal sacrocolpopexy* with total abdominal hysterectomy (TAH) is another reasonable option that has less apical failure, postoperative dyspareunia, and stress incontinence than SSLS, but is associated with longer surgical time, longer patient recovery, and more short- and long-term complications. Laparoscopic and robotic-assisted techniques are the preferred option due to reduced recovery times.
3 *Colpocleisis (Lefort procedure)* is usually reserved for very elderly women or those at high risk for complications. In this limited operation, the anterior and posterior vaginal walls are sutured together, making vaginal intercourse effectively impossible.

Posthysterectomy vaginal vault prolapse
Surgical options
Laparoscopic or *robotic-assisted sacrocolpopexy* has emerged as the preferred option over the abdominal approach for surgeons with advanced minimally invasive surgical skills, but the learning curve is protracted. SSLS is another alternative.

21 Puberty and precocious puberty

Figure 21.1 DIAGNOSTIC WORK-UP OF PRECOCIOUS PUBERTY

History

- Age of onset
- Rapidity
- Family history

↓

Physical examination

- Record of growth
- Height/weight percentiles
- Abdominal–pelvic examination
- Neurological examination
- Tanner staging

Figure 21.2 TANNER STAGING

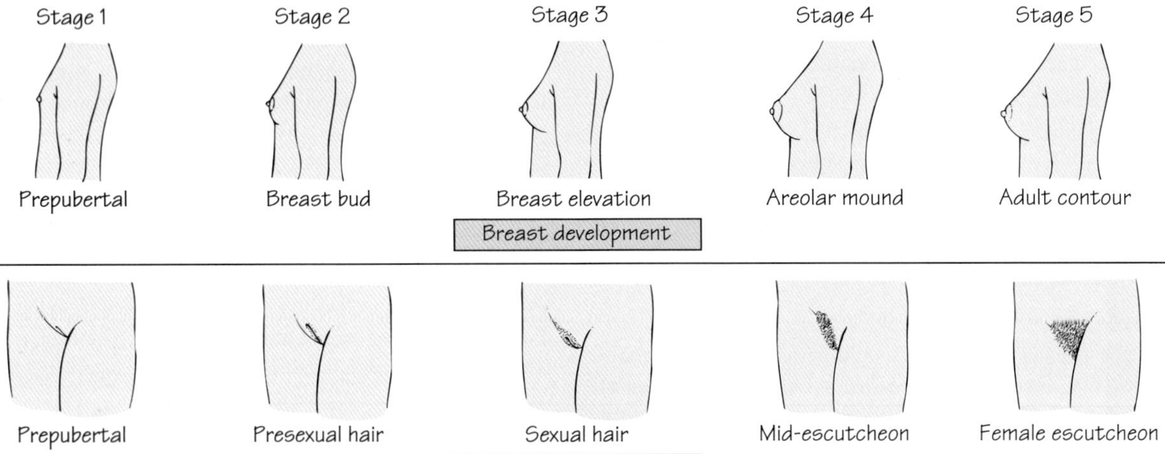
Stage 1
Stage 2
Stage 3
Stage 4
Stage 5
Prepubertal
Breast bud
Breast elevation
Areolar mound
Adult contour
Breast development
Prepubertal
Presexual hair
Sexual hair
Mid-escutcheon
Female escutcheon
Pubic hair development

↓

Laboratory evaluation and imaging studies

- TSH, LH, FSH concentrations
- Sex steroid concentrations
- Abdominal–pelvic ultrasound
- Radiological bone age
- Head CT scan or head MRI

Diagnosis

Central (true) precocious puberty

1 Idiopathic (constitutional) puberty (75%)
2 Central nervous system lesions (5–10%)
- Hypothalamic hamartomas
- Craniopharyngiomas
- Astrocytomas
- Encephalitis
- Cranial irradiation
- Hydrocephalus
- Skull injury
- Tuberculosis
- Neurofibromatosis
- Epilepsy

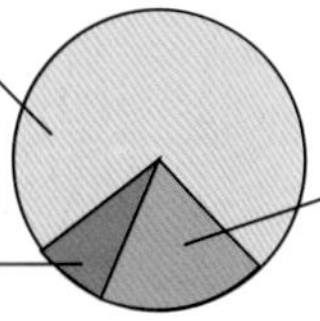

Peripheral precocious puberty

- Granulosa cell tumors(10%)
- Ovarian follicular cysts (10%)
- McCune–Albright syndrome (5%)
- Iatrogenic
- Other
  – hypothyroidism
  – congenital adrenal hyperplasia

Obstetrics and Gynecology at a Glance, Fourth Edition. Errol R. Norwitz and John O. Schorge.

Puberty

- *Puberty* refers to the series of events leading to sexual maturity. It is a time of accelerated growth, skeletal maturation, development of secondary sexual characteristics, and achievement of fertility. The age at which puberty occurs has dropped significantly over the past 150 years due to improved nutrition and living conditions.
- *Adolescence* is the period of psychological and social transition between childhood and adulthood. Adolescence largely overlaps the period of puberty, but its boundaries are less precisely defined and it refers as much to the psychosocial and cultural characteristics of development during the teen years as to the physical changes of puberty.
- *Thelarche* (breast development) is the first sign of puberty. It usually begins between 8 and 13 years of age and is associated with increased estrogen production.
- *Adrenarche* (development of pubic and axillary hair) is the second stage in maturation and typically occurs between 11 and 12 years of age. Axillary hair usually appears after the growth of pubic hair is complete.
- *Menarche* (onset of menstruation) usually occurs 2–3 years after thelarche at an average age of 11–13 years. Initial cycles are often anovulatory and irregular.
- The major determinant of the timing of puberty is genetic. Puberty begins earliest in black girls, followed by Hispanic and white girls. Environmental factors (general health, nutritional status, geographic location) are also important.

Biologic basis of puberty

- Pubertal changes are triggered by the maturation of the hypothalamic–pituitary–ovarian axis.
- The onset of puberty is heralded by hypothalamic pulsatile release of gonadotropin-releasing hormone (GnRH).
- Increased pituitary gonadotropin (luteinizing hormone [LH], follicle-stimulating hormone [FSH]) production in response to pulsatile GnRH is the endocrinologic *hallmark* of puberty.
- The final maturation phase is the development of a cyclic midcycle surge of LH in response to the positive feedback of the steroid hormones, primarily estradiol-17β. This midcycle LH surge induces ovulation and the normal female menstrual cycle (see Chapter 2).

Precocious puberty

Early sexual development deserves evaluation because it may (1) induce early bone maturation and reduce eventual adult height, (2) indicate the presence of a tumor or other serious problem, or (3) cause the child to become an object of adult sexual interest.

- *Definition.* Pubertal changes before 8 years of age.
- *Guidelines for evaluation.* Thelarche or adrenarche should be evaluated if this occurs before age 7 in white girls and before age 6 in black girls.

Diagnostic work-up (Figure 21.1)

Medical evaluation is often necessary to distinguish the few children with serious conditions from the majority who have entered puberty early but are still medically normal.

- *History.* Determining the age of onset, rapidity, and family history is crucial. Coexisting illness (hypothyroidism), medications (estrogen ingestion), or a history of head trauma may be important.
- *Physical examination.* Increased growth is often the first observable change. Abdominal–pelvic examination should focus on examination of the external genitalia, ruling out a pelvic mass, and looking for signs of androgenization. A brief neurologic examination may suggest the presence of an intracranial mass. Premature thelarche and pubarche can be quantified by assessment of the Tanner stage.
- *Laboratory evaluation.* Thyroid function tests, LH/FSH values, and sex steroid levels may support the diagnosis.
- *Imaging studies.* Abdominal–pelvic ultrasound is an accurate way of detecting ovarian tumors. Radiologic bone age may be compared with standards for the chronologic age. A head CT scan or MRI should be performed if an intracranial mass is suspected.

Types of precocious puberty (Figure 21.2)

Central (true) precocious puberty

- *Definition.* Premature maturation of the hypothalamic–pituitary–ovarian axis (gonadotropin dependent).
- *Age of onset.* Between the age of 6 and 8.
- *Sequelae.* The most serious adverse effect is short adult stature. Children are transiently tall for their age, but undergo premature epiphyseal fusion.
- *Etiology:*

  1 *Idiopathic (constitutional) puberty* is most common in girls aged >4 years. This is a benign process and fundamentally a diagnosis of exclusion. The cause is unknown. Follow-up is necessary to rule out slow-growing lesions of the brain, ovary, or adrenal gland. *Treatment*: GnRH agonists in girls with menarche <8 years or those with unusually rapid progression of puberty having bone age >2 years ahead of chronologic age. The goals of therapy are to reduce gonadotropin secretions, decrease the growth rate to normal, and slow skeletal maturation to allow development of maximal adult height. Continuous chronic administration is maintained until the median age of puberty.

  2 *Central nervous system lesions* are often present in girls aged <4 years. Neurologic symptoms (visual disturbance, headaches) commonly precede sexual development. Most lesions are located near the hypothalamus. *Treatment*: surgery, chemotherapy, and/or irradiation may be indicated.

Peripheral precocious puberty

- *Definition.* Premature female sexual maturation that is not based on hypothalamic–pituitary control (gonadotropin independent). The underlying process initiates activation of pubertal development.
- *Etiology:*

  1 *Estrogen-producing ovarian tumors* account for most cases. Granulosa cell tumors are most common, but follicular cysts, thecomas, and Sertoli–Leydig tumors may also occur. *Treatment*: surgical excision.

  2 *McCune–Albright syndrome (polyostotic fibrous dysplasia)* consists of multiple disseminated cystic bone lesions, café-au-lait spots, and sexual precocity. *Treatment*: testolactone (an aromatase inhibitor) prevents the conversion of estrogen precursors to biologically active estrogens and leads to a decreased rate of growth and skeletal maturation. The underlying disease is incurable.

  3 *Iatrogenic causes* result from excessive exogenous hormonal administration. *Treatment*: discontinuation of the medication.

Isolated precocity

- *Definition.* Premature development of a single pubertal event (usually thelarche). *Treatment*: reassurance, because this condition is usually self-limiting and resolves spontaneously.

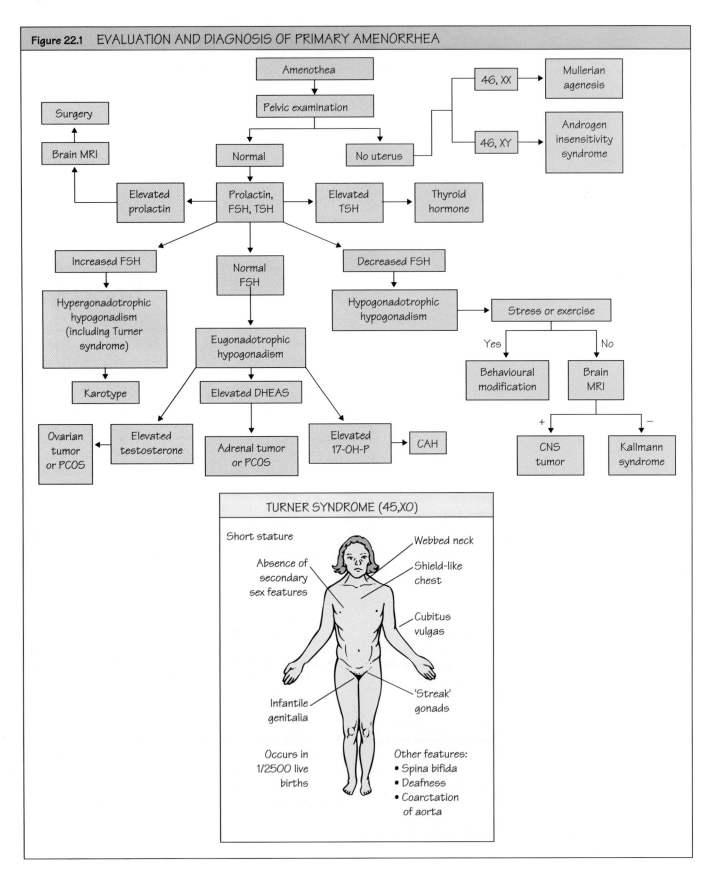

Figure 22.1   EVALUATION AND DIAGNOSIS OF PRIMARY AMENORRHEA

TURNER SYNDROME (45,XO)

Short stature

Absence of secondary sex features

Webbed neck

Shield-like chest

Cubitus vulgas

Infantile genitalia

'Streak' gonads

Occurs in 1/2500 live births

Other features:
• Spina bifida
• Deafness
• Coarctation of aorta

Obstetrics and Gynecology at a Glance, Fourth Edition. Errol R. Norwitz and John O. Schorge.

52   © 2013 John Wiley & Sons, Ltd. Published 2013 by John Wiley & Sons, Ltd.

- *Definition.* (1) No menses by age 14 years and no other evidence of pubertal development, (2) no menses by age 16 despite presence of other pubertal signs, or (3) previous menstrual cycles but now without menses for a time equivalent to three cycles or 6 months.
- Physiologic amenorrhea is seen in prepubescent girls, during pregnancy and lactation (breastfeeding), and after menopause.
- Pathologic (non-physiologic) amenorrhea occurs in 3–4% of reproductive age women and should be investigated to determine the underlying etiology.
- Due to significant overlap, prior categorization of amenorrhea as primary or secondary should be avoided.
- Proper evaluation requires a systematic approach to making a correct diagnosis (Figure 22.1).

Anatomic disorders
Inherited
- Frequent cause in adolescents:
  1 *Müllerian agenesis* (Mayer–Rokitansky–Küster–Hauser syndrome; 1/5,000 female births) involves the congenital absence of all or part of the uterus and vagina. *Treatment*: creation of a neovagina by progressive dilation or surgery (McIndoe operation).
  2 *Imperforate hymen* (1/2,000) and *transverse vaginal septum* (1/70,000 women) are distal outflow tract obstructions. *Treatment*: hymenectomy/excision.

Acquired
1 *Intrauterine synechiae* (Asherman syndrome) after vigorous uterine curettage in early pregnancy may lead to scarring that interferes with normal endometrial growth and shedding. *Treatment*: hysteroscopic lysis of intrauterine adhesions and stimulation of the endometrium with estrogen.
2 *Cervical stenosis* may result from D&C (dilation and curettage), cone biopsy, or infection. *Treatment*: dilation of the cervix.

Endocrine disorders
Hypergonadotropic hypogonadism (premature ovarian failure)
- *Etiology.* Primary ovarian dysfunction – not due to the hypothalamus or pituitary.
- *Definition.* Loss of oocytes before age 40.
- *Diagnosis.* Two serum FSH levels >40 mIU/mL, drawn at least 1 month apart.
- *Incidence.* Occurs in 1/100 women aged <40.
- Gonadal dysgenesis is characterized by streak gonads (bands of fibrous tissue in place of the ovary). Synthesis of ovarian steroids does not occur due to the absence of ovarian follicles. Breast development does not occur because of the very low circulating estradiol levels. *Turner syndrome* (45,XO) accounts for >50% of patients. The remaining causes are commonly due to other non-inherited chromosomal disorders or deletions. *Treatment*: hormone replacement therapy to develop breast tissue and prevent osteoporosis. The presence of a Y chromosome on karyotype requires excision of gonadal tissue to prevent the 25% incidence of malignancy.
- Acquired abnormalities include autoimmune processes (eg, myasthenia gravis), chemotherapy, radiation, or infection. *Treatment*: none, but hormone replacement therapy should be considered.

Hypogonadotropic hypogonadism
- *Etiology.* Primary hypothalamic–pituitary dysfunction.

- *Definition.* Decrease in gonadotropin stimulation of the ovaries leads to loss of ovarian follicle development and results in very low estrogen levels.

1 Hypothalamic disorders
- Inherited hypothalamic disorders are idiopathic. Kallman syndrome is one variant often associated with the inability to smell and other midline facial anomalies. *Treatment*: hormone replacement therapy.
- Acquired hypothalamic dysfunction may be due to brain tumors, physical or emotional stress, weight loss, exercise, or pseudocyesis (the ability of the mind to control physiologic processes). *Treatment*: unless a tumor is present, behavioral modification or hormone replacement therapy may be appropriate, or therapy may be unnecessary if the underlying cause of the amenorrhea is not threatening to her health.

2 Pituitary disorders
- *Inherited pituitary disorders* may result in hypoplasia. *Treatment*: hormone replacement therapy.
- *Acquired pituitary dysfunction* is most commonly due to a prolactin-secreting adenoma, but metastatic tumors or Sheehan syndrome (panhypopituitarism resulting from massive postpartum hemorrhage, pituitary ischemia, and necrosis) is also possible. *Treatment*: surgical resection is usually indicated for patients with pituitary macroadenomas. Other hyperprolactinemic patients should be followed with serial prolactin levels and head imaging to exclude development of a macroadenoma. Sheehan syndrome is managed with hormone replacement therapy.

3 Chronic illnesses
Chronic illnesses such as end-stage kidney disease, AIDS, or advanced liver disease can also result in hypogonadotropic amenorrhea.

Eugonadotropic hypogonadism
- *Etiology.* Disorders that cause amenorrhea, but are not associated with abnormal gonadotropin levels:
  1 *Polycystic ovarian syndrome* (PCOS) (see Chapter 23).
  2 *Congenital adrenal hyperplasia* (CAH; adult onset) resembles PCOS clinically, but is usually due to a gene mutation resulting in patients shunting progesterone precursors to the androgen pathway. *Treatment*: hormone replacement therapy.
  3 *Hyperprolactinemia* and hypothyroidism.

Infertility
- As many of the diagnoses are made during childhood or adolescence, counseling is very important. Insensitivity can be very psychologically devastating to girl who is told that she does not have a uterus, is genotypically male, or is permanently infertile.
- Fortunately, anatomic disorders can usually be corrected to provide an appropriate functional result.
- Hypergonadotropic patients may be able to conceive using a donor oocyte and in vitro fertilization (see Chapter 27).
- Hypogondaotropic patients may become fertile with pulsatile GnRH or gonadotropins (see Chapter 27).
- Eugonadotropic patients, especially those with PCOS, will frequently ovulate with clomiphene citrate (see Chapter 26).

Figure 23.1 APPEARANCE OF POLYCYSTIC OVARIES

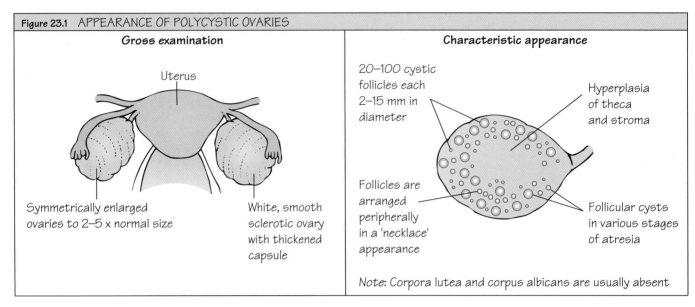

Gross examination

Uterus

Symmetrically enlarged ovaries to 2–5 x normal size

White, smooth sclerotic ovary with thickened capsule

Characteristic appearance

20–100 cystic follicles each 2–15 mm in diameter

Hyperplasia of theca and stroma

Follicles are arranged peripherally in a 'necklace' appearance

Follicular cysts in various stages of atresia

Note: Corpora lutea and corpus albicans are usually absent

Figure 23.2 PATHOPHYSIOLOGY OF POLYCYSTIC OVARIAN SYNDROME (PCOS)

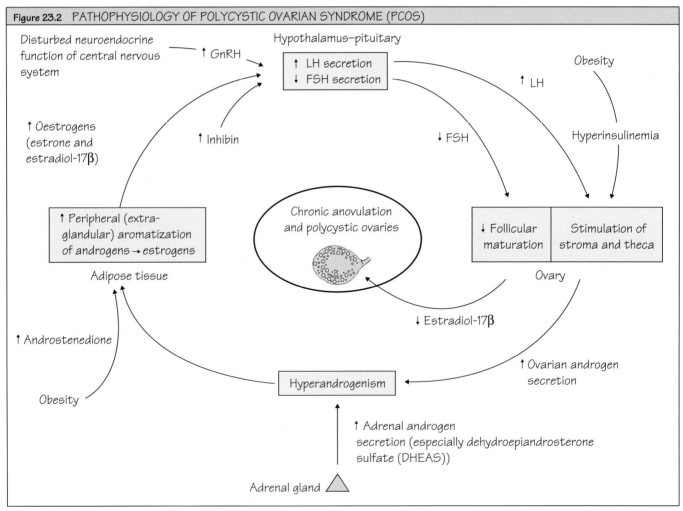

Disturbed neuroendocrine function of central nervous system

↑ GnRH

Hypothalamus–pituitary

↑ LH secretion
↓ FSH secretion

Obesity

↑ LH

↑ Öestrogens (estrone and estradiol-17β)

↑ Inhibin

↓ FSH

Hyperinsulinemia

↑ Peripheral (extra-glandular) aromatization of androgens → estrogens

Chronic anovulation and polycystic ovaries

↓ Follicular maturation

Stimulation of stroma and theca

Adipose tissue

Ovary

↓ Estradiol-17β

↑ Androstenedione

↑ Ovarian androgen secretion

Obesity

Hyperandrogenism

↑ Adrenal androgen secretion (especially dehydroepiandrosterone sulfate (DHEAS))

Adrenal gland

Obstetrics and Gynecology at a Glance, Fourth Edition. Errol R. Norwitz and John O. Schorge.

54 © 2013 John Wiley & Sons, Ltd. Published 2013 by John Wiley & Sons, Ltd.

- *Definition.* A heterogeneous disorder of unexplained hyperandrogenic chronic anovulation in which secondary causes (androgen-secreting neoplasms) have been excluded. PCOS was historically referred to as Stein–Leventhal syndrome.
- *Prevalence.* Five percent of women of reproductive age. It occurs among all races and nationalities, is the most common hormonal disorder of women this age, and is a leading cause of infertility.
- *Etiology.* Unknown: no gene or specific environmental substance has been identified.

Diagnostic evaluation

- *History.* The history should focus on the menstrual pattern, previous pregnancies (if any), concomitant medications, smoking, alcohol consumption, diet, and identification of family members with diabetes and cardiovascular disease.
- *Physical examination* should look for balding, acne, clitoromegaly, body hair distribution, and signs of insulin resistance (obesity, centripetal fat distribution, acanthosis nigricans). Bimanual examination may suggest enlarged ovaries (Figure 23.1).
- *Laboratory tests* such as testosterone or dehydroepiandrosterone sulfate (DHEAS) are useful for documenting ovarian hyperandrogenism. Androgen-secreting tumors of the ovary or adrenal gland are also invariably accompanied by elevated circulating androgen levels, but there is no absolute level that is pathognomonic for a tumor or minimum level that excludes a tumor.
- *Imaging studies* such as a pelvic sonogram can exclude a solid ovarian tumor and may demonstrate the characteristic "polycystic" appearance of the ovaries (Figure 23.1).
- *Criteria.* In 2003, a consensus workshop in Rotterdam indicated that PCOS should be diagnosed if two out of three criteria are met: (1) oligo-ovulation and/or anovulation, (2) excess androgen activity, and (3) polycystic ovaries by sonogram, other endocrine disorders being excluded.

Pathophysiology (Figure 23.2)

- PCOS represents the end-stage of a "vicious cycle" of endocrinologic events that can be initiated at many different entry points.
- It remains unclear whether the primary pathology resides in the ovary or the hypothalamus, but the fundamental defect appears to be "inappropriate" signaling to the hypothalamus and pituitary.
- Elevated luteinizing hormone (LH) levels (the hallmark of PCOS) result from increased peripheral estrogen production (positive feedback) and increased gonadotropin-releasing hormone (GnRH) secretion.
- Suppressed follicle-stimulating hormone (FSH) levels result from increased peripheral estrogen production (negative feedback) and increased secretion of inhibin.
- PCOS is characterized by a "steady state" of chronically elevated LH and chronically suppressed FSH levels, instead of their cyclic rise and fall in a normal menstrual cycle (see Chapter 3).
- Increased LH stimulates ovarian stroma and theca cells to increase production of androgens. Androgens are converted peripherally by aromatization to estrogens, which perpetuate chronic anovulation.
- As a result of suppressed FSH, new follicular growth is continuously stimulated but not to the point of full maturation and ovulation (corpus lutea and corpus albicans are rarely detected). Elevated androgens contribute to the prevention of normal follicular development and induction of premature atresia.
- The *ovary* is the major site of androgen overproduction; the adrenal gland has a minor role.

- Increased adipose tissue in obese patients contributes to the extraglandular aromatization of androgens to estrogens.
- Circulating testosterone is increased (causing hirsutism), because sex hormone-binding globulin (SHBG) levels are decreased in PCOS.

Clinical manifestations

- *Menstrual irregularities* (80%) begin soon after menarche, including secondary amenorrhea and/or oligomenorrhea.
- *Hirsutism* (70%) refers to the presence of excessive male pattern (upper lip, chin, chest, back) hair growth in women.
- *Obesity* (50%) contributes substantially to the metabolic abnormalities of PCOS.
- *Infertility* (75%) is due to chronic anovulation.
- *Acanthosis nigricans* is a dermatologic marker of insulin resistance and hyperinsulinemia which is marked by gray–brown, velvety, sometimes verrucous, discoloration of the skin at the neck, groin, and axillae.
- *HAIR-AN syndrome* (**h**yper**a**ndrogenism, **i**nsulin **r**esistance, and **a**canthosis **n**igricans) represents the extreme effects of hyperandrogenic chronic anovulation.

Long-term sequelae

- Endometrial hyperplasia/adenocarcinoma (see Chapter 32)
- Insulin resistance/type 2 diabetes
- High blood pressure, cardiovascular disease, dyslipidemia
- Strokes
- Weight gain.

Management

Medical treatment of PCOS is tailored to the patient's goals in four main categories: (1) lowering of insulin levels, (2) restoration of fertility, (3) treatment of hirsutism or acne, and (4) restoration of regular menstruation with prevention of endometrial hyperplasia and cancer. There is considerable debate as to the optimal treatment.

- General interventions that help to reduce weight or insulin resistance can be beneficial for all these aims and interrupt the self-perpetuating cycle of hyperandrogenic chronic anovulation.

Medical therapy

1 *Oral contraceptives* have been the mainstay of long-term management of PCOS by decreasing LH and FSH secretion and ovarian production of androgens, increasing hepatic production of SHBG, decreasing levels of DHEA (dehydroepiandrosterone) and preventing endometrial neoplasia. Cyproterone acetate (Dianette/Diane), spironolactone, or topical eflornithine may be especially helpful in patients with excessive hirsutism.

2 *Progestins* have been shown to suppress pituitary LH and FSH and circulating androgens, but breakthrough bleeding is common.

3 *Insulin-sensitizing agents* (metformin) decrease circulating androgen levels, improve the ovulation rate, and improve glucose tolerance.

4 *Clomiphene citrate* (see Chapter 26) has traditionally been the first-line treatment for women desiring pregnancy.

Surgical therapy

1 *Ovarian drilling* with laser or diathermy has few advantages over medical therapy for infertility and does not appear to have significant long-term benefits in improving metabolic abnormalities.

2 *Mechanical hair removal* (laser vaporization, electrolysis, depilatory creams) is often the front line of treatment for hirsutism.

Figure 24.1 EVALUATION OF COUPLES WITH RECURRENT PREGNANCY LOSS

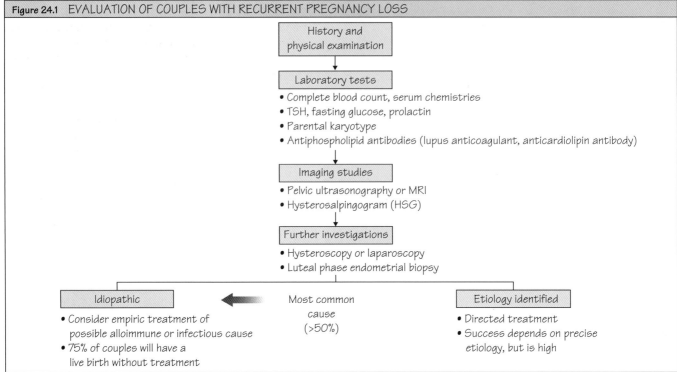

History and physical examination

Laboratory tests
- Complete blood count, serum chemistries
- TSH, fasting glucose, prolactin
- Parental karyotype
- Antiphospholipid antibodies (lupus anticoagulant, anticardiolipin antibody)

Imaging studies
- Pelvic ultrasonography or MRI
- Hysterosalpingogram (HSG)

Further investigations
- Hysteroscopy or laparoscopy
- Luteal phase endometrial biopsy

Idiopathic ← Most common cause (>50%) → Etiology identified

Idiopathic
- Consider empiric treatment of possible alloimmune or infectious cause
- 75% of couples will have a live birth without treatment

Etiology identified
- Directed treatment
- Success depends on precise etiology, but is high

Figure 24.2 ETIOLOGIES OF RECURRENT PREGNANCY LOSS

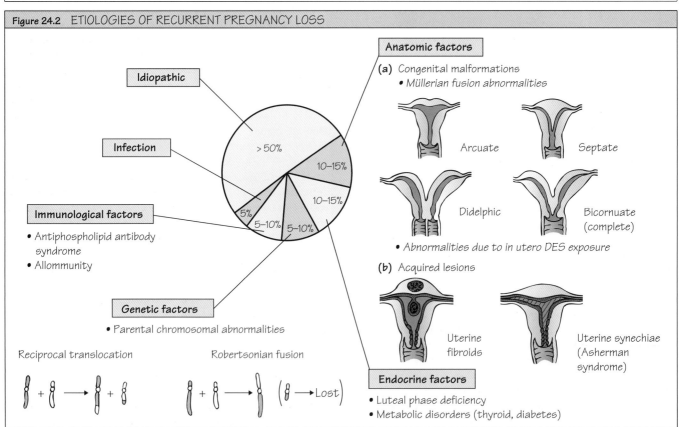

Idiopathic

Infection

Immunological factors
- Antiphospholipid antibody syndrome
- Allommunity

Genetic factors
- Parental chromosomal abnormalities

Reciprocal translocation   Robertsonian fusion

Anatomic factors

(a) Congenital malformations
- Müllerian fusion abnormalities

Arcuate   Septate

Didelphic   Bicornuate (complete)

- Abnormalities due to in utero DES exposure

(b) Acquired lesions

Uterine fibroids   Uterine synechiae (Asherman syndrome)

Endocrine factors
- Luteal phase deficiency
- Metabolic disorders (thyroid, diabetes)

Pie chart percentages: >50%, 10–15%, 10–15%, 5–10%, 5–10%, 5%

- *Definition.* The occurrence of repeated (three or more consecutive) pregnancies that end in miscarriage of the fetus, usually before 20 weeks of gestation.
- *Prevalence.* One percent of women of reproductive age who conceive.

Diagnostic evaluation of couples (Figure 24.1)
- *History.* The pattern, trimester, and characteristics of prior pregnancy losses should be reviewed. Exposure to environmental toxins and drugs, prior gynecologic or obstetric infections, and excluding the possibility of consanguinity are important.
- *Physical examination* may reveal evidence of maternal systemic disease or uterine anomalies.
- *Laboratory tests and imaging studies* should be individually utilized.

Etiology (Figure 24.2)
Most couples will have no clear explanation for their recurrent pregnancy loss (RPL). Several alleged causes are controversial and anxious patients/physicians often explore empiric or alternative treatments with dubious benefit.

Idiopathic (>50%)
- Many couples never have a cause identified, even after extensive investigations. Informative and supportive counseling serves an important role because 60–70% of women with at least one previous live birth will have a successful next pregnancy.

Anatomic factors (10–15%)
- *Uterine anomalies* are most often associated with second-trimester loss. Congenital malformations (see Chapter 10) result from müllerian tube fusion abnormalities and acquired lesions have a more controversial impact. Surgical revision may be helpful in some circumstances.
- *Incompetent cervix* (see Chapter 58) also accounts for mainly second-trimester losses. Cerclage placement may be beneficial in selected patients.

Endocrine factors (10–15%)
- *Luteal phase deficiency* is purported to result from insufficient progesterone secretion by the corpus luteum, resulting in inadequate preparation of the endometrium for implantation and/or an inability to maintain early pregnancy. Two "out-of-phase" endometrial biopsies (in which histologic dating lags behind menstrual dating by ≤2 days) in consecutive cycles are required for the diagnosis. Progesterone supplementation is commonly prescribed, but therapeutic benefit is speculative.
- *Metabolic disorders* (hypothyroidism, poorly controlled diabetes, polycystic ovarian syndrome [see Chapter 23]) require diagnosis and treatment of the underlying disease. Mild or subclinical endocrine diseases are not causative.

Genetic factors (5–10%)
In certain chromosomal situations, although treatment may not be available, in vitro fertilization (IVF, see Chapter 27) with preimplantation genetic diagnosis may be able to identify embryos with a reduced risk of another pregnancy loss which would then be transferred.
- *Parental chromosomal abnormalities* are the *only proven cause* of RPL. The most frequent karyotypic abnormality is a balanced translocation – found most often in the female partner. Two-thirds are reciprocal (exchange of chromatin between any two non-homologous chromosomes without loss of genetic material). A third are robertso-

nian (fusion of chromosomes that have the centromere very near one end of a chromosome [typically 13, 14, 15, 21, or 22] with loss of one centromere and two short arms). The overall risk of spontaneous miscarriage in couples with a balanced translocation is >25%. The only treatment option may be IVF with donor sperm or ova.
- *Recurrent embryonic aneuploidy* may represent non-random events in some predisposed couples. Most aneuploid losses are the result of advanced maternal age. Prenatal diagnosis via amniocentesis or chorionic villous sampling may be useful in some situations – but no treatment is available.

Immunologic factors (5–10%)
- *Antiphospholipid antibody syndrome* is an autoimmune disorder characterized by circulating antibodies against membrane phospholipids and at least one specific clinical syndrome (RPL, unexplained thrombosis, fetal death). The diagnosis requires at least one confirmatory serologic test (lupus anticoagulant, anti-cardiolipin antibody). The treatment of choice is aspirin plus heparin (or prednisone in some circumstances).
- *Alloimmunity* (immunologic differences between individuals) has been proposed as a factor between reproductive partners that causes otherwise unexplained RPL. During normal pregnancy, the mother's immune system is thought to recognize semiallogeneic (50% "nonself") fetal antigens and to produce "blocking" factors to protect the fetus. Failure to produce these blocking factors may play a role, but there is no direct scientific evidence to support this theory and there is no specific diagnostic test. Immunotherapy has been used in an attempt to promote immune tolerance to paternal antigen.

Infection (5%)
Listeria monocytogenes, Mycoplasma hominis, Ureaplasma urealyticum, Toxoplasma gondii, and viruses (herpes simplex, cytomegalovirus, rubella) have been variously associated with spontaneous abortion, but none has been proven to cause RPL. Diagnosis can be made using cervical cultures, viral titers, or serum antibodies. Directed antibiotic therapy may be useful if a causative agent is identified. However, empiric treatment with doxycycline or erythromycin may be more cost-effective and efficient.

Other possible factors
- *Thrombophilia* (propensity for blood clots) increases the risk of RPL. The most common types are factor V Leiden and prothrombin *G2010A* mutation. Anticoagulant therapy may improve the chances of carrying pregnancy to term.
- *Environmental toxins* such as smoking, alcohol, and heavy coffee consumption have been associated with an increased risk of spontaneous miscarriage, but not RPL. Regardless, use should be curtailed if possible.
- *Drugs* such as folic acid antagonists, valproic acid, warfarin, anesthetic gases, tetrachloroethylene, and isotretinoin (Accutane) are also speculative causes.

Prognosis
- If the likely cause can be determined, treatment is to be directed accordingly.
- Close surveillance during pregnancy is generally recommended for RPL patients who become pregnant. Couples are often anxious, frustrated, and on the verge of despair. Fortunately, the possibility of achieving a live birth is high.

25 The infertile couple

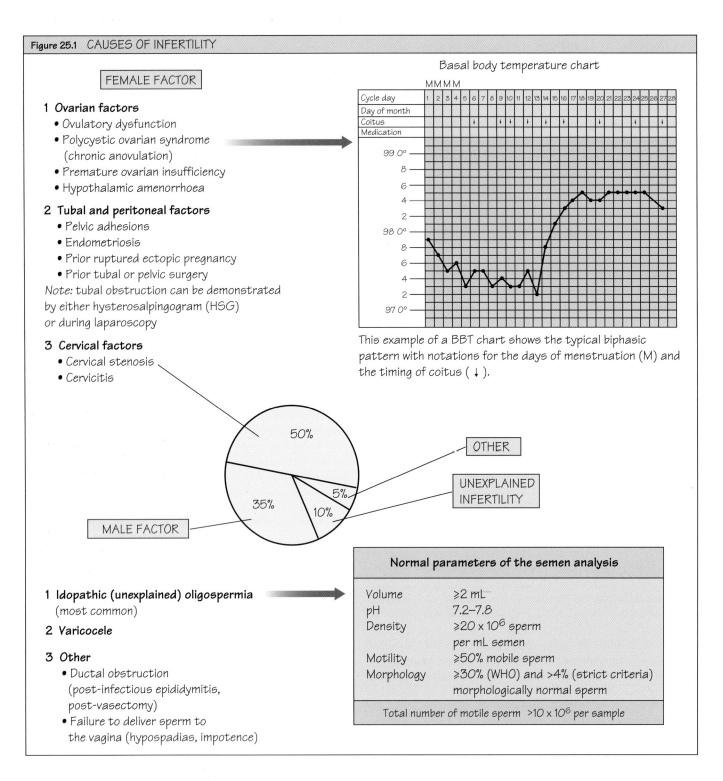

Figure 25.1 CAUSES OF INFERTILITY

FEMALE FACTOR

1 Ovarian factors
- Ovulatory dysfunction
- Polycystic ovarian syndrome (chronic anovulation)
- Premature ovarian insufficiency
- Hypothalamic amenorrhoea

2 Tubal and peritoneal factors
- Pelvic adhesions
- Endometriosis
- Prior ruptured ectopic pregnancy
- Prior tubal or pelvic surgery

Note: tubal obstruction can be demonstrated by either hysterosalpingogram (HSG) or during laparoscopy

3 Cervical factors
- Cervical stenosis
- Cervicitis

Basal body temperature chart

This example of a BBT chart shows the typical biphasic pattern with notations for the days of menstruation (M) and the timing of coitus (↓).

50%

OTHER

5%

UNEXPLAINED INFERTILITY

10%

35%

MALE FACTOR

1 Idopathic (unexplained) oligospermia (most common)

2 Varicocele

3 Other
- Ductal obstruction (post-infectious epididymitis, post-vasectomy)
- Failure to deliver sperm to the vagina (hypospadias, impotence)

Normal parameters of the semen analysis	
Volume	≥2 mL
pH	7.2–7.8
Density	≥20 x 10⁶ sperm per mL semen
Motility	≥50% mobile sperm
Morphology	≥30% (WHO) and >4% (strict criteria) morphologically normal sperm
Total number of motile sperm >10 x 10⁶ per sample	

Definitions

- *Fecundability.* The probability of conceiving during a single monthly cycle. In "normally fertile" couples it is 20–25%, with a cumulative 85–90% chance of pregnancy within 12 months.

- *Infertility.* The inability to conceive after 12 months of appropriately timed intercourse without contraception in women aged <35 years or after 6 months in women aged ≥35 years.
- Primary infertility refers to couples who have never achieved a pregnancy. Secondary infertility implies at least one previous conception.

Obstetrics and Gynecology at a Glance, Fourth Edition. Errol R. Norwitz and John O. Schorge.

Incidence

- 10–15% of reproductive age married couples are infertile.
- The prevalence of infertility has remained constant, but the number of office visits to physicians by "infertile" couples has tripled over the past 20 years. This "infertility epidemic" has been attributed primarily to elective postponement of childbearing and increased insurance coverage of elective fertility therapy.

Risk factors

- Fecundability begins to slowly decline after age 28 and usually declines at a more rapid rate after age 35.
- Cigarette smoking, recreational drug use, and certain occupational and environmental exposures decrease the fertility rate.

Initial assessment

- The primary goals of an infertility evaluation are to provide a rational approach to diagnosis, to present an accurate assessment of ongoing progress and prognosis, and to educate the couple about reproductive physiology.
- *History.* Relevant details include the female patient's age, previous pregnancies, and duration of conception attempts, timing of intercourse, lubricant use, and erectile or ejaculatory dysfunction. A comprehensive gynecologic history should include menarche, menstrual intervals, prior history of sexually transmitted infections, prior tubal or pelvic surgery, prior pelvic infection or ectopic pregnancy, and prior abnormal Pap smears necessitating of the loop electrosurgical excision procedure (LEEP) or cryosurgery.
- *Physical examination.* Features of an endocrine disorder (hirsutism, hepatomegaly, thyromegaly) or gynecologic pathology (fibroids, endometriosis) may be evident.
- *Laboratory tests.* Fertility-related testing includes: day 3 follicle-stimulating hormone (FSH), estradiol, thyroid-stimulating hormone (TSH), prolactin, hysterosalpingogram for the female patient, and semen analysis for the male partner. Additional non-fertility tests usually include complete blood count, Papanicolaou (Pap) smear, and prenatal viral titers (eg, HIV, hepatitis B and C, rubella and varicella) and ethnic specific genetic screening (cystic fibrosis, hemoglobin electrophoresis, Tay–Sachs disease, Canavan disease, spinal muscular atrophy, etc).

Basic work-up

- The common causes of infertility are evaluated by:
  1 Confirmation of predictable ovulation (menstrual intervals, urinary LH kits, basal body temperature)
  2 Ovarian reserve (day 3 FSH, estradiol, clomiphene citrate challenge test, anti-müllerian hormone [emerging evidence])
  3 Semen analysis
  4 Evaluation of tubal patency and uterine factors (hysterosalpingogram, saline sonohysterogram (FemVue)
  5 Endocrinopathies (thyroid dysfunction, hyperprolactinemia, polycystic ovarian syndrome [PCOS])

Causes of infertility (Figure 25.1)

Female factor (50%)

1 Ovarian factor (anovulation, ovulatory dysfunction, premature ovarian insufficiency) (20%)
- *History.* Secondary amenorrhea, irregular menses.
- *Physical examination.* Obesity, hirsutism, galactorrhea, lean body habitus (hypothalamic amenorrhea).

- *Screening tests.* Typical confirmation of ovulation by history (predictable menstrual intervals [21–35 days], urinary kits to detect the midcycle LH surge (indicative of ovulation), recording daily basal body temperature recordings, or mid to late luteal phase serum progesterone concentration.

  Ovarian reserve may be assessed with day 3 FSH, estradiol, anti-müllerian hormone, and/or clomiphene challenge test.
- *Treatment.* Ovulation induction (see Chapter 26).

2 Tubal and peritoneal factors (20%)
- *History.* Prior pelvic infection or ectopic pregnancy may suggest pelvic adhesive disease or tubal disease. Secondary dysmenorrhea or cyclic pelvic pain may prompt suspicion of endometriosis. However, there are no identifiable risk factors in >50% of patients.
- *Physical examination.* Retroverted fixed uterus, rectovaginal nodularity, and uterosacral nodularity are possible clinical signs of endometriosis.
- *Screening tests.* Hysterosalpingogram (HSG) involves injection of a radio-opaque dye through the cervix into the uterus with spillage into the peritoneal cavity. It assesses tubal patency as well the contour of the uterine cavity to exclude filling defects (eg, endometrial polyps, fibroids, synechiae). Recently, newer saline sonohysterogram methods, utilizing echogenic distending fluid (eg, FemVue) have been utilized. Laparoscopy with tubal lavage or fertiloscopy is the "gold standard" diagnostic test because it can exclude adhesions and endometriosis.
- *Treatment.* Tubal surgery (tuboplasty) or in vitro fertilization (see Chapter 27).

3 Male factor (35%)
- *History.* Testicular injury, genitourinary infection, chemotherapy or radiation exposure, genitourinary surgery, erectile or ejaculatory dysfunction, or tobacco or recreational drug use.
- *Physical examination.* Hypospadias, varicocele, cryptorchidism (undescended testes), atropic testicles.
- *Screening test. Semen analysis* is the primary screening test for male infertility. Semen sample should be produced after 2–3 days of abstinence. If a single sample has abnormal parameters (eg, concentration, motility, or morphology) it should be repeated 4 weeks later.
- *Treatment.* Surgical correction of varicocele; intrauterine insemination or in vitro fertilization with or without intracytoplasmic sperm injection (ICSI) depending upon semen parameters.

4 Unexplained (idiopathic) infertility (10–15%)
- *History.* Female patient is ovulatory and all ovarian reserve, endocrine, hysterosalpingogram, and semen analysis testing is normal.
- *Physical examination* and *screening tests* are unremarkable.
- *Treatment.* Ovulation induction and superovulation with intrauterine insemination (IUI) or in vitro fertilization.
- *Prognosis.* About 60% of couples with unexplained infertility who receive no treatment will conceive within 3–5 years.

5 Cervical factor (10%)
- *History.* Prior cervical surgery (cone biopsy, cautery), infection, or *in utero* diethylstilbestrol (DES) exposure.
- *Physical examination.* Cervical abnormalities, lesions.
- *Screening tests.* None is reliable. The postcoital test is a historical method to evaluate sperm–cervical mucus interaction. However, this test is no longer viewed as a standard of care given its significant diagnostic limitations.
- *Treatment.* IUI.

Figure 26.1 WORLD HEALTH ORGANIZATION (WHO) CLASSIFICATION OF OVULATORY DISORDERS

	Group 1	Group 2	Group 3
Mechanism	Hypothalamic–pituitary failure 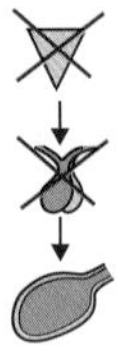	Hypothalamic–pituitary dysfunction 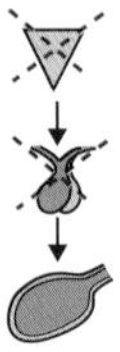	Ovarian (end-organ) failure 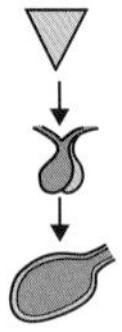
Effect on: 1 LH+FSH	↓↓↓	Normal	↑↑↑
2 Estradiol-17β	↓↓↓	Normal	↓↓↓
Frequency	Common	Most common	Least common
Main diagnosis	Hypothalamic amenorrhea	Polycystic ovarian syndrome (PCOS)	Ovarian failure
Treatment	Gonadotropin (hMG) or GnRH therapy	Clomiphene citrate	Ovum donation

Figure 26.2 OVARIAN HYPERSTIMULATION SYNDROME (OHSS)

	Mild	Moderate	Severe
Frequency	Common	Uncommon	<2%
Symptoms/signs (usually occur 5–7 days after ovulation)	Mild pelvic discomfort	Nausea/vomiting Abdominal distension Weight gain	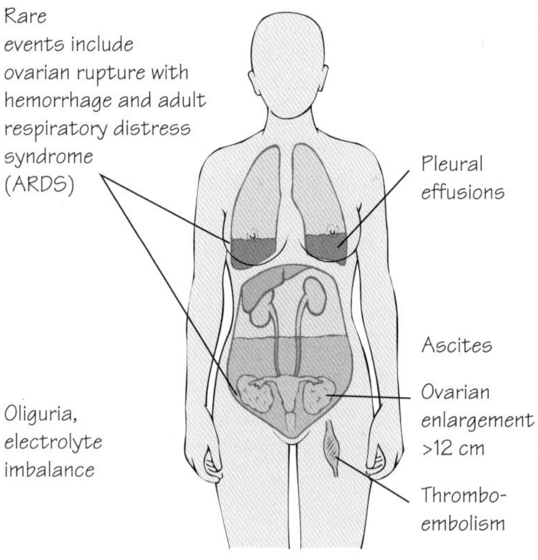 Rare events include ovarian rupture with hemorrhage and adult respiratory distress syndrome (ARDS). Oliguria, electrolyte imbalance. Pleural effusions. Ascites. Ovarian enlargement >12 cm. Thrombo-embolism
Ovarian enlargement	<6 cm	6–12 cm	>12 cm
Estradiol-17β level	2,000–4,000 pg/mL	4,000–6,000 pg/mL	>6,000 pg/mL
Treatment	Observation	Close monitoring, avoid pelvic or abdominal examinations	Hospitalization with supportive care Note: potentially life threatening

Note:
- If no pregnancy occurs, symptoms usually resolve within 7 days
- If pregnancy occurs, symptoms may persist for weeks

Classification of ovulatory disorders

- Ovarian factor infertility (anovulation) is the primary abnormality in 20% of infertile couples.
- Patients are classified into three groups (Figure 26.1).
- Ovulation induction is one of the most successful means of treating infertility. Thoughtful patient selection is essential.

Methods of ovulation induction

Clomiphene citrate (Clomid, Serophene)

- *Indications.* The most common medication used to induce ovulation. The treatment of choice for women with chronic anovulation but adequate levels of estrogen and eugonadotropic eugonadism (WHO group 2). Usually not effective for ovulation induction in WHO group 1 women.
- *Advantages/disadvantages.* Safe, effective, inexpensive, orally administered.
- *Mode of action.* Clomiphene is a selective estrogen receptor modulator (SERM) structurally related to tamoxifen and diethylstilbestrol (DES). It reduces the negative feedback effect of circulating estrogen, thereby triggering hypothalamic gonadotropin-releasing hormone (GnRH) secretion, and increased release of pituitary gonadotropins (follicle-stimulating hormone [FSH], luteinizing hormone [LH]) leading to follicular recruitment, selection, and ovulation 5–12 days after the last dose.
- *Dosage.* The initial dose is 50 mg daily for 5 days beginning on day 3 or 5 of the menstrual cycle. The dose is increased in each cycle in 50-mg increments until ovulation is observed. If there is no response to 150 mg daily dosage, further evaluation is warranted.
- *Monitoring response to therapy.* Follicular development can be monitored ultrasonographically or by urinary LH kits 4–5 days after the last dose of clomiphene. An increased progesterone level 14–17 days after the last clomiphene dose is the hallmark of the luteal phase and implies that ovulation has occurred. At the conclusion of a cycle, either the patient is pregnant or menses occurs, and a further cycle is initiated. Once ovulation has been documented at a given dose of clomiphene, there is no advantage to increasing the dose in subsequent cycles. On average, ovulation usually occurs 5–11 days after the last dose of Clomid.
- *Adjunctive therapy.* The addition of human chorionic gonadotropin (hCG) may be necessary in women who exhibit complete ovarian follicular development but not ovulation. Metformin may also be used in infertile women with oligo-ovulation, hyperandrogenism, glucose intolerance, and insulin resistance.
- *Prognosis.* Of selected women 80% will ovulate on clomiphene, although only 40% will become pregnant. Success is highest in the first few months of therapy. Failure to conceive within six ovulatory clomiphene cycles should prompt the use of other alternatives.
- *Side effects.* Hot flushes, breast tenderness, visual symptoms, and nausea are common, but not dose related.
- *Contraindications.* Liver disease, pregnancy.
- *Complications.* Multiple pregnancies (6%), ovarian hyperstimulation syndrome (OHSS, rare).

Human menopausal gonadotropins (hMGs) or recombinant follicle-stimulating hormone (rFSH)

- *Indications.* Human MG is the treatment of choice for women with ovulatory dysfunction and low levels of estrogen and gonadotropins (hypogonadotropic hypogonadism) (WHO group 1). It is also used in WHO group 1 women who fail to ovulate on clomiphene. Recombinant FSH is typically administered for superovulation in women who have normal ovulatory function (ie, idiopathinc infertility) or for ovulation induction in anovulatory women (WHO group 2).

- *Advantages/disadvantages.* Expensive, requires ultrasound monitoring.
- *Mode of action.* Human MG is a purified preparation of gonadotropins (LH, FSH) extracted from the urine of postmenopausal women. Recombinant FSH is produced from genetically engineered cell lines. Two forms of rFSH include α- and β-follitropin. Administration promotes follicular growth and maturation.
- *Dosage.* Dosage is variable and dependent upon ovarian reserve.
- *Monitoring response to therapy.* Ultrasonography and serial estradiol-17β measurements are required during each cycle to monitor ovarian response to therapy. Ultrasound examinations are initiated to document the number of follicles and their size. The subsequent rise in serum estradiol-17β levels during this active phase is rapid and follicles typically enlarge by 2–3 mm/day.
- *Adjunctive therapy.* When the leading follicle(s) is 16–20 mm in diameter, a single dose of 5,000–10,000 IU of intramuscular purified hCG or 250 µg subcutaneous recombinant hCG is administered to substitute for the endogenous LH surge to trigger ovulation.
- *Prognosis.* Dependent upon female age, ovarian reserve, and underlying infertility diagnoses.
- *Complications.* Multiple pregnancy (10–30%), ectopic pregnancy, OHSS (Figure 26.2). OHSS is rare in the case of gonadotropin therapy. It is usually self-limited, begins 3–5 days after hCG, peaks 7–10 days after hCG, and resolves with menses if conception does not occur. If conception occurs, it may be prolonged and last for up to 10–20 days after hCG.

Bromocriptine mesylate (Parlodel)

- *Indications.* Bromocriptine is indicated only for women with hyperprolactinemic ovulatory dysfunction caused by prolactin-secreting pituitary adenomas or idiopathic hyperprolactinemia.
- *Advantages/disadvantages.* Reduces the size of prolactin-secreting tumors, normalizes hyperprolactinemia-associated menstrual irregularities, or galactorrhea.
- *Mode of action.* Elevated prolactin levels interfere with the normal menstrual cycle by suppressing pulsatile secretion of GnRH by the hypothalamus. Bromocriptine is a dopamine agonist that inhibits the pituitary secretion of prolactin.
- *Dosage.* The ideal maintenance dose is 2.5 mg. It may be increased weekly in 1.25-mg increments until normal menstruation is achieved.
- *Prognosis.* Bromocriptine will restore menstruation in 90% of hyperprolactinemic women.
- *Side effects.* Nausea, vomiting, headaches, postural hypotension (may be minimized by bedtime administration).

GnRH-releasing hormones

- *Indications.* Pulsatile GnRH therapy (subcutaneous pump) may be used in patients with WHO group 1 ovulatory failure. It is used less often now due to emergence of gonadotropin formulations.
- *Advantages/disadvantages.* Portable pump with a catheter must be worn continuously.
- *Mode of action.* Exogenous pulsatile GnRH serves as an artificial hypothalamus to stimulate pituitary gonadotropin release and thus ovulation.
- *Dosage.* GnRH is administered via intravenous (5–10 mg per pulse) or subcutaneous (10–20 mg per pulse) injection.
- *Prognosis.* Of selected patients 80% conceive within six cycles.
- *Complications.* OHSS and multiple gestation are rare, because only "physiologic" levels of FSH are generated by the GnRH pump. Localized, mild, catheter-related complications are common.

Figure 27.1 A TYPICAL STIMULATED *IN VITRO* FERTILIZATION (IVF) CYCLE

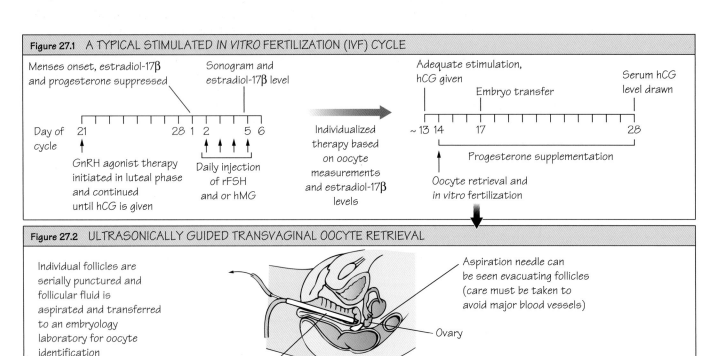

Menses onset, estradiol-17β and progesterone suppressed

Sonogram and estradiol-17β level

Adequate stimulation, hCG given

Embryo transfer

Serum hCG level drawn

Day of cycle: 21 ... 28 1 2 ... 5 6 → ~13 14 ... 17 ... 28

GnRH agonist therapy initiated in luteal phase and continued until hCG is given

Daily injection of rFSH and or hMG

Individualized therapy based on oocyte measurements and estradiol-17β levels

Oocyte retrieval and in vitro fertilization

Progesterone supplementation

Figure 27.2 ULTRASONICALLY GUIDED TRANSVAGINAL OOCYTE RETRIEVAL

Individual follicles are serially punctured and follicular fluid is aspirated and transferred to an embryology laboratory for oocyte identification

Aspiration needle can be seen evacuating follicles (care must be taken to avoid major blood vessels)

Ovary

Transducer

Figure 27.3 TRANSCERVICAL EMBRYO TRANSFER

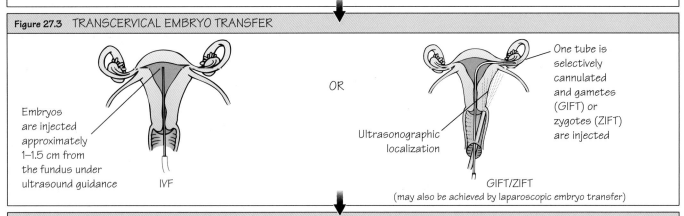

Embryos are injected approximately 1–1.5 cm from the fundus under ultrasound guidance

IVF

OR

One tube is selectively cannulated and gametes (GIFT) or zygotes (ZIFT) are injected

Ultrasonographic localization

GIFT/ZIFT
(may also be achieved by laparoscopic embryo transfer)

Figure 27.4 EFFECT OF ASSISTED REPRODUCTIVE TECHNOLOGY ON MULTIFETAL PREGNANCY

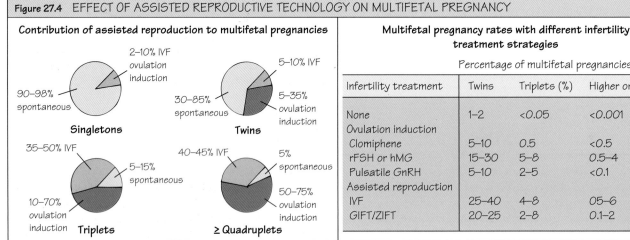

Contribution of assisted reproduction to multifetal pregnancies

Singletons: 90–98% spontaneous, 2–10% IVF ovulation induction

Twins: 30–85% spontaneous, 5–35% ovulation induction, 5–10% IVF

Triplets: 35–50% IVF, 5–15% spontaneous, 10–70% ovulation induction

≥ Quadruplets: 40–45% IVF, 5% spontaneous, 50–75% ovulation induction

Multifetal pregnancy rates with different infertility treatment strategies

Percentage of multifetal pregnancies

Infertility treatment	Twins	Triplets (%)	Higher order (%)
None	1–2	<0.05	<0.001
Ovulation induction			
Clomiphene	5–10	0.5	<0.5
rFSH or hMG	15–30	5–8	0.5–4
Pulsatile GnRH	5–10	2–5	<0.1
Assisted reproduction			
IVF	25–40	4–8	05–6
GIFT/ZIFT	20–25	2–8	0.1–2

- *Definition.* Direct handling and manipulation of oocytes and sperm to facilitate optimal fertilization and maximize the probability of achieving pregnancy. However, IVF is usually performed in Petri dishes.
- *Classification.* IVF is the paradigm of ART procedures. Other examples include gamete or zygote intrafallopian transfer, but these techniques are rarely used.
- *Frequency.* The first baby conceived by IVF was delivered in 1978. Since that historic birth, ART has undergone rapid growth. There are >125,000 IVF cycle initiated in the USA annually.
- *Goal.* To maximize the chance of a successful pregnancy while minimizing the risk of multiple gestations.

In vitro fertilization

Patient selection
- IVF was originally developed for tubal factor infertility. It is now widely utilized for several infertility conditions that have not been successfully treated with other modalities.
- Female age is usually most predictive of IVF success. Most IVF programs limit IVF treatment to women aged up to 43.9 years. Although the menopause has set a natural barrier to further conception, IVF has allowed women to be pregnant in their 50s and 60s using donor egg IVF.
- A serum follicle-stimulating hormone (FSH) level >10 mIU/mL and/or estradiol >80 pg/mL on day 3 of the menstrual cycle is usually indicative of diminished ovarian reserve and suboptimal responsiveness to ovarian stimulation.
- IVF with donor oocytes may be recommended for women with significantly diminished ovarian reserve regardless of age, and for those who have premature ovarian insufficiency or been traditionally considered sterile (eg, Turner syndrome, ovarian dysgenesis).

Ovarian stimulation
- Although unstimulated ("natural cycle") or clomiphene-stimulated IVF cycles are less costly, few oocytes are harvested and success rates are low. These techniques are rarely used. Controlled ovarian hyperstimulation maximizes the retrieval of multiple mature oocytes.
- A typical stimulated IVF cycle (Figure 27.1) is initiated by the administration of a GnRH agonist (eg, leuprolide acetate, nafarelin acetate) in the late luteal phase of the cycle or during pretreatment with combined oral contraceptive pills. A GnRH agonist prevents premature ovulation, decreases cycle cancellation (due to premature luteinization), and increases the number of successful pregnancies per cycle.
- Follicular growth and development are achieved with daily intramuscular administration of rFSH and hMG (see Chapter 26). Once "adequate" ovarian stimulation has been achieved (at least three lead follicles >16–18 mm diameter, a serum estradiol level ≥600 pg/mL), a human chorionic gonadotropin (hCG) trigger is given as a substitute for the luteinizing hormone (LH) surge to promote maturation of the oocytes in preparation for ovulation and oocyte retrieval.
- Of IVF cycles 5–10% are cancelled due to inadequate follicular response.

Oocyte retrieval
- Ultrasound-guided transvaginal oocyte retrieval (Figure 27.2) is performed 35–37 hours after hCG administration.
- The number of harvested oocytes may be correlated to the number of follicles >12 mm. Retrieved oocytes are evaluated for maturity.

Fertilization
- Semen is collected the day of oocyte retrieval. The sperm are "washed" and incubated in supplemented medium.

- Four hours after oocyte retrieval, 25,000–50,000 motile sperm are added to each dish containing a single oocyte.
- Eighteen hours after insemination, the ova are examined microscopically for evidence of fertilization (the presence of two pronuclei). Mature oocytes have a fertilization rate of 50–70%.
- Oocytes that undergo normal fertilization and become embryos are maintained in culture medium and observed for further development. After embryo transfer, supernumerary (remaining appropriate quality) embryos may be cryopreserved.

Embryo culture and transfer
- The fertilized oocytes are placed in growth medium and usually examined daily until day 3 (3 days after oocyte retrieval).
- Embryos are graded by an embryologist based on the number of cells (blastomeres), symmetry of blastomere growth, orientation, and degree of fragmentation.
- The embryo transfer may be performed on day 3 or 5 depending on institutional guidelines.
- The number to be transferred depends on the number available, the age of the woman, and other health and diagnostic factors. In the UK, a maximum of two embryos are transferred except in unusual circumstances.
- Transcervical embryo transfer (Figure 27.3) consists of loading the embryos and a small amount of medium into a flexible catheter, which is then placed through the cervix, and the contents injected with ultrasound guidance.

Luteal phase support
- Progesterone supplementation is started on the day of oocyte retrieval and continued until the 10-week estimated gestational age (EGA) of pregnancy, when the placenta demonstrates autonomous progesterone production. Progesterone supplementation improves pregnancy outcome in IVF.
- A quantitative serum βhCG level may be obtained 12–14 days after transfer to assess for implantation.

Common techniques in ART

Preimplantation genetic diagnosis (PGD)
- "Embryo screening" can be performed on embryos before implantation. Specific genetic mutations or aneuploidy may be detected after analysis of a portion of each embryo.
- PGD is an alternative to prenatal diagnosis that avoids selective pregnancy termination by making it highly likely that the baby will be free of the disease under consideration (eg, cystic fibrosis, sickle cell disease).

Intracytoplasmic sperm injection (ICSI)
- ICSI involves the direct injection of a selected single sperm into the egg. This is typically utilized in cases of male factor infertility (abnormal semen parameters), or suboptimal fertilization or failed fertilization in a prior IVF cycle.

Transfer of cryopreserved embryo(s)
- The major advantage of this option includes: no need for controlled ovarian stimulation and oocyte retrieval, and flexibility in scheduling the embryo transfer,

Pregnancy outcome
- The live birth rate per IVF cycle initiated is dependent upon female age and infertility diagnosis. Typically, those patients aged <35 years or undergoing donor egg IVF have the best live birth pregnancy rates.
- *Effect of ART on multifetal pregnancy* (Figure 27.4). Transfer of multiple embryos may improve the pregnancy rate, but will also increase the number of multiple pregnancies.

28 Menopause and hormone replacement therapy

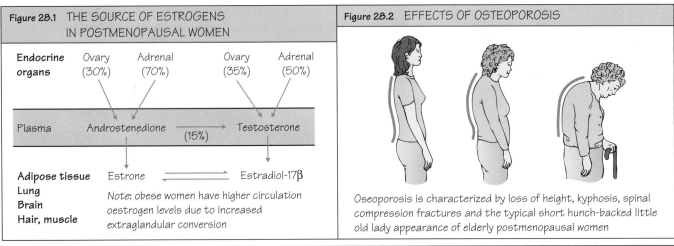

Figure 28.1 THE SOURCE OF ESTROGENS IN POSTMENOPAUSAL WOMEN

Endocrine organs	Ovary (30%)	Adrenal (70%)	Ovary (35%)	Adrenal (50%)

Plasma	Androstenedione	→ (15%)	Testosterone

Adipose tissue
Lung
Brain
Hair, muscle

Estrone ⇄ Estradiol-17β

Note: obese women have higher circulation oestrogen levels due to increased extraglandular conversion

Figure 28.2 EFFECTS OF OSTEOPOROSIS

Oseoporosis is characterized by loss of height, kyphosis, spinal compression fractures and the typical short hunch-backed little old lady appearance of elderly postmenopausal women

Figure 28.3 MANAGEMENT OF THE MENOPAUSE/USE OF HORMONE REPLACEMENT THERAPY

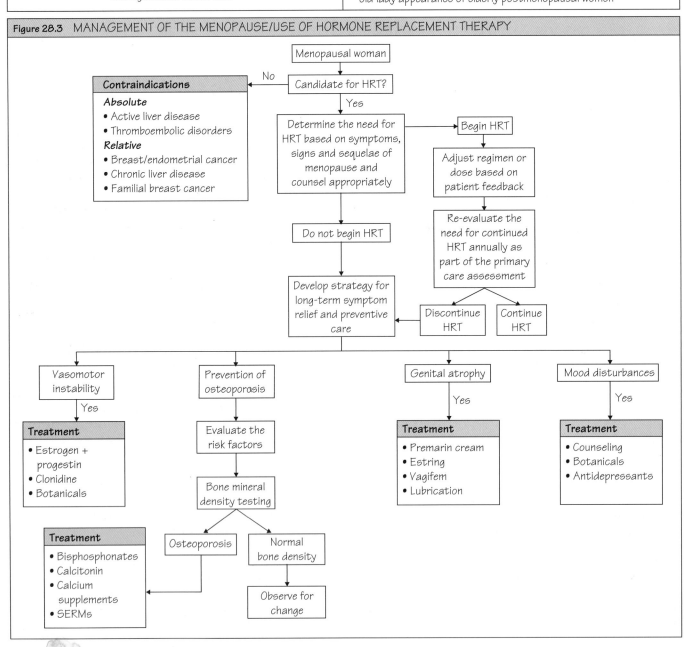

Menopausal woman → Candidate for HRT?

Contraindications

Absolute
- Active liver disease
- Thromboembolic disorders

Relative
- Breast/endometrial cancer
- Chronic liver disease
- Familial breast cancer

No → Contraindications

Yes → Determine the need for HRT based on symptoms, signs and sequelae of menopause and counsel appropriately → Begin HRT → Adjust regimen or dose based on patient feedback → Re-evaluate the need for continued HRT annually as part of the primary care assessment → Discontinue HRT / Continue HRT

Do not begin HRT → Develop strategy for long-term symptom relief and preventive care

Vasomotor instability
Yes

Treatment
- Estrogen + progestin
- Clonidine
- Botanicals

Prevention of osteoporosis → Evaluate the risk factors → Bone mineral density testing → Osteoporosis / Normal bone density → Observe for change

Treatment
- Bisphosphonates
- Calcitonin
- Calcium supplements
- SERMs

Genital atrophy
Yes

Treatment
- Premarin cream
- Estring
- Vagifem
- Lubrication

Mood disturbances
Yes

Treatment
- Counseling
- Botanicals
- Antidepressants

Obstetrics and Gynecology at a Glance, Fourth Edition. Errol R. Norwitz and John O. Schorge.

Menopause

• *Definition.* The permanent cessation of menstruation for 12 months caused by the termination of ovarian follicular recruitment, selection and development in the presence of elevated pituitary gonadotropin (follicle-stimulating hormone [FSH], luteinizing hormone [LH]) levels.
• *Age.* Average age is 51.4 years and may be genetically predetermined.
• *Risk factors* for early menopause include cigarette smoking and surgery (hysterectomy).

Climacteric (perimenopause)

• *Definition.* The transition period before the menopause from the reproductive stage of life to the postmenopausal years. Signs and effects of the menopause transition can begin as early as age 35, although most women who become aware of the transition do so about 10 years later, often in the mid to late 40s. The actual duration and severity of perimenopause in any individual woman cannot be predicted consistently in advance or during the process.
• *Symptoms* include weight gain, especially in the lower abdomen, buttocks, and thighs. This is theorized by some authorities to be bodily adaptation in humans to retain what little estrogen is left in the body (estrogens are fat soluble), and to protect the long bones as estrogen levels decrease and the risk of osteoporosis increases.
• *Menstrual irregularities.* Ten percent of women cease menstruating abruptly, but the vast majority experience 4–5 years of varying cycle length due to progressive ovarian failure.
• *Hormone production.* Initially characterized by elevated FSH and decreased inhibin levels, but normal levels of estradiol-17β and LH. However, there is wide individual variation.

Postmenopausal ovarian physiology

• *Estrogens.* The ovary produces almost no estrogen after the menopause due to the absence of ovarian follicular development. The source of estrogens (Figure 28.1) is derived primarily from peripheral conversion of androgens.
• *Gonadotropins.* There is a 10- to 20-fold increase in FSH and a threefold increase in LH that peaks 1–3 years after the menopause.
• *Androgens.* Elevated gonadotropins drive the ovarian stroma to increase production of androgens.

Hypoestrogenic changes

Estrogen deficiency causes the majority of symptoms, signs, and sequelae of menopause.

1 Vasomotor instability

• Hot flushes affect 70% of perimenopausal women.
• Characterized by the sudden increase in body temperature caused by declining estrogen levels. The "flash" sensation in a "hot flash" occurs as the body temperature peaks and begins a rapid return to normal.
• May also result from acute estrogen withdrawal and not from hypoestrogenism itself. As such, hot flushes lessen in frequency and intensity with advancing age. Obese women may be less symptomatic.

2 Osteoporosis

• Estrogens mitigate bone resorption. Postmenopausal women experience increased bone resorption, diminished formation, and resultant bone fragility that often leads to fracture.
• Defined as a bone mineral density 2.5 standard deviations (SD) or more below the young adult peak mean on the basis of axial skeleton measurements. Osteopenia refers to a bone density 1.0–2.5 SD below the mean.

• Effects of osteoporosis (Figure 28.2) are profound: 50% of women aged >75 years have vertebral fractures and 25% will develop hip fractures by age 80, with devastating health consequences of disability or death.
• Risk factors include European or Asian descent, low body mass index, smoking, and a family history of osteoporosis.
• Bone mineral density testing (dual-energy X-ray absorptiometry, DXA) should be performed on the basis of a patient's risk profile and is not indicated unless the results will influence a treatment or management decision. Osteoporosis most effectively treated with bisphosphonates.

3 Genital atrophy

• The tissues of the lower vagina, labia, urethra, and trigone are all estrogen dependent.
• Dyspareunia, vaginismus, dysuria, urgency, and urinary incontinence are common symptoms.

4 Mood disturbances

• The menopause does not have a measurable effect on mental health.
• Fatigue, anxiety, headaches, insomnia, depression, and irritability are seen more frequently during the perimenopause, and their causal relationship with estrogen withdrawal remains uncertain.

Hormone replacement therapy (HRT) (Figure 28.3)

• *Benefits.* Estrogen given to postmenopausal women will effectively treat hot flashes, osteoporosis, genital atrophy, and perhaps mood disturbances. The risk of Alzheimer disease, osteoarthritis, colon cancer, tooth loss, and skin aging may also be decreased, but has not been consistently proven in prior studies. There is no known reduction in cardiovascular disease.
• *Risks.* Estrogen increases the risk of endometrial hyperplasia and adenocarcinoma (see Chapter 32), unless progestins are added. Women with prior hysterectomy do not need progestins. The risk of breast cancer is moderately increased, depending on the length of use and pre-existing family history.
• *Side effects.* Nausea, erratic vaginal bleeding, headaches, and breast tenderness.
• *Regimens.* Cyclic conjugated equine estrogen (Premarin 0.625 mg, estradiol 0.1 mg) on days 1–25 of the calendar month and Provera (10 mg on days 13–25), continuous daily conjugated equine estrogen (Premarin, estradiol, transdermal estrogen 0.05 mg) and Provera 2.5 mg. There are also vaginal and transdermal patch options.
• *Alternative medications.* Raloxifene (Evista) is a selective estrogen receptor modulator (SERM) that has estrogen agonist effects on bone and cholesterol, but estrogen antagonist effects on breast and endometrium. Gabapentin, antidepressants (paroxetine), and venlafaxine (Effexor) have also been used with some success to treat hot flashes.
• *Botanicals.* Soy products, isoflavones, St John's wort, and black cohosh may be helpful in the short-term treatment of vasomotor symptoms or depression. However, there are limited data to demonstrate equivalent efficacy to HRT and their potential interactions with other medications.
• *Compliance* remains a significant problem with HRT because most of the benefits may be long term (mainly bone protection) and no immediate results (except relief of hot flashes) are evident. Recently, concerns of breast cancer, thromboembolism, and stroke have been a major cause of HRT discontinuation.

Figure 29.1 The 2001 Bethesda System of Cervical Cytology

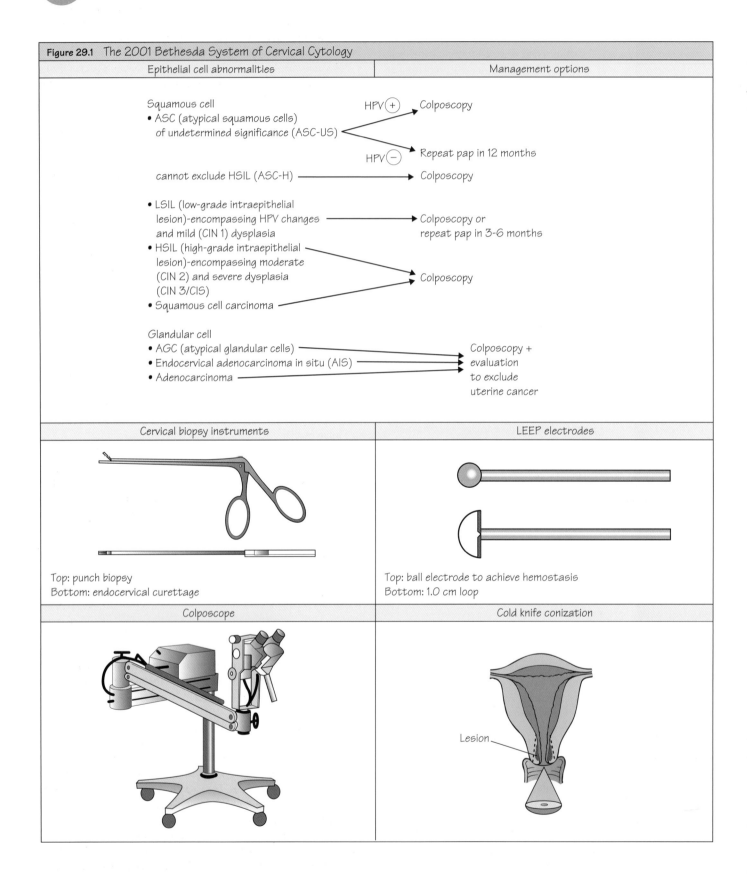

Epithelial cell abnormalities	Management options

Squamous cell
• ASC (atypical squamous cells) of undetermined significance (ASC-US)
  - HPV (+) → Colposcopy
  - HPV (−) → Repeat pap in 12 months

cannot exclude HSIL (ASC-H) → Colposcopy

• LSIL (low-grade intraepithelial lesion)-encompassing HPV changes and mild (CIN 1) dysplasia → Colposcopy or repeat pap in 3-6 months

• HSIL (high-grade intraepithelial lesion)-encompassing moderate (CIN 2) and severe dysplasia (CIN 3/CIS)
• Squamous cell carcinoma → Colposcopy

Glandular cell
• AGC (atypical glandular cells)
• Endocervical adenocarcinoma in situ (AIS)
• Adenocarcinoma
→ Colposcopy + evaluation to exclude uterine cancer

Cervical biopsy instruments

Top: punch biopsy
Bottom: endocervical curettage

LEEP electrodes

Top: ball electrode to achieve hemostasis
Bottom: 1.0 cm loop

Colposcope

Cold knife conization

Lesion

Obstetrics and Gynecology at a Glance, Fourth Edition. Errol R. Norwitz and John O. Schorge.

66 © 2013 John Wiley & Sons, Ltd. Published 2013 by John Wiley & Sons, Ltd.

Cervical intraepithelial neoplasia (CIN)

Cervical smear screening

• *Purpose*. The "Pap" smear has substantially decreased the incidence and mortality from cervical cancer because precursor lesions (dysplasia) can be identified and treated.

• *Natural history*. CIN usually originates at the transformation zone (TZ), a circumferential ring of metaplasia at the squamocolumnar junction of the cervix.

• *Abnormal smears*. Nine out of ten smear results are normal. One out of 20 shows equivocal or mild cell changes, 1 of 100 smears shows moderate cell changes, 1 of 200 shows severe changes, and <1 of 1,000 shows an invasive cancer.

• *Technique*. Performing a cervical smear is simple to perform and painless (see Chapter 1).

• *Sensitivity*. Of lesions 10–25% will be missed on a single cervical smear due to errors in sampling or interpretation.

• *Types*. Conventional Pap smears were prepared by manually smearing the cervical cells on to a glass slide and spraying fixative. Liquid-based cytology (LBC) is an increasingly popular preparation that requires collection of the cells into a vial where cells are better preserved and sensitivity is increased.

• *Frequency*:

USA. Screening should be every 3 years starting at age 21. The interval may be extended to every 5 years in women aged 30+ with the addition of human papillomavirus (HPV) testing. Screening may be discontinued in low-risk women older than 65 years.

UK. Screening should be every 3 years starting at age 25. The interval is extended to every 5 years in women aged 50+. Women aged 65 or over are screened only if they have not been screened since they were 50 or if they have had recent abnormal test results.

• *Classification*:

USA. The 2001 Bethesda System (Figure 29.1) was developed to standardize cervical smear interpretation. Atypical squamous cell diagnoses are now further designated as "undetermined significance" or cannot exclude a "high-grade" lesion. Glandular lesions now consist of "atypical glandular cells" or a more targeted diagnosis of endocervical adenocarcinoma *in situ* (AIS) or adenocarcinoma to help guide management.

UK. Cervical smears are reported as CIN 1, CIN 2, CIN 3, or cervical glandular intraepithelial lesion (CGIN). This classification is not strictly accurate because CIN can only really be diagnosed with a biopsy.

Human papillomavirus testing

• *Method*. Hybrid Capture II detects the presence of at least 1 of 13 high- and intermediate-risk HPV types (eg, 16).

• *Utility*. Primary triage of cervical cytology tests read as ASC-US (atypical squamous cells of undetermined significance) in the USA. More than 80% of LSIL (low-grade intraepithelial lesion) and HSIL (high-grade intraepithelial lesion) cervical smears are HPV positive, making the test less useful as an adjunct.

• *Requirement*. Residual LBC sample or a separate conventional Pap slide.

Colposcopy

• *Indications*

USA. ASC-US (HPV positive or repeated smears), ASC-H, LSIL (first or repeated smear), HSIL, and AGC.

UK. CIN 1 (first or repeated smear), CIN 2, CIN 3, and CGIN.

• *Purpose*. Colposcopy is a microscopic evaluation of the transformation zone (TZ) to identify the most worrisome areas (aceto-white epithelium, mosaicism, punctation, and/or atypical vessels) for directed, diagnostic cervical biopsies.

• *Colposcope* (Figure 29.1). A binocular instrument allowing stereoscopic inspection of the cervix at 5–40× magnification. A green filter is helpful to emphasize vascular patterns by giving red vessels a black color against a pale-green background.

• *Procedure*. The cervix is cleaned and 3–5% acetic acid liberally applied with cotton swabs. Dysplastic epithelium turns white within 1–2 minutes. If the TZ and the extent of the lesion cannot be fully visualized, the examination is called "unsatisfactory."

• *Biopsies* should be performed at the areas appearing most abnormal. Sedation or local anesthesia is rarely needed and bleeding can be quickly controlled with cauterization using silver nitrate or ferrous subsulfate (Monsel solution). An endocervical curettage (ECC) can also be performed if endocervical disease or extension is a possibility.

Management of CIN

• *Treatment* is generally indicated for biopsy-proven CIN 2, CIN 3, and persistent CIN 1 (does not resolve after 1 year). However, overtreatment of innocuous sites is one reason why current recommendations have lengthened the interval of screening because many CIN 1–2 lesions will resolve without treatment if left alone.

• *Loop electrosurgical excision procedure (LEEP)* is the most common method (Figure 29.1). The procedure is done under local anesthesia and removes, rather than destroys, the affected tissue – allowing for diagnosis and treatment during a single visit.

• *Cold knife conization* (Figure 29.1) is indicated for AIS or squamous lesions that extend up the canal.

• *Laser vaporization* and *cryotherapy* destroy the dysplastic cells, but do not provide tissue for diagnosis and to rule out invasive disease.

Vaginal intraepithelial neoplasia (VAIN)

• Patients typically have antecedent or coexistent CIN.

• Should be suspected in patients with persistently abnormal Pap smears and no cervix or a negative cervical colposcopy. It arises most commonly at the vaginal apex and is often multifocal.

• *Treatment*. Local excision, intravaginal 5-fluorouracil cream, or laser.

HPV vaccine

• *Purpose*. Vaccination prevents infection with certain species of HPV associated with the development of cervical cancer, genital warts, and some less common cancers (anal, vulvar, vaginal, penile).

• *Mechanism*. Hollow virus-like particles (VLPs) assembled from recombinant HPV coat proteins.

• *Types*. Two HPV vaccines are currently on the market: Gardasil and Cervarix. Both protect against HPV-16 and HPV-18 which cause 70% of cervical cancer, in addition to some other genital cancers. Gardasil also protects against two of the HPV types that cause genital warts (HPV-6 and -11).

• *Target populations*. The HPV vaccine is recommended for girls/women who are 9–25 years old, ideally before they have been exposed. Public health officials in both the UK and the USA recommend vaccination because of high HPV infection rates, and a desire to reduce the incidence of cervical dysplasia, genital warts, and cervical cancer.

• *UK*. Girls aged 12 and 13 are currently vaccinated after completion of a "catch-up" campaign of all girls up to age 18.

• *USA*. Either HPV vaccine is recommended for 11- and 12-year-old girls. It is also recommended for girls and women aged 13–26 years of age who have not yet been vaccinated or completed the vaccine series.

Figure 30.1 STAGING OF CERVICAL CARCINOMA

Cancer is confined to the cervix and identified only microscopically with invasion up to 5.0 mm and width up to 7.0 mm

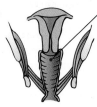

- Stage Ia-1: up to 3.0 mm depth and 7.0 mm width
- Stage Ia-2: 3.1–5.0 mm depth and up to 7.0 mm width

Stage Ia

Cancer is confined to the cervix and larger than stage Ia-2 OR associated with a visible lesion

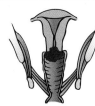

- Stage Ib-1: up to 4.0 cm cervical tumor diameter
- Stage Ib-2: >4.0 cm cervical tumor diameter

Stage Ib

Involvement of the upper two-thirds of the vagina, but no evidence of parametrial involvement

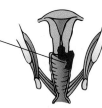

- Stage IIa-1: tumor up to 4.0 cm in greatest dimension
- Stage IIa-2: tumor >4.0 cm in greatest dimension

Stage IIa

Infiltration of the parametria, but not out to the sidewall

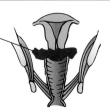

Stage IIb

Involvement of the lower third of the vagina, but not out to the pelvic sidewall if the parametria are involved

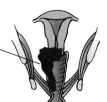

Stage IIIa

Ureter

Ureteral obstruction by tumor

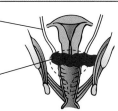

Extension to the pelvic sidewall and/or hydronephrosis or non-functional kidney (unless known to be attributable to other causes)

Stage IIIb

Extension outside the reproductive tract with involvement of the mucosa of the bladder

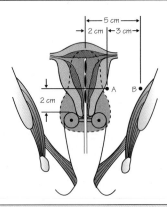

OR rectum

Stage IVa

Distant metastases, including supraclavicular, brain, subcutaneous, or pulmonary sites

Stage IVb

Figure 30.2 Brachytherapy

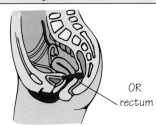

5 cm
2 cm | 3 cm
A B
2 cm

Tandem and ovoid

- Pear-shaped distribution of radiation delivered

Interstitial implant

- Used for advanced disease with anatomical distortion

Obstetrics and Gynecology at a Glance, Fourth Edition. Errol R. Norwitz and John O. Schorge.

Cervical cancer

Epidemiology and risk factors

• *Incidence (annual).* The USA: 12,000 new cases and 4,200 deaths; the UK: 3,400 new cases and 950 deaths. Cervical cancer is the most frequent cause of cancer death in developing nations because of a lack of effective screening. Worldwide it is estimated that there are 530,000 cases of cervical cancer, and 275,000 deaths per year.

• *Median age.* Early 50s in USA/UK.

• *Risk.* Cervical cancer is a disease of sexually active women. It is more prevalent in women of lower socioeconomic status and is correlated with early age at first coitus and having multiple sexual partners.

• *Human papillomavirus* (HPV) is the primary causative agent in cervical cancer. HPV-6 and -11 predispose to benign condylomas. HPV-16, -18, -31, and -45 account for 80% of all invasive cervical cancers.

Prevention and diagnosis

• *Screening.* Regular Pap smear screening reduces a woman's chance of dying of cervical cancer by 90%. HPV vaccines (see Chapter 29) have great potential to eradicate this highly preventable disease.

• *Symptoms.* The early stages of cervical cancer may be completely asymptomatic. Postcoital bleeding is a common early symptom. Menorrhagia or metrorrhagia occurs later. Symptoms of advanced disease may include loss of appetite, weight loss, fatigue, pelvic pain, back pain, leg pain, single swollen leg, and leaking of urine or feces.

• *Physical examination.* The cervical lesion may appear exophytic, barrel shaped, or ulcerative. A small tumor may be entirely visible. Larger lesions that extend beyond the cervix are usually too difficult to assess completely in the office for potential involvement of the bladder, rectum, or parametrium.

Pathology

• *Squamous cell carcinoma* (75–80%) is the most common type, but the incidence is decreasing in countries with widespread Pap smear screening.

• *Adenocarcinomas* (20–25%) are more difficult to detect and appear to be increasing in incidence, especially among younger women.

Staging (Figure 30.1)

• *Note.* Cervical cancer is *clinically* staged.

• Direct local extension is the primary mode of disease spread. Lymphatic and hematogenous spread become more likely as tumor size increases.

• Stage Ia cancer is most commonly diagnosed by cone biopsy.

• Stage Ib-1 cancer is usually diagnosed by visualizing a small gross lesion.

• Stage Ib-2 to IVa cases require formal staging with an examination under anesthesia, chest radiograph, cystoscopy, proctoscopy, and, in some cases, an intravenous urogram or barium enema. Computed tomography (CT), magnetic resonance imaging (MRI), and/or positron emission tomography (PET) is NOT used for staging. However, when the technology is available, one or more such test is usually obtained to help guide therapy.

Treatment

• Primary therapy by stage:

1 Stage Ia-1 disease is treated by cone biopsy or simple hysterectomy in the absence of high-risk features.

2 Stage Ia-2/Ib-1 disease is usually treated by radical hysterectomy. This procedure differs from simple hysterectomy by removal of parametrial tissue to the pelvic side wall, resection of the uterine artery at its origin, removal of the upper third of the vagina, and resection of half the uterosacral ligaments to achieve negative margins. Pelvic ± para-aortic lymphadenectomy is also routinely performed. Historically, the operation was performed via laparotomy, but recently, laparoscopic or robotic-assisted techniques have become increasingly popular. A Schauta radical vaginal hysterectomy is another much less common route.

3 Stage Ib2/IIa disease is usually treated by primary chemoradiation therapy: weekly or triweekly cisplatin and external beam radiation (teletherapy) followed by local radiation implants (brachytherapy: either low-dose rate tandem and ovoids [Figure 30.2] or high-dose rate). Radical hysterectomy may also be appropriate in selected cases, but most patients will require postoperative chemoradiation for high-risk features (lymph node metastases, deep cervical invasion).

4 Stage IIb/IIIa/IIIb/IVa disease is treated by primary chemoradiation because there is minimal likelihood of safely performing an operation that will achieve negative margins.

5 IVb cervical cancer is treated with palliative intent using chemotherapy ± directed radiation.

• *Adjuvant therapy.* Patients with high-risk early stage disease (positive lymph nodes, deep invasion) benefit from postoperative chemoradiation. Postradiation hysterectomy is not universally advocated.

• *Recurrent disease.* Patients who develop recurrence after surgery alone are candidates for radiation therapy. Pelvic exenteration (removal of bladder, uterus, rectum, and other involved structures) is the only curable option for postradiation recurrence with central pelvic disease.

• *Palliative therapy.* Most patients with recurrent cervical cancer are not candidates for exenteration due to pelvic side-wall disease or distant metastases. The combination of cisplatin, paclitaxel and bevacizumab is the most effective palliative chemotherapy regimen, particularly in patients who did not receive prior cisplatin. Regional radiotherapy may be effective in reducing pain symptoms from lesions outside the original radiation field.

• *Quality of life.* Patients with progressive cervical cancer frequently experience unrelenting bone or nerve pain that requires increasing doses of opiates. Most will develop renal failure from bilateral ureteral obstruction unless they are diverted. Frequently, vesicovaginal or rectovaginal fistulas also develop as the tumor destroys tissue planes.

Prognosis

• Lymph node metastases are the most significant pathologic variable (excluding clinical stage).

• With treatment, 80–90% of women with stage I cancer and 50–65% of those with stage II cancer are alive 5 years after diagnosis. Only 25–35% of women with stage III cancer and 15% or fewer of those with stage IV cancer are alive after 5 years.

Vaginal cancer

• *Incidence (annual).* The USA: 2,700 new cases and 850 deaths; the UK: 280 new cases and 100 deaths. Extension of cervical cancer and secondary metastases from other gynecologic malignancies are far more common.

• *Staging.* Similar to cervical cancer.

• *Pathology.* Squamous cell carcinoma (85–90%) is the most common histologic type, followed by adenocarcinoma (5%). Maternal use of diethylstilbestrol (DES) in the 1960s was followed by a dramatic increase in the incidence of *clear cell vaginal adenocarcinoma* among exposed female fetuses. However, this is largely of historical interest because the last DES dose was given in the 1970s.

• *Treatment.* Radiation therapy is the treatment of choice because anatomic distortion makes primary surgical management more difficult.

31 Vulvar cancer

Figure 31.1 STAGING OF VULVAR CANCER

Ia Lesions 2 cm or less in size confined to the vulva or perineum and with stromal invasion no greater than 1.0 mm (no nodal metastasis)

Ib Lesions >2 cm in size or with stromal invasion >1.0 mm confined to the vulva or perineum (no nodal metastasis)

II Tumor of any size with extension to lower urethra, lower vagina, or anus (no nodal metastasis)

IIIa 1 nodal metastasis (at least 5 mm) or 1–2 nodes metastasis(es) up to 5 mm

IIIb 2 or more nodal metastases (at least 5 mm) or 3 or more nodal metastases up to 5 mm

IIIc Positive nodes having extracapsular spread

IVa Tumor invades any of the following: upper urethra, bladder, mucosa, rectal mucosa, bone, or fixed or ulcerated inguino-femoral nodes

IVb Any distant metastasis including pelvic lymph nodes

Figure 31.2 SURGERY FOR EARLY-STAGE VULVAR CANCER

Partial radical vulvectomy and sentinel node mapping

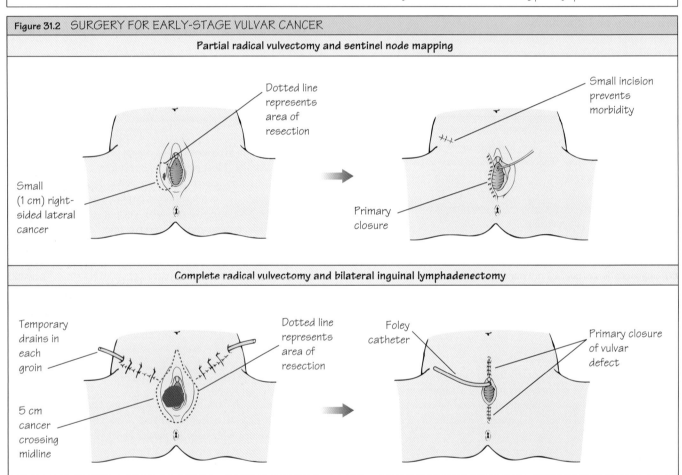

Dotted line represents area of resection

Small incision prevents morbidity

Small (1 cm) right-sided lateral cancer

Primary closure

Complete radical vulvectomy and bilateral inguinal lymphadenectomy

Temporary drains in each groin

Dotted line represents area of resection

Foley catheter

Primary closure of vulvar defect

5 cm cancer crossing midline

Figure 31.3 MANAGEMENT ADVANCED OF VULVAR CANCER

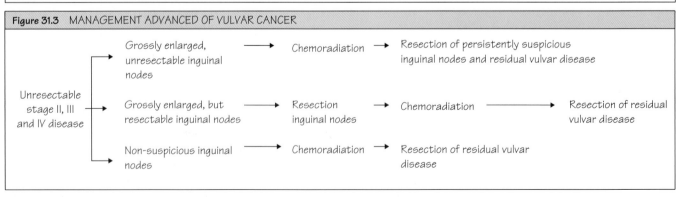

Unresectable stage II, III and IV disease

Grossly enlarged, unresectable inguinal nodes → Chemoradiation → Resection of persistently suspicious inguinal nodes and residual vulvar disease

Grossly enlarged, but resectable inguinal nodes → Resection inguinal nodes → Chemoradiation → Resection of residual vulvar disease

Non-suspicious inguinal nodes → Chemoradiation → Resection of residual vulvar disease

Obstetrics and Gynecology at a Glance, Fourth Edition. Errol R. Norwitz and John O. Schorge.

70 © 2013 John Wiley & Sons, Ltd. Published 2013 by John Wiley & Sons, Ltd.

Vulvar intraepithelial neoplasia (VIN)

- Half of patients are asymptomatic, but others have local discomfort including itching, burning, and pain.
- Twenty percent have a coexistent invasive vulvar cancer.
- *Risk factors.* Patients infected with HIV or other immunodeficient medical conditions tend to be most susceptible. Smokers are also at higher risk.
- *Diagnosis.* Careful inspection of the vulva during routine gynecologic examinations is the most effective diagnostic "technique." VIN has multiple possible appearances. It can resemble a wart, a mole, or condylomas, or be practically invisible. Application of acetic acid using soaked cotton balls for at least 5 minutes is necessary before many lesions are colposcopically apparent. Keyes dermatologic punch biopsies should be performed liberally under local anesthesia for any abnormality. Premenopausal women are more likely to have human papillomavirus (HPV)-related, multifocal lesions.
- *Surgical treatment.* Wide local excision (simple partial vulvectomy) is usually the treatment of choice for a small, solitary lesion. It provides tissue to rule out invasive disease, but can disrupt the anatomy for larger lesions. Carbon dioxide (CO_2) laser ablation is particularly useful for scattered, multifocal lesions, as is Cavitron ultrasonic aspiration (CUSA). "Skinning" vulvectomy is indicated for large, confluent lesions, but rarely required.
- *Medical treatment.* Imiquimod (Aldara) locally stimulates the immune system to attack HPV-affected areas. 5-Fluorouracil (5-FU) is another topical chemotherapeutic agent, but it results in considerable local irritation and is not consistently successful – most likely related to poor patient compliance.

Vulvar cancer

Epidemiology and risk factors

- *Incidence (annual).* The USA: 4,500 new cases and 950 deaths; the UK: 1,000 new cases and 350 deaths – accounts for 5% of all gynecologic cancers.
- *Median age.* Sixty-five years.
- *Risk factors.* HPV exposure is a risk factor – especially in younger women – and condylomas or VIN often precedes the cancer. Vulvar dystrophies, such as lichen sclerosis, or chronic inflammation due to inadequate personal hygiene contributes more in older women.

Prevention and diagnosis

- *Screening.* Annual vulvar examination is the most effective prevention. Many women do not seek medical evaluation for months or years despite noticing an abnormal "lump."
- *Symptoms and signs.* Typically a lesion is present in the form of a lump or ulceration, often associated with itching, irritation, sometimes local bleeding, and discharge. Dysuria, dyspareunia, and pain may also be noted. Due to modesty or embarrassment, even obvious advanced disease may not be detected in a timely fashion.

Pathology

- *Squamous cell carcinoma* (90%) is the most common histologic type, followed by melanoma (5%).
- Primary disease can occur anywhere on the vulva; 70% of lesions arise on the labia, most commonly the labia majora.
- Vulvar cancer spreads primarily via the lymphatics to the superficial inguinal lymph nodes. Metastases to the intra-abdominal pelvic nodes almost never occur if the inguinal nodes are negative. Direct extension to the vagina, urethra, and anus is another common method of disease growth.

Staging (Figure 31.1)

- *Note.* Vulvar cancer is *surgically* staged.
- Of patients 30–40% present with stage III or IV disease.

Management of vulvar cancer

- *Surgery* (Figure 31.2) depends primarily on the size of the lesion and is designed to achieve widely negative margins. Radical excisions should provide at least 2 cm gross lateral margins and dissection deep to the underlying pelvic fascia.
- *Lymph node assessment* is an important adjunct. Classically, inguinal lymphadenectomy is performed and drains are left in place for about 2 weeks. Recently, sentinel lymph node biopsy (SLNB) for tumors <4 cm in size has been shown to decrease postoperative morbidity:
  1 Stage Ia disease is treated by wide local excision.
  2 Stage Ib disease is treated by radical partial vulvectomy and SLNB or lymphadenectomy.
  3 Stage II–III clinically resectable disease is treated by a combination of radical surgery and lymph node assessment.
- *Chemoradiation.* Unresectable stage II, III, and IV disease requires a sequence of external beam radiation (teletherapy) with concurrent chemotherapy (usually cisplatin with or without 5-FU), followed by surgical evaluation to resect any residual disease. Skin grafts, myocutaneous flaps, or other reconstructive procedures may be required to close the surgical defect in some cases.
- *Surgical morbidity.* The incidence of surgical wound breakdown is high (>50%) after radical vulvectomy due to the difficulty in keeping the postoperative area clean and dry. Patients are often elderly and in frail health. Chronic lower extremity lymphedema is a permanent sequela in many patients who undergo lymphadenectomy – especially if postoperative radiation is performed.
- *Adjuvant therapy.* Metastasis to the inguinal lymph nodes is the primary indication for adjuvant teletherapy. The utility of concomitant sensitizing chemotherapy is under investigation.
- *Recurrent disease.* Most recurrences occur near the site of the primary lesion and can be surgically resected. Distant metastases rarely respond to palliative chemotherapy.

Prognosis

- The *number of positive inguinal lymph nodes* is the single most important prognostic variable.
- Overall, vulvar cancer has a 75% 5-year survival rate, but it varies widely by stage, type of lesion, age, and general medical health. The 5-year survival rate is down to about 20% when pelvic lymph nodes are involved but better than 90% for patients with stage I lesions.

Vulvar melanoma

- Occurs predominantly in postmenopausal white women.
- Most are located on the labia minora or clitoris.
- Tends to display the typical dark discoloration.
- The FIGO staging system is not applicable: prognosis is primarily related to the depth of invasion. The Clark or Breslow classification is used and the prognosis decreases considerably with level of extension.
- *Treatment.* Radical excision with at least 2 cm gross lateral margins – SLNB has largely replaced inguinal lymphadenectomy.

Paget disease of the vulva

- A rare intraepithelial neoplasm.
- Predominantly affects postmenopausal white women.
- Twenty percent have a coexisting adenocarcinoma.
- *Treatment.* Wide local excision, but positive margins and recurrent disease are very common.

Figure 32.1 UNOPPOSED ESTROGEN

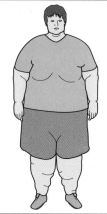

1 Obesity
 • Increased adipose tissue causes
  aromatization of androgens – estrogens
2 Tamoxifen
 • Estrogenic effect on uterus
 • Anti-estrogen effect on breast tissue
3 Polycystic ovarian syndrome
 • Chapter 21
4 Exogenous estrogen
 • Postmenopausal estrogen without progestin
 • Alternative medications (ie, St. John's Wort)
  with 'natural' hormones

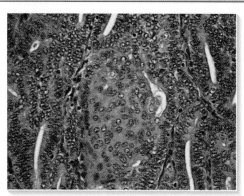

Grade 1 endometrial cancer

Figure 32.2 STAGING OF ENDOMETRIAL CANCER

Endometrium

Tumor limited to the uterus
with no or less than half
myometrial invasion

Stage Ia

Myometrium

Invasion equal to or more
than half of myometrium

Stage Ib

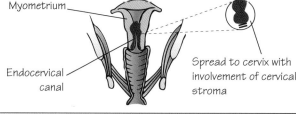

Myometrium

Endocervical
canal

Spread to cervix with
involvement of cervical
stroma

Stage II

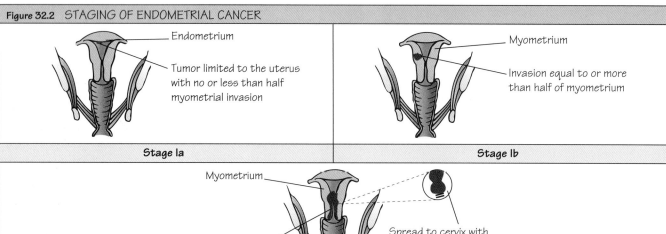

Tumor invades
uterine serosa
and/or adnexae

Stage IIIa

Vaginal
metastases or
parametrial
involvement

Stage IIIb

IIIc-2
Para-aortic nodes

IIIc-1
Pelvic nodes

Spread to
retroperitoneal
lymph nodes

Stage IIIc

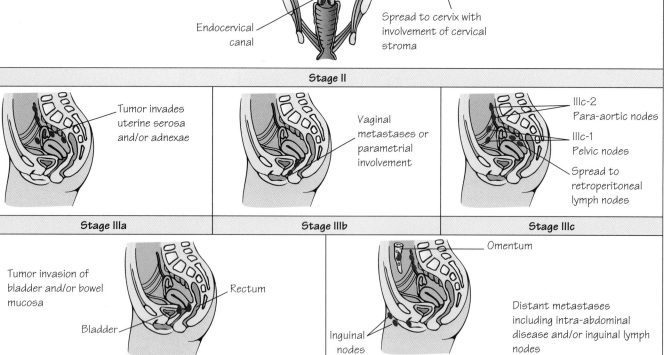

Tumor invasion of
bladder and/or bowel
mucosa

Rectum

Bladder

Stage IVa

Omentum

Inguinal
nodes

Distant metastases
including intra-abdominal
disease and/or inguinal lymph
nodes

Stage IVb

Obstetrics and Gynecology at a Glance, Fourth Edition. Errol R. Norwitz and John O. Schorge.

Endometrial hyperplasia

- *Definition.* abnormal endometrial glandular proliferation.
- *Etiology.* prolonged unopposed estrogenic stimulation due to endogenous (obesity) or exogenous (unopposed estrogen) sources.
- *Classification:*
  1 *Hyperplasia with cytologic atypia* exhibits an increased nuclear/cytoplasmic ratio, hyperchromasia, and loss of cell polarity. More than 40% of patients with this biopsy result will already have an early endometrial adenocarcinoma.
  2 *Hyperplasia without cytologic atypia* is clinically benign, but accurate diagnosis is dependent on the sampling.
- *Diagnosis.* Patients typically present with abnormal uterine bleeding or a Pap smear having atypical glandular cells. An office endometrial biopsy (see Chapter 4) makes the diagnosis.
- *Treatment.* Fertility sparing treatment involves oral contraceptives, progestins, or insertion of a progesterone intrauterine device (IUD; see Chapter 12), followed by a repeat endometrial biopsy in 3–6 months to confirm resolution. Hysterectomy is recommended for most women with cytologic atypia.

Endometrial cancer (>95%)

Epidemiology and risk factors

- *Incidence (annual).* The USA: 47,000 new cases and 8,000 deaths; the UK: 7,700 new cases and 2,000 deaths – lifetime risk is 2% in the general population.
- *Median age.* Sixty years.
- *Etiology.* Exposure to unopposed estrogen increases the risk of endometrial cancer. Protective factors include high parity, pregnancy, and smoking.
- *Hereditary factors.* Women with a hereditary non-polyposis colorectal cancer (HNPCC) gene mutation (*MLH1*, *MSH2*) have a 40–60% lifetime risk of developing endometrial cancer.

Prevention and diagnosis

- *Screening.* Endometrial biopsy is NOT recommended for routine screening, even in patients on tamoxifen. Pap smear screening is not a sensitive means of detection either.
- *Chemoprevention.* Oral contraceptive use decreases the risk of developing endometrial cancer. Hormonal treatment of endometrial hyperplasia will usually slow down or prevent progression to cancer.
- *Symptoms and physical findings.* Abnormal uterine bleeding occurs frequently. Intermenstrual or heavy, prolonged bleeding in premenopausal women and any postmenopausal bleeding should be evaluated.
- *Diagnostic work-up.* Initial evaluation should include a pelvic examination, Pap smear, and endometrial biopsy.

Pathology

- Endometrioid adenocarcinoma (>80%) is by far the most common and most curable histologic type.
- Uterine papillary serous carcinoma and clear cell carcinomas often present with extensive intra-abdominal disease despite minimal or absent myometrial invasion. Mixed müllerian mesodermal tumors (carcinosarcoma) have malignant elements that are usually inherent to the uterus (homologous), but may include bone, cartilage, or skeletal muscle (heterologous). Any high-risk cell type on biopsy indicates the need for preoperative imaging of the chest, abdomen, and pelvis.

Advanced disease is treated like epithelial ovarian cancer (see Chapter 33), but prognosis is very poor.
- The histologic grade is based on tumor architecture and reflects the amount of non-gland-forming (solid) tumor. Grades 1, 2, and 3 indicate solid growth patterns in ≤5%, 6–50%, and >50% of the tumor, respectively.
- Endometrial carcinoma spreads by lymphatic or hematologic dissemination, direct extension, and transtubal passage.

Staging (Figure 32.2)

- Endometrial cancer is *surgically* staged.
- Of patients 75% present with stage I disease.

Treatment

- *Primary therapy.* Historically, exploratory laparotomy, peritoneal washings, total abdominal hysterectomy, and bilateral salpingo-oophorectomy were the most common treatment, but increasingly laparoscopic or robotic-assisted techniques are being employed. Rarely, primary radiation therapy is used in women with unacceptable surgical risks but the cure rate is diminished by 10–15%.
- *Lymph nodes.* The decision of when to perform staging lymphadenectomy is not consistently applied. Historically, the decision to remove nodes hinged on (1) the tumor grade on preoperative biopsy and (2) the depth of myometrial invasion (as determined at the time of surgery) – yet both were shown to be inaccurate measures. More recently, specific algorithms or sentinel node mapping is being prospectively analyzed.
- *Adjuvant therapy.* Vaginal brachytherapy is indicated for "intermediate-risk" disease (IA grade 3, IB grade 1–2). Higher risk (IB grade 3, II, and above) tumors receive teletherapy ± chemotherapy.
- *Recurrent disease.* Radiation or rarely pelvic exenteration may be curative options for locally recurrent endometrial cancer. Combination chemotherapy with paclitaxel, doxorubicin, and cisplatin (TAP), or paclitaxel and carboplatin, has the highest response rates for more systemic disease.
- *Palliation.* Hormonal therapy (progestin, tamoxifen) has minimal toxicity and reasonable response rates – especially in grade 1 tumors.

Prognosis

- Endometrial cancer characteristically has an excellent prognosis because, early in its course, abnormal bleeding occurs.
- The 5-year survival rate for endometrial cancer after appropriate treatment is: 85% for stage I disease, 50% for stage II, 30% for stage III, and <5% for stage IV.

Uterine sarcomas (<5%)

- Aggressive tumors with a poor prognosis.
- Surgical resection is the only treatment of any proven curative value.
  1 *Leiomyosarcomas* are uterine smooth muscle tumors that are distinguished from benign fibroids by the increased number of cellular mitoses. Hematogenous spread to the lungs is very common.
  2 *Endometrial stromal tumors* are rare, soft, fleshy, usually polypoid masses that protrude into the endometrial cavity. Endometrial stromal sarcoma (previously referred to as "low grade") has a relatively good prognosis compared with the high-grade undifferentiated sarcoma variant. These are distinguished mainly by the mitotic count of the tumor.

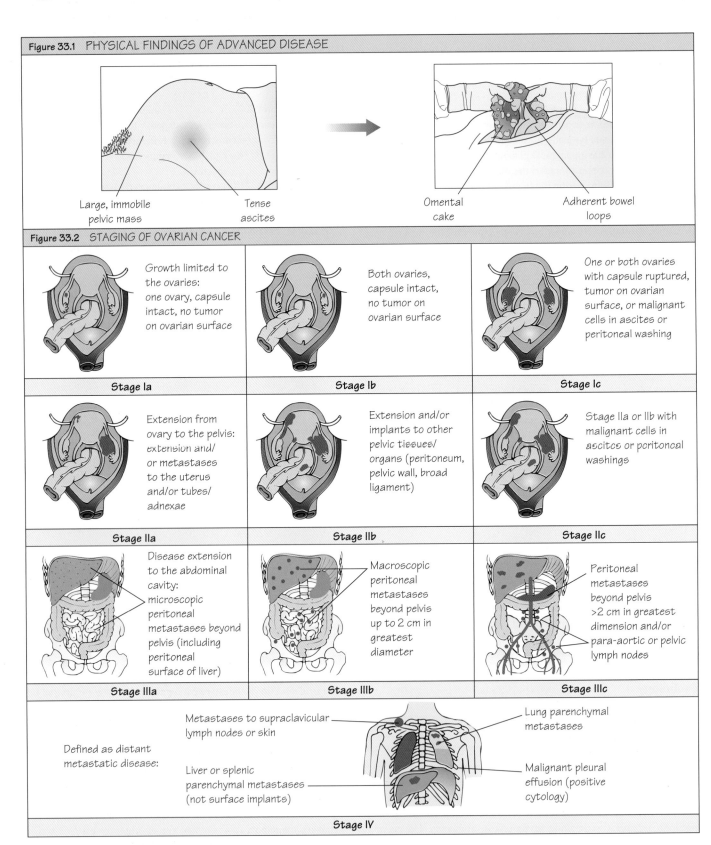

Figure 33.1 PHYSICAL FINDINGS OF ADVANCED DISEASE

Large, immobile pelvic mass

Tense ascites

Omental cake

Adherent bowel loops

Figure 33.2 STAGING OF OVARIAN CANCER

Growth limited to the ovaries: one ovary, capsule intact, no tumor on ovarian surface

Stage Ia

Both ovaries, capsule intact, no tumor on ovarian surface

Stage Ib

One or both ovaries with capsule ruptured, tumor on ovarian surface, or malignant cells in ascites or peritoneal washing

Stage Ic

Extension from ovary to the pelvis: extension and/or metastases to the uterus and/or tubes/adnexae

Stage IIa

Extension and/or implants to other pelvic tissues/organs (peritoneum, pelvic wall, broad ligament)

Stage IIb

Stage IIa or IIb with malignant cells in ascites or peritoneal washings

Stage IIc

Disease extension to the abdominal cavity: microscopic peritoneal metastases beyond pelvis (including peritoneal surface of liver)

Stage IIIa

Macroscopic peritoneal metastases beyond pelvis up to 2 cm in greatest diameter

Stage IIIb

Peritoneal metastases beyond pelvis >2 cm in greatest dimension and/or para-aortic or pelvic lymph nodes

Stage IIIc

Defined as distant metastatic disease:

Metastases to supraclavicular lymph nodes or skin

Liver or splenic parenchymal metastases (not surface implants)

Lung parenchymal metastases

Malignant pleural effusion (positive cytology)

Stage IV

Obstetrics and Gynecology at a Glance, Fourth Edition. Errol R. Norwitz and John O. Schorge.

Epithelial ovarian cancer (90–95%)

- *Incidence (annual).* The USA: 22,000 new cases and 15,500 deaths; the UK: 7,000 new cases and 4,300 deaths. More patients die from this malignancy in industrialized western countries than all other gynecologic cancers combined.
- *Median age.* Sixty years.
- *Risk factors.* Low parity, family history of breast or ovarian cancer, and living in industrialized western countries. Protective factors include multiparity, breastfeeding, and chronic anovulation.
- *Hereditary factors* account for 5–10% of all cases. Women with two first- or second-degree relatives having premenopausal breast or ovarian cancer (any age) should be referred to genetic counseling. Testing can identify *BRCA-1* or *BRCA-2* mutation carriers.
- *Screening.* No combination of CA-125 ± transvaginal sonography has been shown to reliably detect early disease or decrease mortality.
- *Chemoprevention.* Oral contraceptive use decreases the incidence of ovarian cancer by up to 50%.
- *Surgical prophylaxis.* High-risk women (*BRCA* mutation carriers) may be offered prophylactic bilateral salpingo-oophorectomy (BSO) beginning at age 35 or upon completion of childbearing. This reduces their ovarian cancer risk by 90% and their breast cancer risk by 50%. Primary peritoneal carcinoma can still occur rarely.
- *Signs and symptoms.* Women with early stage ovarian cancer frequently report symptoms such as bloating, increased abdominal size, and urinary symptoms. Most often these are vague symptoms that are overlooked by the doctor or patient. Early satiety, recent bowel changes, or "indigestion" is a common complaint of advanced disease.
- *Physical findings.* Early ovarian cancer may be suspected by detection of an adnexal mass on pelvic examination. Advanced disease (Figure 33.1) is more clinically obvious.
- *Diagnostic work-up.* Transvaginal sonography is the most sensitive method to evaluate an adnexal mass. Computed tomography (CT) of the abdomen/pelvis and a chest radiograph are most helpful for treatment planning in advanced disease. Diagnostic paracentesis is mainly indicated in the absence of an ovarian mass.

Staging (Figure 33.2)

- Ovarian cancer is *surgically* staged.
- Two-thirds of patients present with stage III–IV disease.

Treatment

- *Early stage* disease that is clinically confined to the ovary requires hysterectomy, BSO, staging (peritoneal cytology, random biopsies, omentectomy, and pelvic and para-aortic node dissection) and may be performed laparoscopically. Patients with stage Ia–Ib, grade 1–2 disease do not require postoperative chemotherapy.
- *Advanced ovarian cancer* treatment has recently become more controversial. In the USA, most patients still undergo laparotomy, total abdominal hysterectomy (TAH), BSO, and primary cytoreductive surgery to remove all visible disease. Much of the UK and Europe give neoadjuvant platinum-based chemotherapy followed by an "interval" debulking after three to four courses of treatment due to data demonstrating similar outcomes with decreased morbidity.
- *Adjuvant therapy.* The global standard for stage IC–IV disease is six cycles of intravenous carboplatin ± paclitaxel. Selected patients may achieve better results with the "dose-dense" (weekly) paclitaxel variation or platinum-based intraperitoneal chemotherapy. The majority will achieve remission. Second-look laparotomy to look for residual cancer does not improve survival and should be infrequently done

outside of clinical trials. Continuation of "maintenance" chemotherapy in an attempt to prevent relapse is also of dubious benefit.
- *Prognostic factors* include surgical stage, extent of residual disease, volume of ascites, patient age, and clinical performance status.
- *Surveillance.* Once in remission, patients are regularly seen for symptom review and physical examination. Serum CA-125 levels are also routinely drawn in the USA, but due to unproven clinical value they are not monitored in the UK. When an abnormality is detected by any method, imaging is performed to confirm recurrence.
- *Relapse* eventually occurs in 80% of patients with advanced disease. Patients with a prolonged clinical response to initial platinum-based therapy should be re-evaluated for "secondary" tumor cytoreduction and/or re-treatment with a platinum regimen. Otherwise, second-line chemotherapy should be considered.
- *Palliation.* Most patients eventually develop several areas of small bowel obstruction and subsequent malnutrition from intraperitoneal tumor spread. Palliative therapy aimed at temporary relief of symptoms is critical to maximize patient comfort. Gastrostomy tube placement and intravenous hydration may be appropriate in terminal cases.

Borderline (low malignant potential) ovarian tumors

- Ten to fifteen percent of epithelial ovarian cancers.
- Younger age at diagnosis (mean: 35 years).
- Treatment includes hysterectomy, BSO (or fertility-sparing unilateral salpingo-oophorectomy [USO]), and surgical staging. Postoperative chemotherapy is rarely indicated. Prognosis is excellent: 95% will survive at least 10 years.

Malignant germ cell ovarian tumors (<5%)

- Younger age at diagnosis (mean: 20 years).
  1 Dysgerminomas (50%) are most common. Lactate dehydrogenase may be a useful tumor marker, up to 20% of tumors are bilateral and two-thirds are stage I. Highly curable.
  2 Yolk-sac (endodermal sinus) tumors (20%) have characteristic microscopic Schiller–Duval bodies. α-Fetoprotein (AFP) is a highly accurate tumor marker. The most lethal variant.
  3 Immature teratomas (15–20%) are distinct from dermoids by the presence of immature neural elements.
- *Treatment.* Fertility-sparing USO and surgical staging are usually indicated due to patient age (otherwise hysterectomy and BSO). Bleomycin, etoposide, and cisplatin (BEP) chemotherapy is indicated for all patients except stage IA dysgerminomas or immature teratomas.

Sex cord-stromal tumors (<5%)

- Mean age at diagnosis is 50 years, but the range is very broad.
  1 Granulosa cell tumors (70%) are the most common type. Microscopic Call–Exner bodies are pathognomonic; 80–90% are stage I at diagnosis. Inhibin A/B or estradiol may be a useful tumor marker.
  2 Sertoli–Leydig tumors (10–20%) present with progressive virilization and >95% are stage I at diagnosis.
- *Treatment.* Hysterectomy, BSO (or fertility-sparing USO), and staging. Postoperative therapy is not usually needed.

Fallopian tube cancer

- Historically thought to be very rare, but the distal tubal fimbria is increasingly emerging as a potential site of origin for many "ovarian cancers," especially hereditary (*BRCA-1/BRCA-2*) types.
- The staging, treatment, and prognosis are similar to ovarian cancer.

34 Gestational trophoblastic disease (GTD)

Figure 34.1 CHROMOSOMAL ORIGIN OF HYDATIDIFORM MOLE

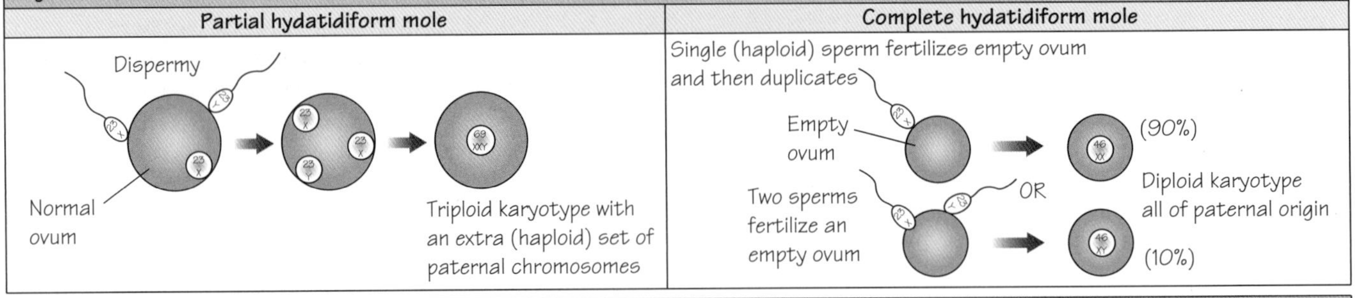

Partial hydatidiform mole	Complete hydatidiform mole

Partial hydatidiform mole:
Dispermy
Normal ovum
Triploid karyotype with an extra (haploid) set of paternal chromosomes

Complete hydatidiform mole:
Single (haploid) sperm fertilizes empty ovum and then duplicates
Empty ovum → (90%)
Two sperms fertilize an empty ovum OR → (10%)
Diploid karyotype all of paternal origin

Figure 34.2 FEATURES OF HYDATIDIFORM MOLES

Features	Partial moles	Complete mole
Karyotype	69,XXX or 69,XXY	46,XX or 46,XY
Pathology		
Fetus	Present	Absent
Chorionic villi	Focal, variable edema	Diffusely hydropic
Trophoblastic hyperplasia	Focal, minimal	Diffuse, severe
Clinical presentation		
Symptoms/signs	Missed abortion	Molar gestation
Uterine size	Appropriate	28% large for dates
GTN		
Non-metastatic	3–4%	15%
Metastatic	0	4%

Figure 34.3 FIGO STAGING OF GESTATIONAL TROPHOBLASTIC NEOPLASIA (GTN)

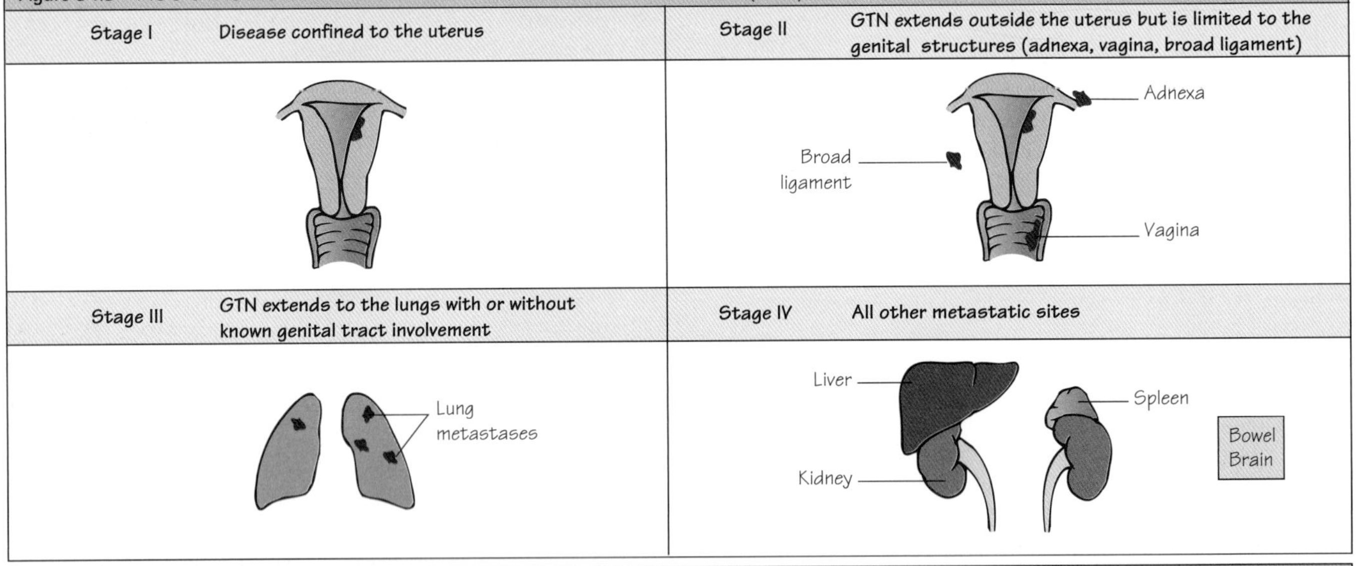

Stage I	Disease confined to the uterus	Stage II	GTN extends outside the uterus but is limited to the genital structures (adnexa, vagina, broad ligament)

Stage II labels: Adnexa, Broad ligament, Vagina

Stage III	GTN extends to the lungs with or without known genital tract involvement	Stage IV	All other metastatic sites

Stage III: Lung metastases
Stage IV: Liver, Kidney, Spleen, Bowel, Brain

Figure 34.4 Modified WHO prognostic scoring system

Scores	0	1	2	4
Age	<40	≥40	–	–
Antecedent pregnancy	Mole	Abortion	Term	–
Interval months from index pregnancy	<4	4–<7	7–<13	≥13
Pretreatment serum hCG (IU/mL)	$<10^3$	10^3–$<10^4$	10^4–$<10^5$	$\geq10^5$
Largest tumor size (including uterus)	–	3–<5 cm	≥5 cm	–
Site of metastases	Lung	Spleen, kidney	Gastrointestinal	Liver Brain
Number of metastases	–	1–4	5–8	>8
Previous failed chemotherapy	–	–	Single Drug	2 or more drugs

Obstetrics and Gynecology at a Glance, Fourth Edition. Errol R. Norwitz and John O. Schorge.

- *Definition.* A spectrum of histologically distinct diseases originating from the placenta: partial and complete hydatidiform mole, choriocarcinoma, and placental-site trophoblastic tumor (PSTT).
- *Tumor marker.* Serum levels of βhCG (β-human chorionic gonadotropin) are extremely accurate.

Hydatidiform moles

- *Incidence.* Japan has the highest incidence of molar pregnancy (2.0/1,000 pregnancies versus 0.6–1.1 for Europe and North America). Variations in the worldwide incidence rates result in part from discrepancies between population-based data and hospital-based data.
- *Risk factors* include maternal age >35 years (>2× increase), prior molar pregnancy (10× increase), long-term use of oral contraceptives (2× increase), and dietary deficiency (β-carotene, vitamin A).
- *Chromosomal origin* (Figure 34.1).
- *Clinical presentation.* Partial moles usually present as a missed abortion during the first or early second trimester. Normal or marginally elevated βhCG levels are common. Complete moles typically have abnormal vaginal bleeding (85%) that prompts a healthcare visit. Due to earlier detection, fewer than 10% of women will have anemia, hyperemesis gravidarum, or pre-eclampsia. Markedly elevated βhCG levels (>>100,000 mIU/mL) are characteristic.
- *Sonographic findings.* Partial moles may be suspected by visualizing a fetus with focal cystic spaces in the placenta and an increase in the transverse diameter of the gestational sac. Complete moles classically have a "snowstorm" appearance of diffuse hydropic swelling without a fetus. First-trimester sonograms may be too early to distinguish small molar villi from degenerating chorionic villi.
- *Diagnosis* of hydatidiform moles is made by histopathologic analysis. Partial moles have a non-viable fetus with malformations (syndactyly, hydrocephalus, growth restriction), variably hydropic (swollen) villi, and minimal trophoblastic hyperplasia. Complete moles have no fetal tissue and consist of diffusely hydropic villi (grape-like vesicles) with widespread trophoblastic hyperplasia. Immunostaining with p57 or ploidy analysis may be indicated in some equivocal cases.
- *Treatment.* Electric vacuum aspiration (EVA; see Chapter 16) is generally the initial treatment for molar pregnancy because patients are commonly young and desirous of future fertility. Hysterectomy is an alternative in selected patients who desire surgical sterilization.
- *Prophylaxis.* Anti-D immunoglobulin should be administered to appropriate rhesus-negative patients.
- *Surveillance.* βhCG levels should be monitored post-evacuation until they are undetectable.
- *Hormonal contraception* should be encouraged to prevent pregnancy and reduce the potential for complicating βhCG interpretation.
- *Future pregnancies.* Patients may expect normal reproductive outcome of subsequent conceptions. The risk of developing another hydatidiform mole is increased 10-fold to approximately 1%.

Gestational trophoblastic neoplasia (GTN)

- *Antecedent gestation.* Most commonly occurs after a molar pregnancy, but may occur after any gestational event (termination or spontaneous miscarriage [see Chapter 15], ectopic pregnancy [see Chapter 5], term pregnancy).
- *Diagnosis* is not uniform worldwide, but includes one of these criteria:

  1 βhCG plateau of four measurements over a period of at least 3 weeks
  2 βhCG rise of three measurements over a period of at least 2 weeks

  3 βhCG level remains elevated for more than 6 months
  4 Histologic diagnosis of choriocarcinoma.
- *Choriocarcinoma* consists of sheets of anaplastic cytotrophoblast and syncytiotrophoblast cells without chorionic villi. Invasive moles may have the histologic features of either choriocarcinoma or hydatidiform mole, but metastases are always choriocarcinoma.
- *PSTT* (placental-site trophoblastic tumor) is a rare variant of choriocarcinoma that is insensitive to chemotherapy and usually requires hysterectomy.

Staging (Figure 34.3)

- GTN is anatomically staged.
- The combination of a chest radiograph, abdominal/pelvic computed tomography (CT) scan, and pelvic examination is an effective strategy to determine the extent of disease. Chest and head CT scans are indicated if the chest radiograph is abnormal.
- Biopsy of suspected metastatic lesions is not recommended and may cause hemorrhage.
- The modified World Health Organization (WHO) prognostic scoring system (Figure 34.4) is used to categorize patients with GTN into low-risk (score: 0–6) or high-risk (score: ≥7) groups.

Treatment

- Low-risk GTN (WHO score 0–6) is most frequently treated by single-agent methotrexate using a variety of intramuscular or intravenous regimens. If the tumor is resistant, the patient may be switched to intravenous "pulse" dactinomycin. Recently, methotrexate has been shown to have a lower response rate than dactinomycin, but most clinicians still use it preferentially due to its very mild toxicity.
- High-risk GTN (WHO score >6) and patients who fail single-agent low-risk GTN therapy are best managed by combination chemotherapy (etoposide, methotrexate, dactinomycin, cyclophosphamide, vincristine [EMA/CO]) due to the increased risk of tumor resistance to a single agent. Patients who progress through EMA/CO may be switched to EMA/EP (where EP is etoposide and cisplatin) or a paclitaxel regimen with alternating etoposide and cisplatin.
- *Surveillance.* βhCG levels are measured until undetectable and therapy is completed. Follow-up should continue for 12 (stage I–III) to 24 months (stage IV).
- *Prognosis.* Of patients 98–100% of stage I–III patients and 75–80% of stage IV patients will be cured. Few women die from GTN in the USA or the UK, but those who do generally present moribund with stage IV disease and quickly succumb.

Placental-site trophoblastic tumor (PSTT)

- Rare variant of GTN that has intermediate cytotrophoblasts.
- Diagnosis is not usually very straightforward due to lower βhCG levels and less dramatic bleeding symptoms.
- Hysterectomy is almost mandatory because the tumor tends to be insensitive to chemotherapy.

Phantom hCG

- *Definition.* Persistent mild elevations of hCG leading physicians to treat patients for GTN when in reality no true hCG or trophoblast disease is present.
- *Cause.* Some individuals have circulating factors in their serum (heterophilic antibodies) that interact with the hCG antibody and cause false-positive results using some laboratory assays.
- *Diagnosis.* Negative urine test or serial dilutions of the serum hCG.
- *Treatment.* Recognition of the false-positive test. No treatment is needed.

35 Embryology and early fetal development

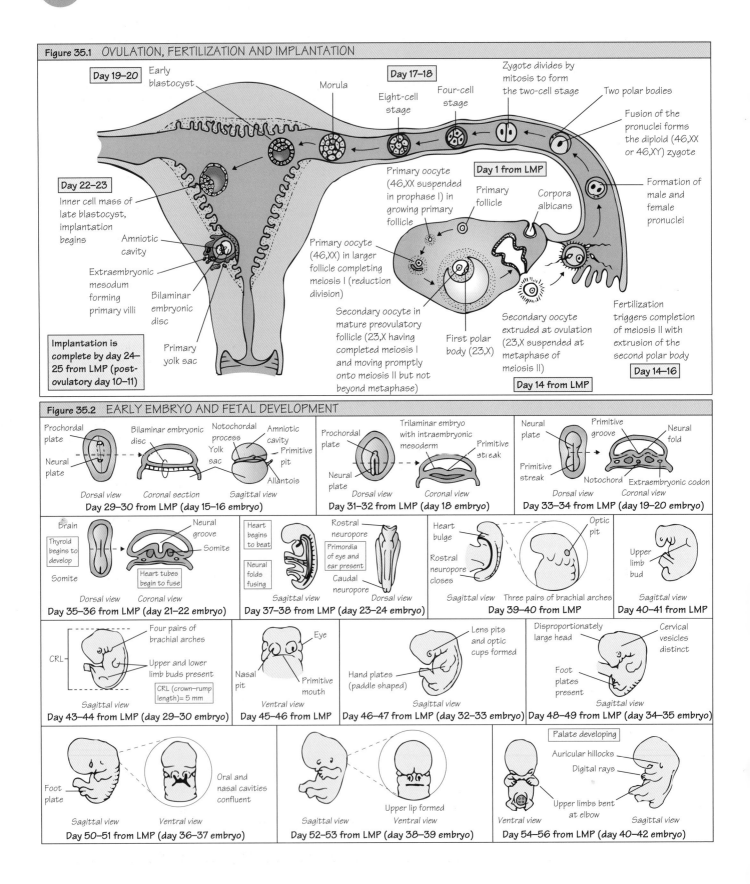

Figure 35.1 OVULATION, FERTILIZATION AND IMPLANTATION

Figure 35.2 EARLY EMBRYO AND FETAL DEVELOPMENT

Obstetrics and Gynecology at a Glance, Fourth Edition. Errol R. Norwitz and John O. Schorge.

78 © 2013 John Wiley & Sons, Ltd. Published 2013 by John Wiley & Sons, Ltd.

Ovulation, fertilization, and implantation
(Figure 35.1)
Definitions
• Gestational age refers to the duration of pregnancy dated from the first day of the last menstrual period (LMP), which precedes ovulation and fertilization by around 2 weeks.
• From fertilization to 10 weeks' gestation (8 weeks post-conception), the conceptus is called an embryo. From 10 weeks to birth, it is a fetus.

Follicular development and ovulation
• Primitive germ cells are present in the female embryo by the end of the third week of intrauterine life. The number of germ cells in the fetal ovary peak at around 7 million at 5 months. Degeneration occurs thereafter, with only 2 million primary oocytes surviving in the ovary at birth and as few as 300,000–400,000 in the ovary of prepubertal women.
• Primary oocytes have a diploid number of chromosomes (46,XX) which are suspended in prophase of meiosis I. During the follicular phase of the menstrual cycle, several primary oocytes mature under the influence of follicle-stimulating hormone (FSH), with completion of meiosis I. This results in formation of the secondary oocyte with a haploid number of chromosomes (23,X) and extrusion of the first polar body. The mature follicle is known as a graafian follicle (described by de Graaf in 1677). Secondary oocytes enter meiosis II but become suspended in metaphase. Selection of a single dominant follicle occurs at this time.
• The midcycle surge of luteinizing hormone (LH) results in ovulation and extrusion of the secondary oocyte into the abdominal cavity.

Fertilization
• Fertilization of a mature ovum by a single spermatozoon (23,X or 23,Y) occurs in the fallopian tube within the first few hours after ovulation. The genetic composition of the spermatozoon thus determines the gender of the conceptus.
• Fertilization serves as a trigger for the secondary oocyte to complete meiosis II. The male and female pronuclei (each haploid) fuse to form the zygote, which has a diploid number of chromosomes (46,XX or 46,XY).

Preimplantation embryo development
• Mitotic division of the zygote (known as segmentation or cleavage) gives rise to daughter cells called blastomeres. The initial division results in a two-cell stage followed by a four-cell stage and an eight-cell stage. Such divisions continue while the embryo is still in the fallopian tube. As the blastomeres continue to divide, a solid ball of cells is produced known as the morula.
• The morula enters the uterine cavity around 3–4 days after fertilization. The accumulation of fluid between blastomeres results in formation of a fluid-filled cavity, converting the morula to a blastocyst.
• A compact mass of cells (the inner cell mass) collects at one pole of the blastocyst. These cells are destined to produce the embryo. The outer rim of trophectoderm cells is destined to become the trophoblast (placenta).

Implantation
• Implantation usually occurs in the upper part of the uterus and more often on the posterior uterine wall.
• Before implantation, the collection of cells surrounding the blastocyst (known as the zona pellucida) disappears and the blastocyst adheres to the endometrium. This is known as apposition.
• The blastocyst then proceeds to invade the endometrium. Implantation is usually completed by day 24–25 of gestation (day 10–11 post-conception).

Early embryo and fetal development
(Figure 35.2)
Embryonic development after implantation
• By day 24–26 of gestation, the embryonic disc is bilaminar, consisting of embryonic ectoderm and endoderm.
• Cellular proliferation in the embryonic disc results in midline thickening known as the primitive streak. Cells then spread out laterally from the primitive streak between the endoderm and ectoderm to form the mesoderm. This results in a trilaminar embryonic disk.
• These three germ layers give rise to all the organs of the embryo. The nervous system and epidermis along with its derivatives (lens of the eye, hair) are derived from ectoderm. The gastrointestinal tract and derivatives (pancreas, liver, thyroid) arise from endoderm. The skeleton, dermis, muscles, and vascular and urogenital systems are derived from mesoderm.

Early fetal development
The embryonic period ends after 10 weeks' gestation (8 weeks post-conception). The crown–rump length (CRL) of the embryo is now 4 mm. The fetal period is characterized by growth and maturation of structures formed during the embryonic period.

Gestational age (weeks)		CRL (mm)	Fetal weight (g)	Main external features
Menstrual	Fertilization			
12	10	8	14	Fingers, toes visible; intestines in umbilical cord
16	14	12	110	Sex is distinguishable; well-defined neck; head erect
20	18	16	320	Vernix caseosa present
24	22	21	630	Skin red and wrinkled; lanugo (body hair) present; limit of fetal survival
28	26	25	1,100	Eyes partly open; eyebrows, eyelashes present
32	30	28	1,800	Body filling out; intact fetal survival >95%
36	34	32	2,500	Skin pink and smooth; body plump; testes descending
40	38	36	3,400	Prominent chest; testes in scrotum; breasts protrude

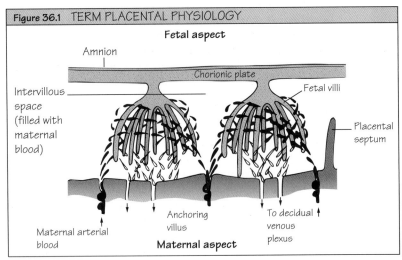

Figure 36.1 TERM PLACENTAL PHYSIOLOGY

Fetal aspect

Amnion

Chorionic plate

Intervillous space (filled with maternal blood)

Fetal villi

Placental septum

Maternal arterial blood

Anchoring villus

To decidual venous plexus

Maternal aspect

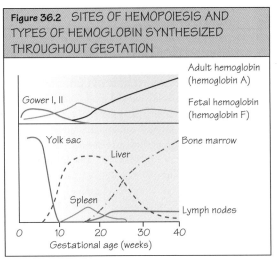

Figure 36.2 SITES OF HEMOPOIESIS AND TYPES OF HEMOGLOBIN SYNTHESIZED THROUGHOUT GESTATION

Adult hemoglobin (hemoglobin A)

Gower I, II

Fetal hemoglobin (hemoglobin F)

Yolk sac

Liver

Bone marrow

Spleen

Lymph nodes

Gestational age (weeks)

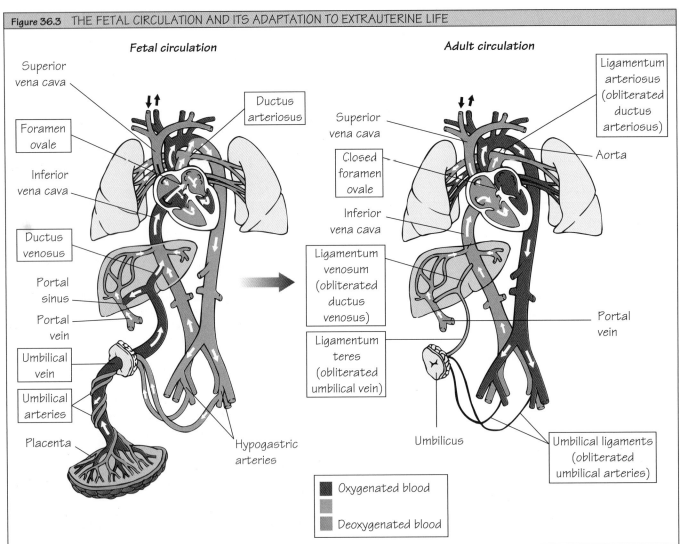

Figure 36.3 THE FETAL CIRCULATION AND ITS ADAPTATION TO EXTRAUTERINE LIFE

Fetal circulation

Adult circulation

Superior vena cava

Foramen ovale

Inferior vena cava

Ductus venosus

Portal sinus

Portal vein

Umbilical vein

Umbilical arteries

Placenta

Ductus arteriosus

Hypogastric arteries

Ligamentum arteriosus (obliterated ductus arteriosus)

Superior vena cava

Closed foramen ovale

Inferior vena cava

Ligamentum venosum (obliterated ductus venosus)

Ligamentum teres (obliterated umbilical vein)

Aorta

Portal vein

Umbilicus

Umbilical ligaments (obliterated umbilical arteries)

Oxygenated blood

Deoxygenated blood

Obstetrics and Gynecology at a Glance, Fourth Edition. Errol R. Norwitz and John O. Schorge.

80 © 2013 John Wiley & Sons, Ltd. Published 2013 by John Wiley & Sons, Ltd.

Placental physiology

• The placenta has several functions, including the maternal–fetal transfer of nutrients and oxygen, the clearance of fetal waste, and the synthesis of proteins and hormones.

• The human placenta is classified as *hemochorioendothelial*, because only three cell layers separate the maternal and fetal circulations: fetal trophoblast, fetal villous stroma, and fetal capillary endothelium. Fetal villi are suspended in intervillous spaces bathed with maternal blood (Figure 36.1).

• Placental villi create a high surface area/volume ratio with a total surface area at term of around $10\,m^2$.

• Transfer across the placenta occurs by passive diffusion (oxygen, CO_2, electrolytes, simple sugars), active transport (iron, vitamin C), or carrier-mediated facilitated diffusion (immunoglobulins).

• There is a large placental reserve; 30–40% of placental villi can be lost without evidence of placental insufficiency.

Fetal physiology

Nutrition

• The embryo consists almost entirely of water. After 10 weeks, however, the fetus is dependent on nutrients from the maternal circulation via the developing placenta.

• The average term fetus weighs 3,400 g. Birthweight is influenced by race, socioeconomic status, parity, genetic factors, diabetes, smoking, and fetal gender. At term, the fetus grows around 30 g/day.

Cardiovascular system

• The fetal heart starts beating at 4–5 weeks' gestation.

• The fetoplacental blood volume at term is 120 mL/kg (or a total of approximately 420 mL).

• After birth, the fetal circulation undergoes profound hemodynamic changes (Figure 36.3). The umbilical vessels, ductus arteriosus, foramen ovale, and ductus venosus constrict. This is thought to be due to a change in oxygen tension within minutes of birth. The distal portions of the umbilical arteries atrophy within 3–4 days to become the *umbilical ligaments*, and the umbilical vein becomes the *ligamentum teres*. The ductus venosus is functionally closed within 10–90 hours of birth, but anatomic closure and formation of the *ligamentum venosum* is achieved only by 2–3 weeks of life.

Respiratory system

• Within minutes of birth, the fetal lungs must be able to provide oxygen and eliminate CO_2 if the fetus is to survive.

• Movements of the fetal chest can be detected at 11 weeks. The ability of the fetus to "breathe" amniotic fluid into the lungs at 16–22 weeks appears to be important for normal lung development. Pulmonary hypoplasia may result if this does not occur.

• Surfactant is a heterogeneous detergent-like substance that lowers alveoli surface tension and prevents alveoli collapse after birth. It is made in the lungs by type II pneumocytes.

• Functional maturation results in an increase in surfactant in the lungs. Respiratory compromise due to surfactant deficiency is known as *hyaline membrane disease* (HMD) or *respiratory distress syndrome* (RDS), and is seen primarily in premature infants. Antenatal *corticosteroid therapy* promotes surfactant production and decreases the risk of RDS by 50%.

Fetal blood

• Sites of hemopoiesis change with gestational age (Figure 36.2).

• The hemoglobin of fetal blood rises to the adult level of 15 g/dL by mid-pregnancy, and increases to 18 g/dL at term. The average fetal hematocrit is 50%.

• Hemoglobin F (fetal hemoglobin) has a higher affinity for oxygen than hemoglobin A (adult hemoglobin). Hemoglobin A is present in the fetus from 11 weeks and increases linearly with increasing gestational age (Figure 36.2). A switch from hemoglobin F to hemoglobin A begins at around 32–34 weeks. By term, 75% of total hemoglobin is hemoglobin A.

• The average fetal hematocrit is 50%.

Gastrointestinal system

• The small intestine is capable of peristalsis by 11 weeks. By 16 weeks, the fetus is able to swallow.

• The fetal liver absorbs drugs rapidly but metabolizes them slowly because the hepatic pathways for drug detoxification and inactivation are poorly developed until late in fetal life.

• During the last trimester, the liver stores large amounts of glycogen and the enzyme pathways responsible for glucose synthesis mature.

Genitourinary system

• Fetal urination starts early in pregnancy, and fetal urine is a major component of amniotic fluid, especially after 16 weeks.

• Renal function improves slowly as pregnancy progresses.

Nervous system

• Neuronal development continues throughout gestation and at least into the second year of extrauterine life. Development of the central nervous system requires normal thyroid activity.

• The fetus is able to perceive sounds at 24–26 weeks. By 28 weeks, the fetal eye is sensitive to light.

• Gonadal steroids are the major determinant of sexual behavior.

Immune system

• Fetal IgG (immunoglobulin G) is derived almost exclusively from the mother. Receptor-mediated transport of IgG from mother to fetus begins at 16 weeks' gestation, but the bulk of IgG is acquired in the last 4 weeks of pregnancy. As such, preterm infants have very low circulating IgG levels. IgM (immunoglobulin M) is not actively transported across the placenta. As such, IgM levels in the fetus accurately reflect the response of the fetal immune system to infection.

• B lymphocytes appear in the fetal liver by 9 weeks, and in the blood and spleen by 12 weeks. T cells leave the fetal thymus at around 14 weeks.

• The fetus does not acquire much IgG (passive immunity) from colostrum, although IgA (immunoglobulin A) in breast milk may protect against some enteric infections.

Endocrine system (see Chapter 37)

• Both oxytocin and vasopressin are secreted by the fetal neurohypophysis by 10–12 weeks.

• The fetal thyroid begins functioning at 12 weeks. Very little fetal thyroid hormone is derived from the mother (see Chapter 47).

Figure 37.1 SERUM CONCENTRATIONS OF SELECT HORMONES DURING PREGNANCY

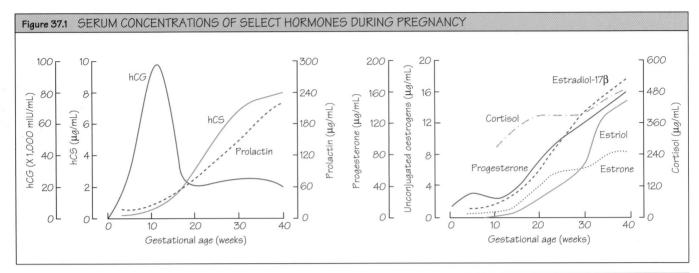

Figure 37.2 FACTORS RESPONSIBLE FOR MAINTAINING UTERINE QUIESCENCE THROUGHOUT GESTATION

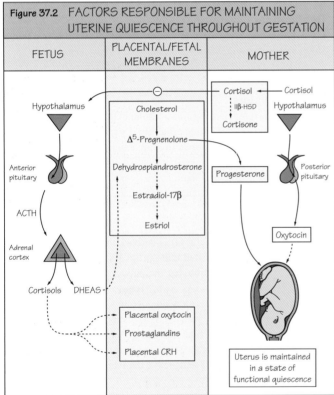

Figure 37.3 FACTORS RESPONSIBLE FOR ONSET OF LABOR AT TERM

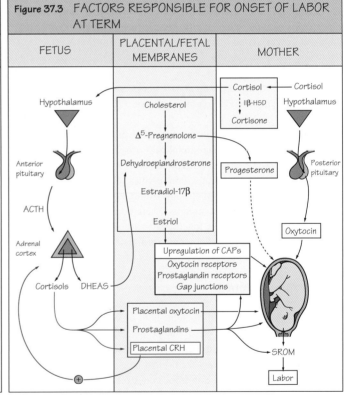

Obstetrics and Gynecology at a Glance, Fourth Edition. Errol R. Norwitz and John O. Schorge.

82 © 2013 John Wiley & Sons, Ltd. Published 2013 by John Wiley & Sons, Ltd.

Endocrinology of pregnancy

The placenta is a rich source of hormones, including human chorionic gonadotropin, human chorionic somatolactotropin, steroid hormones, oxytocin, growth hormone, corticotropin-releasing hormone, pro-opiomelanocortin, prolactin, and gonadotropin-releasing hormone. A few are discussed here.

Human chorionic gonadotropin

• Human chorionic gonadotropin (hCG) is a heterodimeric protein hormone that shares a common α-subunit with luteinizing hormone (LH), follicle-stimulating hormone (FSH), and thyroid-stimulating hormone (TSH), but has a unique β-subunit. It is most closely related to LH.

• Human CG is produced exclusively by the syncytiotrophoblast cells and can be detected in maternal serum 8–9 days after conception. It is the basis of all standard pregnancy tests.

• Human CG levels double every 48 hours in the first several weeks of pregnancy, reaching a peak of 80,000–100,000 mIU/mL at around 8–10 weeks' gestation. Thereafter, hCG concentrations fall to 10,000–20,000 mIU/mL, and remain at that level for the remainder of pregnancy.

• The primary function of hCG appears to be maintenance of progesterone production from the corpus luteum of the ovary, until the placenta can take over progesterone production at around 6–8 weeks' gestation. Progesterone is essential for early pregnancy success, eg, surgical removal of the corpus luteum or administration of a progesterone receptor antagonist (such as RU 486, mifepristone) before 7 weeks (49 days) of gestation will cause abortion.

• Human CG also has thyrotropic activity (0.025% of TSH), which only becomes clinically significant if hCG levels are markedly elevated such as in complete molar pregnancies.

Human chorionic somatolactotropin

• Human chorionic somatolactotropin (hCS) – previously known as human placental lactogen (hPL) – is a family of protein hormones produced exclusively by the placenta which are closely related to both prolactin and growth hormone.

• Human CS production is directly proportional to placental mass and levels rise steadily throughout pregnancy.

• The function of hCS is not known, but it has anti-insulin-like activity and may be involved in the development of insulin resistance, which characterizes pregnancy.

Steroid hormones

• The placenta is the major source of progesterone and estrogen production during pregnancy.

• In the placenta, estrogen is synthesized from androgen precursors and is important for preparing the uterus for labor. Progesterone is derived primarily from maternal substrate (cholesterol) and may be important for maintaining uterine quiescence before labor.

Endocrine control of labor

• Reproductive success is critical for survival of the species. Each species has solved the problem of labor in a different way. Such differences may reflect the evolutionary status of the organism in question or may represent solutions to inherent obstacles to reproduction faced by each species (such as differences in placentation, gestational length, and the number of offspring per pregnancy).

• The slow progress in our understanding of the mechanisms responsible for the process of labor in humans reflects the lack of an adequate animal model and the difficulty of extrapolating from endocrine mechanisms in many animal species to the paracrine/autocrine mechanisms of parturition in humans.

Initiation of labor

• Considerable evidence suggests that, in most viviparous animals, the fetus is in control of the timing of labor. It is likely that this is achieved through activation of the fetal hypothalamic–pituitary–adrenal (HPA) axis before the onset of labor, and that this is common to all viviparous species.

• A proposed "parturition cascade" is outlined in Figures 37.1 and 37.2.

• The human placenta is an incomplete steroidogenic organ, and estrogen production by the placenta has an obligatory need for androgen precursor. This excess androgen is supplied by the fetus in the form of dehydroepiandrosterenedione sulfate (DHEAS).

• Activation of the fetal HPA axis at term results in excess DHEAS release from the intermediate (fetal) zone of the fetal adrenal. DHEAS is 16-hydroxylated in the fetal liver and passes via the fetal circulation to the placenta where it is converted almost exclusively to estriol (16-hydroxyestradiol-17β).

• Human pregnancy is characterized by a hyperestrogenic state of unparalleled magnitude in the entire mammalian kingdom. The placenta is the primary source of estrogens. The concentration of estrogens in the maternal circulation increases with gestational age. Placental estrone and estradiol-17β are derived primarily from maternal C19 androgens (testosterone and androstenedione), whereas estriol is derived almost exclusively from fetal DHEAS. Estrogens do not cause uterine contractions, but do promote a series of myometrial changes (including increasing the number of prostaglandin receptors, oxytocin receptors, and gap junctions) that enhance the capacity of the myometrium to generate contractions.

• In addition to DHEAS, the enlarged fetal adrenal glands also produce cortisol, which has two actions:

  1 It prepares fetal organ systems for extrauterine life.

  2 It promotes expression of a number of placental products, including corticotropin-releasing hormone (CRH), oxytocin, and prostaglandins (especially prostaglandin E_2 – PGE_2).

• Placental CRH initiates a *positive feedback loop* by stimulating the fetal HPA axis to produce more DHEAS and more cortisol, which then further upregulates placental CRH expression. (This stimulatory effect of cortisol on placental CRH should be contrasted with the feedback inhibition of cortisol on maternal CRH.)

• Placental oxytocin acts directly on the myometrium to cause contractions and indirectly by upregulating prostaglandin production (especially prostaglandin $F_{2\alpha}$ – $PGF_{2\alpha}$) by the decidua.

• $PGF_{2\alpha}$ is produced primarily by the maternal decidua and acts on the myometrium to upregulate oxytocin receptors and gap junctions, and thereby promote uterine contractions.

• PGE_2 is primarily of fetoplacental origin and is probably more important in promoting cervical "ripening" (maturation) and spontaneous rupture of the fetal membranes (SROM).

38 Maternal adaptations to pregnancy

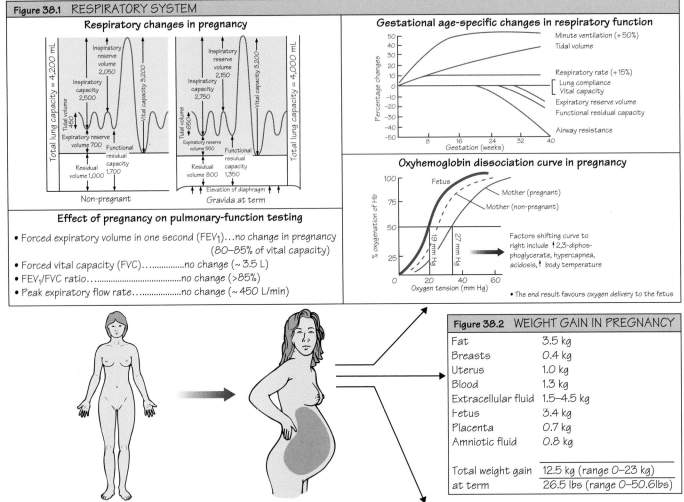

Figure 38.1 RESPIRATORY SYSTEM

Respiratory changes in pregnancy

Non-pregnant — Total lung capacity = 4,200 mL; Inspiratory capacity 2,500; Inspiratory reserve volume 2,050; Vital capacity 3,200; Tidal volume 450; Expiratory reserve volume 700; Functional residual capacity 1,700; Residual volume 1,000

Gravida at term — Total lung capacity = 4,000 mL; Inspiratory capacity 2,750; Inspiratory reserve volume 2,150; Vital capacity 3,200; Tidal volume 650; Expiratory reserve volume 550; Functional residual capacity 1,350; Residual volume 800; Elevation of diaphragm

Effect of pregnancy on pulmonary-function testing

- Forced expiratory volume in one second (FEV_1)...no change in pregnancy (80–85% of vital capacity)
- Forced vital capacity (FVC)..................no change (~ 3.5 L)
- FEV_1/FVC ratio.......................................no change (>85%)
- Peak expiratory flow rate...................no change (~ 450 L/min)

Gestational age-specific changes in respiratory function

Minute ventilation (+50%); Tidal volume; Respiratory rate (+15%); Lung compliance; Vital capacity; Expiratory reserve volume; Functional residual capacity; Airway resistance

Oxyhemoglobin dissociation curve in pregnancy

Fetus; Mother (pregnant); Mother (non-pregnant); 19 mm Hg; 27 mm Hg

Factors shifting curve to right include ↑2,3-diphosphoglycerate, hypercapnea, acidosis, ↑ body temperature

- The end result favours oxygen delivery to the fetus

Figure 38.2 WEIGHT GAIN IN PREGNANCY

Fat	3.5 kg
Breasts	0.4 kg
Uterus	1.0 kg
Blood	1.3 kg
Extracellular fluid	1.5–4.5 kg
Fetus	3.4 kg
Placenta	0.7 kg
Amniotic fluid	0.8 kg
Total weight gain at term	12.5 kg (range 0–23 kg)
	26.5 lbs (range 0–50.6lbs)

Figure 38.3 CARDIOVASCULAR SYSTEM

Central hemodynamic changes induced by pregnancy

Measurement	Non-pregnant	Term pregnant	Change
• Blood volume (mL)	3,500	5,000	+40%
• Mean arterial BP (mmHg)	86 ± 8	90 ± 6	no change
• Cardiac output (L/min)	4.3 ± 1	6.2 ± 1	+44%
• Heart rate (bpm)	71 ± 10	83 ± 10	+17%
• Central venous pressure (mmHg)	4 ± 3	4 ± 3	no change
• Pulmonary capillary wedge pressure (mmHg)	6 ± 2	8 ± 2	no change
• Systemic vascular resistance (dyne/s per cm⁻⁵)	1,530 ± 520	1,210 ± 266	−21%
• Pulmonary vascular resistance (dyne/s per cm⁻⁵)	119 ± 47	78 ± 22	−35%
• Left ventricular stroke work index (g/m per m²)	41 ± 8	48 ± 6	no change

Blood volume changes during pregnancy

Blood volume; Plasma volume; RBC mass; Delivery

Gestational age-specific changes in mean arterial pressure

Nadir at 20–24 weeks; Back to baseline at term; 20% increase in labor; Rapid resolution postpartum; First trimester; Second trimester; Third trimester; Labor; Puerperium

- Physiologic adaptations in the mother occur in response to demands created by pregnancy. These include:
  1 support of the fetus (volume, nutritional and oxygen support, clearance of fetal waste)
  2 protection of the fetus (from starvation, drugs, toxins)
  3 preparation of the uterus for labor
  4 protection of the mother from potential cardiovascular injury at delivery.
- Maternal age, ethnicity, genetic factors, and maternal comorbidities affect the ability of the mother to adapt to pregnancy.
- All maternal organ systems are required to adapt to the demands of pregnancy. The quality, degree, and timing of the adaptation vary from one individual to another and from one organ system to another.

Respiratory system (Figure 38.1)
- Respiratory adaptations during pregnancy are designed to optimize maternal and fetal oxygenation, and to facilitate transfer of CO_2 waste from the fetus to the mother.
- Many pregnant women report a subjective perception of shortness of breath (dyspnea) in the absence of pathology. The reason for this is unclear.
- The mechanics of respiration change with pregnancy. The ribs flare outward and the level of the diaphragm rises 4 cm.
- During pregnancy, tidal volume increases by 200 mL (40%), resulting in a 100–200 mL (5%) increase in vital capacity and a 200 mL (20%) decrease in the residual volume, thereby leaving less air in the lungs at the end of expiration. The respiratory rate does not change. The end-result is an increase in minute ventilation and a drop in arterial PCO_2 (see table below). Arterial PO_2 is essentially unchanged. A compensatory decrease in bicarbonate enables the pH to remain unchanged. Pregnancy thus represents a state of *compensated respiratory alkalosis*.

	pH	PO_2 (mmHg)	PCO_2 (mmHg)
Non-pregnant	7.40	93–100	35–40
Pregnant	7.40	100–105	28–30

Cardiovascular system (Figure 38.3)
- Progesterone decreases systemic vascular resistance early in pregnancy, leading to a decline in blood pressure. In response, cardiac output increases by 30–50%.
- Activation of the renin–angiotensin system results in increased circulating angiotensin II, which encourages sodium and water retention (leading to a 40% increase in blood volume) and directly constricts the peripheral vasculature.

Gastrointestinal tract
- Nausea ("morning sickness") occurs in >70% of pregnancies. Symptoms usually resolve by 17 weeks.
- Progesterone causes relaxation of gastrointestinal smooth muscle, resulting in delayed gastric emptying and increased reflux.
- Pregnancy predisposes to cholelithiasis (gallstones). Most gallstones in pregnancy are cholesterol stones.
- Pregnancy is a "diabetogenic state" with evidence of insulin resistance and reduced peripheral uptake of glucose (due to increased levels of placental anti-insulin hormones, primarily human chorionic soma-

tolactotropin [hCS]). These mechanisms are designed to ensure a continuous supply of glucose to the fetus.

Genitourinary system
- Glomerular filtration rate (GFR) increases by 50% early in pregnancy, leading to an increase in creatinine clearance and a 25% decrease in serum creatinine and urea concentrations.
- Increased GFR results in an increase in filtered sodium. Aldosterone levels increase two- to threefold to reabsorb this sodium.
- Increased GFR also results in decreased resorption of glucose. As such, 15% of normal pregnant women exhibit glycosuria.
- Mild hydronephrosis and hydroureter are common sonographic findings that are due to high progesterone levels and partial obstruction from the gravid uterus.
- Five percent of pregnant women have bacteria in their urine. Pregnancy does not increase the incidence of asymptomatic bacteriuria, but such women are more likely to develop pyelonephritis (20–30%).

Hematologic system
- Increased intravascular volume results in dilutional anemia. Elevated erythropoietin levels lead to a compensatory increase in total red cell mass, but never fully correct the anemia.
- A modest increase in white blood cell count (leukocytosis) can be seen during pregnancy, but the differential count should not change.
- Mild thrombocytopenia (<150,000 platelets/mL) is seen in 10% of pregnant women. This is probably dilutional and rarely clinically significant.
- Pregnancy represents a hypercoagulable state with increased circulating levels of factors II (fibrinogen), VII, IX, and X. These changes protect the mother from excessive blood loss at delivery, but also predispose to thromboembolism.

Endocrine system (see Chapter 37)
- Estrogen increases hepatic production of thyroid-binding globulin, leading to an increase in total thyroid hormone concentration. However, thyroid-stimulating hormone (TSH), free triiodothyronine (T_3), and free thyroxine (T_4) levels remain unchanged.
- Serum calcium levels decrease in pregnancy leading to an increase in parathyroid hormone, which encourages conversion of cholecalciferol (vitamin D_3) to its active metabolite, 1,25-dihydroxycholecalciferol (DHCC), by 1α-hydroxylase in the placenta. This leads to increased intestinal absorption of calcium.
- Aldosterone and cortisol are increased in pregnancy.
- Prolactin increases in pregnancy, but its function is unknown. It is probably more important for lactation after delivery.

Immune system
Cellular immunity is depressed during pregnancy. As a result, pregnant women may be at increased risk for contracting viral infections and tuberculosis.

Musculoskeletal and dermatologic systems
- A shift in posture (exaggerated lumbar lordosis) and lower back strain are common in pregnancy.
- Increased estrogens and melanocyte-stimulating hormone may cause hyperpigmentation (darkening) of the umbilicus, nipples, abdominal midline (linea nigra), and face (chloasma).
- Increased estrogen may also lead to skin changes such as spider angioma and palmar erythema.

39 Prenatal diagnosis

Figure 39.1 ROUTINE PRENATAL SCREENING

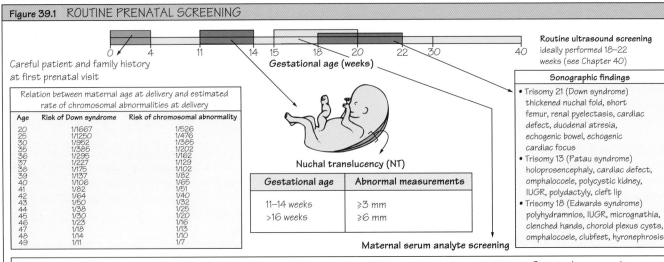

Careful patient and family history at first prenatal visit

Routine ultrasound screening
ideally performed 18–22 weeks (see Chapter 40)

Relation between maternal age at delivery and estimated rate of chromosomal abnormalities at delivery

Age	Risk of Down syndrome	Risk of chromosomal abnormality
20	1/1667	1/526
25	1/1250	1/476
30	1/952	1/385
35	1/385	1/202
36	1/295	1/162
37	1/227	1/129
38	1/175	1/102
39	1/137	1/82
40	1/106	1/65
41	1/82	1/51
42	1/64	1/40
43	1/50	1/32
44	1/38	1/25
45	1/30	1/20
46	1/23	1/16
47	1/18	1/13
48	1/14	1/10
49	1/11	1/7

Nuchal translucency (NT)

Gestational age	Abnormal measurements
11–14 weeks	≥3 mm
>16 weeks	≥6 mm

Maternal serum analyte screening

Sonographic findings

- Trisomy 21 (Down syndrome) thickened nuchal fold, short femur, renal pyelectasis, cardiac defect, duodenal atresia, echogenic bowel, echogenic cardiac focus
- Trisomy 13 (Patau syndrome) holoprosencephaly, cardiac defect, omphalocoele, polycystic kidney, IUGR, polydactyly, cleft lip
- Trisomy 18 (Edwards syndrome) polyhydramnios, IUGR, micrognathia, clenched hands, choroid plexus cysts, omphalocoele, clubfeet, hyronephrosis

- AFP is fetal glycoprotein related to albumin. It is produced sequentially by yolk sac, gastrointestinal tract, and liver
- AFP levels peak in fetus at the end of the first trimester and in the mother at around 30 weeks' gestation
- Elevated MS-AFP will detect 85% of all open neural tube defects. Other causes include ventral wall defects, twins, placental abnormalities, congenital nephrosis

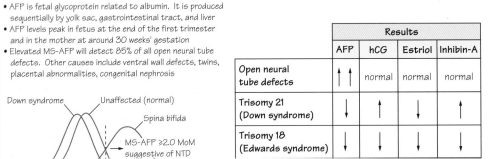

Down syndrome   Unaffected (normal)

Spina bifida

MS-AFP ≥2.0 MoM suggestive of NTD

Maternal serum AFP (MoM)

Results

	AFP	hCG	Estriol	Inhibin-A
Open neural tube defects	↑↑	normal	normal	normal
Trisomy 21 (Down syndrome)	↓	↑	↓	↑
Trisomy 18 (Edwards syndrome)	↓	↓	↓	↓

Down syndrome screening

- 20% of Down syndrome births occur to women >35 years of age at delivery
- Use of serum analyte screening will increase the detection rate to 60% with a false-positive rate of ~5% (MS-AFP alone will detect 20–25% of Down syndrome conceptions. hCG is the most sensitive maternal marker for Down syndrome)
- Ultrasound can increase detection of Down syndrome fetuses to ~85%
- 15% of Down syndrome pregnancies will be missed by maternal age, serum screening, and ultrasound screening
- Karyotype provides a definitive diagnosis
- cfDNA is increasingly being used as an alternative screening test

Figure 39.2 INDICATIONS FOR FURTHER PRENATAL SCREENING

Maternal		Fetal
• Maternal age ≥35 years at delivery • Prior child with neural tube defect • Previous child with chromosomal abnormality • Chromosomal abnormality in either parent • Family history of chromosome abnormality	• Abnormal maternal serum analyte screening • Teratogen exposure • Maternal medical conditions	• Abnormal nuchal translucency • Abnormal fetal structural survey

Figure 39.3 FURTHER PRENATAL TESTING

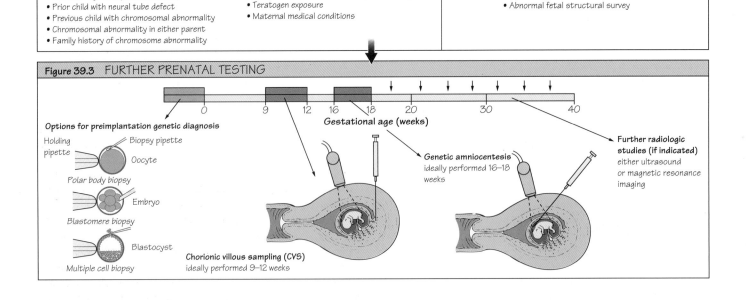

Options for preimplantation genetic diagnosis

Holding pipette   Biopsy pipette
Oocyte
Polar body biopsy
Embryo
Blastomere biopsy
Blastocyst
Multiple cell biopsy

Gestational age (weeks)

Chorionic villous sampling (CVS)
ideally performed 9–12 weeks

Genetic amniocentesis
ideally performed 16–18 weeks

Further radiologic studies (if indicated) either ultrasound or magnetic resonance imaging

Obstetrics and Gynecology at a Glance, Fourth Edition. Errol R. Norwitz and John O. Schorge.

Congenital disorders and the fetus

• Congenital anomalies refer to structural defects present at birth. Major congenital anomalies (those incompatible with life or requiring major surgery) occur in 2–3% of live births, and 5% have minor malformations.

• Of congenital anomalies 30–40% have a known cause, including chromosomal abnormalities (0.5% of live births), single gene defects (1% of births), multifactorial disorders, and teratogenic exposures; 60–70% have no known cause.

Classification of chromosomal abnormalities
Autosomal disorders

• *Trisomy 21 (Down syndrome)*. The most common autosomal disorder. Overall incidence is 1/800 live births, but it is strongly associated with maternal age (Figure 39.1). Long-term prognosis depends largely on the presence of cardiac anomalies.

• *Trisomy 18 (Edward syndrome)*. One in 3,500 births. It is characterized by intrauterine growth restriction (IUGR), single umbilical artery, overlapping clenched fingers, and "rocker-bottom" feet. Fewer than 10% of infants survive to age 1.

• *Trisomy 13 (Patau syndrome)*. One in 5,000 births. IUGR with facial clefts, ocular anomalies, and polydactyly. Fewer than 3% survive to age 3.

• *5p- (cri-du-chat syndrome)*. One in 20,000 births. Round facies, epicanthal folds, learning disability, and a high-pitched, monotonous cry. Variable survival.

Sex chromosomal disorders

• *47,XXY (Klinefelter syndrome)*. The most common sex chromosome disorder; 1/500 births. Male phenotype, but with female adipose distribution and breast development. Normal pubic and axillary hair, scant facial hair. Twentyfold increase in breast cancer. Usually infertile.

• *45,X (Turner syndrome)*. One in 2,500 live births (but accounts for around 25% of early miscarriage). Short female with a webbed neck, primary amenorrhea, renal anomalies, cardiac defect (aortic coarctation). Affected individuals are infertile.

• *47,XYY*. One in 800 births. Tall male with normal genitalia and testosterone levels, but intellectually limited. Usually fertile.

Classification of genetic disorders
Autosomal dominant (70%)

• Inherited from either parent or a new mutation.

• *Examples.* Huntington disease, neurofibromatosis, achondroplasia, Marfan syndrome.

Autosomal recessive (20%)

• Genetic screening is difficult as many different mutations may result in the same clinical disorder.

• *Examples.* Sickle cell disease (African carrier rate 1/10), cystic fibrosis (1/20 in white people), Tay–Sachs disease (1/30 in Ashkenazi Jews), β-thalassemia (1/25 in women of Mediterranean origin).

X-linked recessive (5%)

Examples. Duchenne muscular dystrophy, hemophilia.

X-linked dominant (rare)

Examples. Vitamin D-resistant rickets, hereditary hematuria.

Multifactorial inheritance

• May be isolated or part of a clinical syndrome.

• *Examples.* Neural tube defect, talipes equinovarus (club feet), hydrocephaly, cleft lip, cardiac anomalies.

Routine prenatal screening (Figure 39.1)

• *Patient history* may identify a fetus at risk for aneuploidy (genetic anomalies), eg, the risk of recurrent neural tube defect is 1% (compared with a baseline risk of 0.1%).

• The risk of fetal aneuploidy (primarily Down syndrome) increases with *maternal age*. "Advanced maternal age" refers to women aged ≥35 years at their due date. Such women account for 5–8% of deliveries and 20–30% of Down syndrome births.

• *Nuchal translucency (NT)* in early pregnancy correlates with fetal aneuploidy. A measurement of >2.5 mm at 8–12 weeks is seen in 2–6% of fetuses, of which 50–70% will have a chromosomal anomaly. *First trimester aneuploidy screening* incorporates NT and the serum analyte markers, PAPP-A and β-human chorionic gonadotropin (βhCG).

• Second trimester *maternal serum analyte screening* uses a panel of biochemical markers to adjust the maternal age-related risk for fetal aneuploidy. The standard "quadruple panel" test at 15–20 weeks uses four markers: α-fetoprotein (AFP), βhCG, inhibin A, and estriol. The most important variable is gestational age which accounts for most false-positive results.

Further prenatal testing

• *Amniocentesis* involves sampling amniotic fluid from around the fetus. The fluid itself or fetal cells can be used for karyotyping, DNA analysis, or enzyme assays. When performed at 16–18 weeks, the procedure-related loss rate is quoted at 1 in 400. US practice favors offering all women aged ≥35 years at delivery elective amniocentesis, because the risk of fetal aneuploidy approximately equals the procedure-related loss rate. Early amniocentesis (<15 weeks) is associated with a higher rate of pregnancy loss, and should not be performed.

• *Chorionic villous sampling (CVS)* involves sampling of placental tissue at 9–12 weeks. Tissue can be used for DNA analysis, cytogenetic testing, or enzyme assays. Advantages include earlier diagnosis. Disadvantages include high procedure-related loss rate (1%), potential for maternal cell contamination, and sampling of cells destined to become placenta rather than fetus. CVS performed at <9 weeks is associated with a threefold increase in limb reduction defects.

• *Percutaneous umbilical blood sampling (PUBS)* involves ultrasound-guided aspiration of fetal blood from the umbilical cord. Advantages include the ability to get a rapid fetal karyotype and to measure several hematologic, immunologic, and acid–base parameters in the fetus. Fetal blood transfusions can also be performed, but have a procedure-related fetal loss rate of 1–5%.

• *Other studies* may include magnetic resonance imaging or invasive procedures (fetoscopy, fetal tissue biopsy).

• *Future options:*

1 *Preimplantation genetic diagnosis* (Figure 39.3) involves genetic analysis of a cell(s) removed before embryo transfer at in vitro fertilization.

2 *Fetal cells* exist in the maternal circulation (approximately 1 fetal cell per 10,000 maternal cells). The ability to isolate such cells (or DNA) may provide an option for fetal genetic analysis.

• *Non-invasive prenatal testing (NIPT)* involves sequencing of cell-free DNA in the maternal circulation, 4–10% of which comes from the fetus (placenta). A sample of maternal blood can be sent as early as 9 weeks. NIPT can detect fetal trisomy 21 and 18 with a sensitivity of >99% and false-positive rate of 0.2%, but it is not considered diagnostic; confirmation by CVS/amniocentesis is recommended at this time.

40 Obstetric ultrasound

Figure 40.1 INDICATIONS FOR OBSTETRIC ULTRASOUND

Maternal
- Pelvic mass
- Uterine size > dates
- Follow fibroid growth
- Cervical length evaluation in women at risk for cervical insufficiency, preterm birth

Fetal
- Estimation of gestational age
- Evaluation of fetal growth
- Determine fetal presentation
- Suspected multiple gestation
- Suspected fetal death
- Follow-up fetal anomaly
- Biophysical profile
- Suspected ectopic pregnancy

Uteroplacental
- Vaginal bleeding of unclear etiology, suspected abruption
- Suspected molar pregnancy
- Suspected uterine anomaly
- Suspected polyhydramnios or oligohydramnios
- Follow-up on placental location in previously identified previa

Other
- Amniocentesis or CVS
- Abnormal MS-AFP
- Adjuvant to cervical cerclage placement
- External cephalic version
- Adjunct to surgical procedure (embryo transfer, intrauterine transfusion, fetoscopy)

Figure 40.2 FIRST TRIMESTER SONOGRAPHY

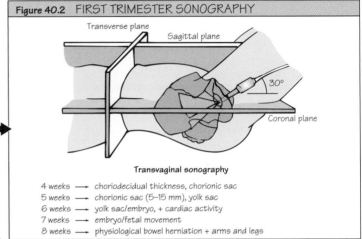

Transvaginal sonography

4 weeks ⟶ choriodecidual thickness, chorionic sac
5 weeks ⟶ chorionic sac (5–15 mm), yolk sac
6 weeks ⟶ yolk sac/embryo, + cardiac activity
7 weeks ⟶ embryo/fetal movement
8 weeks ⟶ physiological bowel herniation + arms and legs

Figure 40.3 SECOND AND THIRD TRIMESTER SONOGRAPHY

Fetal biometry and estimated fetal weight (EFW)

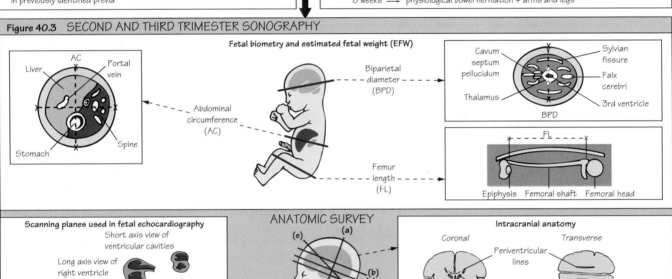

ANATOMIC SURVEY

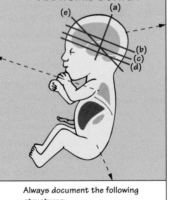

Scanning planes used in fetal echocardiography

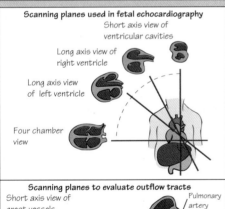

- Short axis view of ventricular cavities
- Long axis view of right ventricle
- Long axis view of left ventricle
- Four chamber view

Scanning planes to evaluate outflow tracts

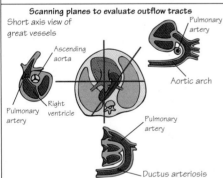

Short axis view of great vessels

Always document the following structures:

- Stomach bubble
- Kidneys
- Face (view of upper lip to exclude cleft)
- Spine in its entirety
- Nuchal thickness
- Bladder
- Genitalia
- Limbs (if possible)
- Umbilical cord insertion and cross-section

Intracranial anatomy

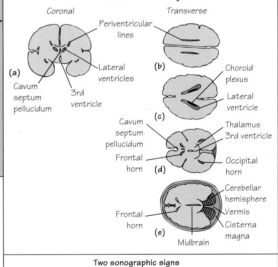

Two sonographic signs seen in spina bifida/NTD

Scalloping of frontal bones ('lemon sign')

Flattening of cerebellar hemispheres ('banana sign')

Obstetrics and Gynecology at a Glance, Fourth Edition. Errol R. Norwitz and John O. Schorge.

Principles of ultrasonography

- Ultrasound uses sound waves delivered at high frequency (3.5–5 MHz for transabdominal and 5–7.5 MHz for transvaginal transducers). The higher the frequency the better the resolution, but the less the tissue penetration.
- Interpretation of images requires operator experience.

Indications (Figure 40.1)

Routine use of obstetric ultrasound can improve detection of fetal anomalies, accurately determine gestational age, and facilitate early diagnosis of multiple pregnancies. However, it is expensive and has not consistently been shown to improve perinatal outcome.

Complications

There are no confirmed adverse effects of ultrasound on the fetus. The major complication is false-positive and false-negative diagnoses.

Guidelines for obstetric ultrasound

First trimester sonography (Figure 40.2)

- Evaluate the uterus for the presence of a *gestational sac*. An intrauterine gestational sac should be seen at a serum βhCG (β-human chorionic gonadotropin) level of ≥1,000–1,200 mIU/mL by transvaginal scan and ≥6,000 mIU/mL by transabdominal ultrasound. If no intrauterine pregnancy is seen, the possibility of an ectopic pregnancy should be considered.
- If a gestational sac is identified, it should be examined for a *yolk sac* (usually evident at a βhCG of 7,000 mIU/mL) and *embryo* (at 11,000 mIU/mL).
- *Gestational age* should be documented. Crown–rump length (CRL) in the early first trimester is an accurate determinant of gestational age to within 3–5 days (compared with an error of ±2 weeks by second trimester measurements and ±3 weeks by third trimester ultrasound).

CRL (in mm) + 6.5 = Approximate gestational age in weeks

In the late first trimester, measurement of the biparietal diameter (BPD) can be used to estimate gestational age.

- Fetal *cardiac activity* is usually evident once the fetal pole is seen. If the CRL is 3–5 mm but no cardiac activity is seen, a follow-up ultrasound is indicated in 3–5 days to evaluate fetal viability. Once fetal cardiac activity has been documented, the fetal loss rate decreases to around 5%.
- Document *fetal number*. If a multiple pregnancy is identified, chorionicity should be determined (see Chapter 55).
- Measure *nuchal translucency* (see Chapter 39).
- Evaluate the uterus, adnexal structures, and cul-de-sac for anomalies unrelated to pregnancy.

Second trimester sonography (Figure 40.3)

- Document fetal cardiac activity and fetal number.
- Estimate *amniotic fluid volume* (see Chapter 50).
- Document *placental location*. Overdistension of the maternal bladder or a lower uterine contraction can give a false impression of placenta previa. If placenta previa is identified at 18–22 weeks, serial ultrasound examinations should be performed to follow placental location. Only 5% of placenta previa identified in the second trimester will persist to term.

- The *umbilical cord* should be imaged, and the number of vessels (a single umbilical artery may suggest fetal aneuploidy, especially if associated with other structural anomalies), placental insertion (if possible), and insertion into the fetus (to exclude an anterior abdominal wall defect) should be noted. Extra-abdominal herniation of the midgut into the umbilical cord occurs normally at 8–12 weeks' gestation and should not be misdiagnosed as an abdominal wall defect.
- *Cervical length* should be documented. A shortened cervix is associated with an increased risk for preterm birth.
- Assessment of *gestational age.*
- *Anatomic survey* (Figure 40.3) is best done at 18–22 weeks.
- Evaluation of uterus and adnexae.

Third trimester sonography

- As for second trimester sonography.
- Determine *estimated fetal weight* (EFW) using the average of three readings for each of the following three measurements: femur length (FL), abdominal circumference (AC), and BPD. Each of these measurements has been standardized to specific fetal landmarks (Figure 40.3). Of the three measurements, the AC is the most important because it is disproportionately weighted in the calculation of EFW. It is also the most difficult to measure. A small difference in AC will result in a large difference in EFW. As a result, sonographic EFW estimations have an error of 15–20%.
- A detailed *anatomic survey* should be performed with each ultrasound even if a prior anatomic survey was reported as normal. Certain fetal anomalies will only become evident later in gestation (such as achondroplastic dwarfism).

Doppler velocimetry

- Doppler velocimetry shows the direction and characteristics of blood flow, and can be used to examine the uteroplacental or fetoplacental circulations.
- Doppler velocimetry should not be performed routinely. Indications include intrauterine growth restriction, cord malformations, unexplained oligohydramnios, pre-eclampsia, and possibly fetal cardiac anomalies.

Fetal echocardiography (Figure 40.3)

Fetal echo is indicated for pregnancies at high risk of a fetal cardiac anomaly (such as pregnancies complicated by maternal diabetes or maternal congenital cardiac disease).Use of ultrasound to detect fetuses with aneuploidy

- Fetuses with trisomy 13 or 18 tend to have major structural anomalies that can be detected on ultrasound.
- Fetuses with trisomy 21 (Down syndrome) may have no anomalies, structural malformations that can only reliably be detected late in pregnancy (duodenal atresia), or very subtle biometric or morphologic abnormalities (shortened femurs, renal pyelectasis). Only 30–50% of Down syndrome fetuses will be detected by routine ultrasound (see Chapter 39). A normal anatomic survey decreases the risk of Down syndrome by approximately 50%.

Ultrasound and hydrops fetalis

Hydrops fetalis is a pathologic condition characterized by excessive fluid accumulation in the fetus. It is a sonographic diagnosis (see Chapter 53).

Figure 41.1 TIMING AND INDICATIONS FOR TESTS DURING PREGNANCY

Test	Indication for test	Timing of test	Who is eligible	Comments
First prenatal visit				
Complete blood count (CBC)	√ for anemia √ platelet count	First prenatal visit, repeat in 3rd trimester	Everyone	• Prescribe iron supplementation for women with hemoglobin <11 g/dL
Blood group type and screen (T&S)	√ Rh status √ for autoantibodies	First prenatal visit, repeat in 3rd trimester	Everyone	• If Rh-negative, check father • If Rh-negative, administer anti-[D] immunoglobulin within 72 hours of vaginal bleeding, at 28 weeks, and after delivery, if indicated • If Rh isoimmunized, check titers every month and refer to MFM; no anti-[D] immunoglobulin
Rubella antibodies	√ rubella immunity status	First prenatal visit	Everyone	• Vaccination if negative (but not during pregnancy)
VDRL (or RPR)	√ for syphilis	First prenatal visit, repeat in 3rd trimester	Everyone	• VDRL and RPR are screening tests; a definitive test is required to confirm the diagnosis (e.g., FTA, MHA-TP)
HIV	√ for HIV infection	First prenatal visit	Everyone	• Diagnosis requires a positive ELISA and western blot • Consider repeating in third trimester in high-risk patients
PAP smear	√ for cervical cancer	First prenatal visit	Everyone	• Not needed if the patient is up to dat with screening
Hepatitis B	√ for infection	First prenatal visit	Everyone	• Hepatitis B immunoglobulin and vaccine can prevent infestion in baby
Urinalysis, culture and sensitivity	√ for proteinuria √ for glycosuria √ for infection	First prenatal visit, repeat in 3rd trimester	Everyone	• Repeat monthly in high-risk patients (sickle cell trait/disease, diabetes, history of recurrent UTI)
Cystic fibrosis (CF) screening	√ CF carrier status	Anytime	Everyone	• All women should be offered testing to determine their CF carrier status • If the mother is positive, then the father should be tested and the couple offered genetic counseling
Genetic counseling	√ for genetic syndromes by getting a detailed family pedigree	First prenatal visit	High-risk patients	• Ashkenazi Jewish ethnicity: Tay-Sachs, Canavan disease, familial dysautonomia • Family history of unexplained mental retardation in males: fragile X • Consider α-thalassemia testing in Mediterranean (Italian) women, esp. in presence of severe anemia
Hemoglobin electrophoresis	√ for hemoglobinopathies	First prenatal visit	High-risk patients	• African-American women should be offered screening for sickle cell trait • Consider in Mediterranean women with anemia to exclude β-thalassemia
Chlamydia	√ for infection	First prenatal visit	High-risk patients	• DNA-based test superior to culture-based test
Gonorrhea	√ for infection	First prenatal visit	High-risk patients	• DNA-based test superior to culture-based test
Urine toxicology screen	√ for illicit drug use	Every prenatal visit	High-risk patients	
Weight (kg/m²) BMI Blood pressure, proteinuria	√ weight gain √ for pre-eclampsia (720w)	Every prenatal visit	Everyone	• Check baseline liver/renal function tests, 24 hour urine collection in high-risk patients
First trimester				
Ultrasound	√ pregnancy dating √ fetal viability √ multiple pregnancy	First prenatal visit	As clinically indicated	• An early ultrasound for pregnancy dating is routinely recommended in Europa, but not in the U.S.
First trimester risk assessment for fetal aneuploidy	Estimate risk of fetal aneuploidy	11–14 weeks	Everyone	• Uses serum markers (β-hCG, PAPP-A) and ultrasound (nuchal translucency) to adjust a patient's age-related risk of fetal aneuploidy
Second trimester				
PPD test	√ for TB exposure	Anytime, but done most often in second trimester	Everyone	• If positive, check chest x-ray • If chest x-ray positive, exclude active TB and give INH chemoprophylaxis
Chorionic villous sampling (CVS)	√ fetal karyotype	11–14 weeks	High-risk patients	• Diagnostic test for fetal aneuploidy • CVS not performed <9 weeks (due to association with limb reduction defects)
Second trimester serum analyte screening for fetal aneuploidy	Estimate risk of fetal aneuploidy	15–20 weeks	Everyone	• Quadruple ("quad") screen uses four serum markers (β-hCG, estriol, AFP, inhibin A) to adjust a patient's age-related risk of fetal aneuploidy • It does not include ultrasound
Maternal serum alfa-fetoprotein (MS-AFP)	Estimate risk of fetal neural tube defect (NTD)	15–20 weeks	Everyone	• One of the markers in the "quad" screen • High levels of MS-AFP (>2.0 MoM) are associated with open NTD • Ultrasound is diagnostic
Genetic amniocentesis	√ fetal karyotype	15–20 weeks	High-risk patients	• Diagnostic test for fetal aneuploidy • Amniocentesis not performed <15 weeks (due to increased procedure-related pregnancy loss rate)
Fetal anatomic survey (genetic ultrasound)	√ for fetal anomalies √ for 'soft markers' of fetal aneuploidy	18–22 weeks	Everyone	• Screening test for fetal aneuploidy (can detect most cases of trisomy 13 & 18, but only 50% of trisomy 21) • Diagnostic test for fetal anomalies
Fetal echocardiography	√ for fetal cardiac anomalies	20–22 weeks	High-risk patients	• Diagnostic test for fetal cardiac anomalies
Cervical length (CL) and fetal fibronectin (fFN)	Assess risk for preterm birth	CL can be measured 16–32 weeks; fFN can be tested 22–34 weeks	High-risk patients	• CL is best measured by transvaginal ultrasound • These 2 tests can be used together to identify women at risk of preterm birth
Early glucose load test (GLT)	√ for GDM	16–20 weeks	High-risk patients	• 1-hour GLT is a screening test • If early GLT is negative, repeat at 24–28 weeks
Routine glucose load test (GLT)	√ for GDM	24–28 weeks	Everyone	• 1-hour GLT is a screening test; 3-hour GTT is required for diagnosis
Glucose tolerance test (GTT)	√ for GDM	After GLT	Only if GLT is positive	• 3-hour GTT is a diagnostic test for GDM
Third trimester				
Group B β-hemolytic streptococcus (GBS)	√ GBS perineal carrier status	35–36 weeks	Everyone	• If positive, treat intrapartum with IV penicillin to prevent early-onset neonatal GBS sepsis
Ultrasound	√ fetal growth √ follow progression of fetal anomalies	After 24 weeks	High-risk patients	• Only check estimated fetal weight (EFW) q 3–4 weeks given error of 15–20% in measurements
Ultrasound	√ amniotic fluid √ fetal presentation √ placental location	After 24 weeks	As clinically indicated	
Fetal testing	√ fetal wellbeing	After 24 weeks	As clinically indicated	• BPP/AFV can be done after 24 weeks • NST after 32 weeks, usually weekly

Obstetrics and Gynecology at a Glance, Fourth Edition. Errol R. Norwitz and John O. Schorge.

Table 41.1 Levels of perinatal care

Level of care	Responsibility	Appropriate provider
Basic (level I)	Risk-oriented prenatal record, physical exam, laboratory data, and interpretation of findings. Determine gestational age. Provide ongoing risk assessment with referral to a specialist, if indicated. Provide psychosocial support, childbirth education, and overall care coordination	Obstetricians, family practitioners, certified nurse midwives, other advance-practice nurses
Specialty (level II)	Basic care plus fetal diagnostic testing (eg, basic ultrasound, amniocentesis, genetic counseling). Expertise in the management of medical and obstetric complications	Obstetricians
Subspecialty (level III)	Basic and specialty care plus advanced fetal diagnosis (eg, targeted fetal ultrasound, fetal echo), genetic counseling, and advanced fetal diagnosis and therapy (eg, chorionic villous sampling, percutaneous umbilical cord blood sampling, intrauterine transfusion). Able to serve as a consultant to generalist obstetricians, surgeons, internists, and pediatricians. Expertise in the management of severe maternal complications	Subspecialists in maternal–fetal medicine, clinical genetics

Objectives of perinatal care
- To promote the health and wellbeing of the pregnant woman, fetus, infant, and family up to 1 year after birth.
- The major components of perinatal care include: (1) early and continuing risk assessment, including preconception assessment; (2) continued health promotion; and (3) both medical and psychosocial assessment and intervention.
- Three levels of perinatal care are described (in Table 41.1).

Issues that should be addressed routinely
- Establish accurate gestational age.
- Folate (400 μg daily for all reproductive age women).
- Identify and treat sexually transmitted infections (STIs), diabetes, thyroid disease, HIV, hepatitis B.
- Identify maternal phenylketonuria (PKU).
- Stop Coumadin (warfarin), vitamin A, and other teratogenic agents.
- Counsel on risks of smoking, alcohol, and illicit drug use.
- Counsel about appropriate use of seatbelts during pregnancy.
- Reassure about the safety of sexual intercourse and moderate exercise in uncomplicated pregnancy.
- Review symptoms/signs of pregnancy complications, including preterm labor and pre-eclampsia.
- Check rubella immunity status.
- Ask about chickenpox (consider checking varicella immunity status if no history of chickenpox).
- Counsel about toxoplasmosis prevention (transmitted in cat feces, uncooked meats, soil).
- Counsel about influenza vaccination in pregnancy.
- Counsel about food safety: avoid raw or undercooked meat, poultry, fish, shellfish, pâté, raw/unpasteurized dairy (listeriosis, toxoplasmosis); avoid large amounts of large fish (mercury).
- Prescribe multivitamins (especially for smokers, women with multiple pregnancies, poor diet, vegetarians).
- Encourage breastfeeding.

What makes your pregnancy high risk?
- Twenty percent (1 in 5) of pregnancies are high risk. Risk factors for adverse pregnancy outcome may exist before pregnancy or develop during pregnancy or labor (Figure 41.1).
- The content and timing of prenatal visits should vary depending on the risk status of the pregnant woman and her fetus (Figure 41.1). In low-risk women, prenatal visits are typically every 4 weeks to 28 weeks' gestation, every 2–3 weeks to 36 weeks' gestation, and then weekly until delivery.

High-risk pregnancies
Maternal factors
- Pre-existing medical conditions (pregestational diabetes, chronic hypertension, maternal cardiac disease, chronic renal disease, chronic pulmonary disease)
- Pre-eclampsia
- Gestational diabetes
- Morbid obesity
- Active venous thromboembolic disease
- Poor obstetric history (prior preterm birth, PPROM, IUGR, placental abruption, pre-eclampsia, recurrent miscarriage)
- Extremes of maternal age

Fetal factors
- Toxic exposure during pregnancy (to known environmental toxins, medications, illicit drugs)
- Known fetal structural or chromosomal anomaly
- Prior baby with a structural or chromosomal anomaly
- Family history of a genetic syndrome
- Multiple pregnancy (especially if monochorionic)
- IUGR
- Fetal macrosomia
- Isoimmunization
- Intra-amniotic infection
- Non-reassuring fetal testing ("fetal distress")

Uteroplacental factors
- Preterm premature rupture of fetal membranes
- Unexplained oligohydramnios
- Large uterine fibroids
- Prior uterine surgery, especially a "classic" hysterotomy
- Placental abruption
- Uterine anomaly
- Placenta previa
- Abnormal placentation (placenta accreta, increta, or percreta)
- Vasa previa
- Prior cervical insufficiency

Ob/Gyn is a primary care specialty
For some women, visiting obstetrics/gynecology (Ob/Gyn) for their annual physical exam may be their only interaction with the medical profession. As such, Ob/Gyn as a primary care specialty. An annual visit is an opportunity to screen for potential medical and psychosocial problems, such as:
- Screening for cervical cancer (Pap smear)
- Screening for breast cancer (self-examination, mammography)
- Screening for colon cancer (stool guaiac, colonoscopy)
- Screening for hypertension and hyperlipidcholesterolemia
- Screening for diabetes and thyroid disease, if indicated
- Discussing contraception
- Screening for domestic violence and depression
- Ensuring that vaccinations are up to date.

42 Infections in pregnancy: bacteria and protozoa

Figure 42.1 BACTERIAL AND PROTOZOAN INFECTIONS IN PREGNANCY

	Diagnosis	Organism	Maternal signs and symptoms	Fetal/neonatal effects
Bacteria	Group B streptococcus	Streptococcus agalactiae	Asymptomatic colonization Urinary tract infection Chorioamnionitis Endomyometritis	Early onset: neonatal sepsis Late onset: meningitis
	Chorioamnionitis	Polymicrobial • Bacteroides sp. • Streptococcus agalactiae • E. coli	Presents with fever; tachycardia, uterine tenderness, leukocytosis, and/or malodorous discharge	Neonatal sepsis
	Listeriosis	Listeria monocytogenes from unpasteurized cheese, processed meats	Asymptomatic (most common) Flu-like symptoms Fatigue (similar to infectious mononucleosis) Meningitis (rare)	Early onset: neonatal sepsis Late onset: meningitis
	Tuberculosis	Mycobacterium tuberculosis	Asymptomatic (most common) Active disease: cough, night sweats, weight loss, hemoptysis	Congenital tuberculosis may be fatal (especially tuberculous meningitis)
	Bacterial vaginosis	Overgrowth of normal vaginal bacteria	Preterm labor Vaginal discharge	Prematurity Low birthweight
	Gonorrhea	Neisseria gonorrhoeae	Preterm labor Chorioamnionitis Disseminated gonococcal infection Vaginal discharge	Neonatal sepsis Neonatal gonococcal ophthalmia
	Chlamydia	Chlamydia trachomatis	Asymptomatic Preterm labor Chorioamnionitis	Conjunctivitis Pneumonia
Protozoa	Toxoplasmosis	Toxoplasma gondii	Asymptomatic Fatigue Lymphadenopathy, myalgia	Abortion Intracranial calcifications Hepatosplenomegaly Chorioretinitis, convulsions
	Trichomoniasis	Trichomonas vaginalis	Vaginal discharge Premature rupture of fetal membranes	Low birthweight

Figure 42.2 PROTOCOLS FOR PREVENTION OF EARLY-ONSET NEONATAL GROUP B STREPTOCOCCUS (GBS) INFECTION

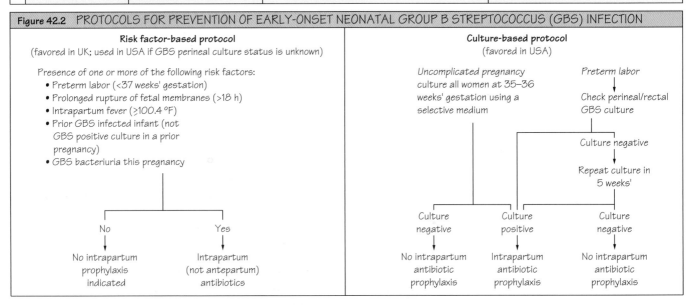

Risk factor-based protocol
(favored in UK; used in USA if GBS perineal culture status is unknown)

Presence of one or more of the following risk factors:
- Preterm labor (<37 weeks' gestation)
- Prolonged rupture of fetal membranes (>18 h)
- Intrapartum fever (≥100.4 °F)
- Prior GBS infected infant (not GBS positive culture in a prior pregnancy)
- GBS bacteriuria this pregnancy

No → No intrapartum prophylaxis indicated

Yes → Intrapartum (not antepartum) antibiotics

Culture-based protocol
(favored in USA)

Uncomplicated pregnancy culture all women at 35–36 weeks' gestation using a selective medium

Preterm labor → Check perineal/rectal GBS culture → Culture negative → Repeat culture in 5 weeks'

Culture negative → No intrapartum antibiotic prophylaxis

Culture positive → Intrapartum antibiotic prophylaxis

Culture negative → No intrapartum antibiotic prophylaxis

Bacterial infection (Figure 42.1)

Group B streptococcus

• *Incidence.* In developed countries, neonatal group B streptococcus (GBS) sepsis complicates 1.8/1,000 live births.
• *Maternal signs/symptoms.* Of all pregnant women 20% are asymptomatically colonized in the vaginal or perianal region.
• *Fetal/neonatal effects.* Two clinically distinct neonatal GBS infections have been identified:

1 *Early onset*, neonatal GBS infection (80%) results from transmission during labor or delivery. Signs of serious infection (respiratory distress, septic shock) usually develop within 6–12 hours of birth. The mortality rate is 25% and surviving infants frequently exhibit neurologic sequelae.

2 *Late-onset* GBS infection (20%) is a nosocomial or community-acquired infection. It presents more than a week after birth, usually as meningitis. The mortality rate is lower than for early onset disease, but neurologic sequelae are equally common.

• *Prevention.* Strategies to prevent early onset neonatal GBS infection vary. In the UK, a risk factor-based protocol is used. Patients are treated in labor if one of the following risk factors is present: a prior affected infant (not GBS positive in a prior pregnancy), GBS urinary tract infection (UTI) in index pregnancy, preterm labor, fever, or rupture of membranes ≥18 hours. This protocol results in the treatment of 15–20% of pregnant women and prevents 65–70% of early onset GBS sepsis. US practice favors a universal screening protocol. All women are screened for GBS carrier status at 35–37 weeks. Women who are GBS carriers receive intrapartum antibiotics. The latter protocol results in the treatment of 25–30% of pregnant women and prevents 85–90% of cases of early onset GBS sepsis. Patients with unknown GBS carrier status in labor should be treated according to the risk factor-based protocol.
• *Treatment.* Intrapartum penicillin (second-generation cephalosporin, erythromycin, or clindamycin if penicillin allergy and sensitivities available; vancomycin if penicillin allergy and no sensitivities available).

Chorioamnionitis

• *Incidence.* One to ten percent of pregnancies.
• *Maternal signs/symptoms.* Chorioamnionitis is a clinical diagnosis. Definitive diagnosis requires a positive amniotic fluid culture. Maternal complications may include sepsis, adult respiratory distress syndrome (ARDS), pulmonary edema, and death.
• *Fetal/neonatal effects.* Neonatal sepsis, pneumonia, death.
• *Prevention.* Avoidance of rupture of membranes >18 hours.
• *Treatment.* Prompt administration of broad-spectrum antibiotics and expedite delivery. Chorioamnionitis is not an indication for cesarean section delivery; however, the cesarean section rate is increased due to dysfunctional labor dystocia and non-reassuring fetal testing.

Listeriosis

• Listeriosis is an uncommon cause of neonatal sepsis that may be acquired transplacentally. Cervical and blood cultures should be obtained in women with suspicious symptoms. Listeriosis is a common cause of intrauterine fetal demise and neonatal mortality rate is high.
• *Treatment.* Ampicillin and gentamicin.

Tuberculosis

• *Incidence.* Tuberculosis (TB) in pregnant women is rare in developed countries. Cases occur most commonly among recent immigrants.
• *Maternal signs/symptoms.* Most infected women are asymptomatic. Active disease at presentation is rare.

Table 42.1 Interpretation of the PPD screening test for TB

Very high risk	High risk	No risk factors
HIV positive Abnormal chest radiograph Recent contact with an active case of TB ↓	Foreign born Intravenous drug use Medical condition increasing the risk of TB ↓	↓
≥5 mm is positive	≥10 mm is positive	≥15 mm of induration (not redness) is positive

• *Fetal/neonatal effects.* Congenital or neonatal TB is a highly morbid condition that may be fatal if misdiagnosed.
• *Prevention.* Intradermal placement of purified protein derivative (PPD) is an accurate way to screen for TB. Interpretation of the PPD test depends on the risk status of the patient (Table 42.1).
• *Treatment.* A positive PPD necessitates a chest radiograph. If the radiograph is normal, 6 months of isoniazid (INH) is recommended in women aged <35 years (can be deferred until after delivery). If the chest radiograph is abnormal, immediate treatment with INH and ethambutol is indicated, and three early morning sputum cultures should be sent to exclude active pulmonary TB.

Bacterial vaginosis (see Chapter 7)

Bacterial vaginosis (BV) is the most common cause of vaginal discharge in pregnancy. It is associated with preterm delivery in high-risk women. However, it remains unclear whether treatment for asymptomatic BV will reduce the risk of preterm delivery.

Chlamydia infection and gonorrhea (see Chapters 7 and 8)

• *Incidence.* Very prevalent sexually transmitted infections.
• *Maternal signs/symptoms.* Usually asymptomatic.
• *Fetal/neonatal effects.* Untreated maternal chlamydia and gonorrhea infections are associated with increased neonatal morbidity.
• *Prevention.* Cervical cultures in early pregnancy in high-risk women reliably detect infection. Instillation of prophylactic antibiotic ointment into the eyes of all newborns prevents eye infection.
• *Treatment.* *Chlamydia*: oral erythromycin or azithromycin; gonorrhea: intramuscular ceftriaxone, oral cefuroxime, or ceftriaxone.

Protozoan infections (Figure 42.1)

Toxoplasmosis

• *Incidence.* Acute toxoplasmosis during pregnancy is rare.
• *Maternal signs/symptoms.* Most patients are asymptomatic, but some have flu-like symptoms.
• *Fetal/neonatal effects.* Only acute toxoplasmosis in pregnancy is capable of being transmitted to the fetus; 10% of infected newborns will have clinical evidence of disease.
• *Prevention.* Toxoplasmosis is acquired through ingestion of encysted organisms in raw or undercooked meat or through contact with infected cat feces. Avoid cleaning litter box. Strict hygiene.
• *Treatment.* Sulfadiazine with pyrimethamine.

Trichomoniasis (see Chapter 7)

• *Vaginal trichomoniasis* is very common.
• *Treatment.* Metronidazole.

Infections in pregnancy: viruses and spirochetes

Figure 43.1 VIRAL AND SPIROCHETE INFECTIONS IN PREGNANCY

	Organism	Maternal signs and symptoms	Fetal/neonatal effects	Prevention	Management
Viruses	Rubella	Mild illness (rash, arthralgia, diffuse lymphadenopathy)	*Congenital rubella syndrome* • Deafness, eye lesions (cataracts), heart disease (patent ductus arteriosus), mental retardation, IUGR	MMR to children and non-immune (non-pregnant) adults	None
	Cytomegalovirus	• Asymptomatic (common) • Mild viral illness • Infectious mononucleosis-like syndrome • Hepatitis (rare)	*CMV inclusion disease* • Hepatosplenomegaly, intracranial calcification, chorioretinitis, learning disability, interstitial pneumonitis • 30% mortality • Hearing loss	None	None
	HIV	• Asymptomatic • Mild viral illness • AIDS	Childhood AIDS	Barrier contraception, abstinence, avoid IV drug use	Zidovudine (AZT) and possibly elective cesarean delivery to prevent vertical transmission. HAART if indicated.
	Varicella-zoster	• "Chickenpox" (most common) • Pneumonitis (10–20%) • Meningitis (rare) • Shingles	*Congenital varicella syndrome* • Chorioretinitis, cerebral cortical atrophy, hydronephrosis, longbone defects • Exposure <20 weeks' gestation *Near-term infection* • Benign chickenpox • Fulminant disseminated infection can be fatal	• VZV vaccine to non-immune (non-pregnant) adults • VZIG within 96 hours of VZV exposure and to neonates, if indicated	Acyclovir
	Herpes simplex virus (HSV)	*First-episode primary* • Systemic illness, fever, arthralgias, painful genital lesions, adenopathy *Recurrent infection* • Painful genital lesions (blister, ulcer)	• Herpetic lesions of the skin and mouth • Viral sepsis • Herpes encephalitis • Disseminated herpes simplex virus infection (long-term neurological sequelae, high mortality rate)	Cesarean section delivery if HSV lesion or symptoms are present in labor	Prophylactic acyclovir from 35–36 weeks to decrease incidence of active lesions in labor
	Hepatitis B and C	Mild/moderate viral illness (nausea, vomiting, hepatosplenomegaly, jaundice, right upper quadrant pain)	Chronic hepatitis carrier	• Avoid sexual contact with infected partners, IV drug abuse, infected blood • Hepatitis B vaccine (no vaccine for HCV)	Hepatitis B immune globulin (HBIG) and hepatitis B vaccine to neonate. Consider antiretroviral therapy if hepatitis B viral load is high.
Spirochetes	Syphilis (*Treponema pallidum*)	• Primary (solitary genital tract lesion or gumma) • Secondary (rash, snail-track ulcers in the mouth, adenopathy, condylomata lata) • Tertiary neurosyphilis or meningovascular syphilis	• Stillbirth *Early congenital syphilis* • Maculopapular rash • 'Sniffles' • Hepatosplenomegaly • Chorioretinitis *Late congenital syphilis* • Hutchinson teeth • Mulberry molars • Saber shins • Cardiovascular anomalies • Sensorineural deafness	• Avoid sexual contact with infected partners • Treat infected women to prevent vertical transmission	Penicillin (in pregnancy, women who are allergic to penicillin should undergo penicillin desensitization and then be treated with penicillin)
	Lyme disease (*Borrelia burgdorferi*)	• Local infection (fever, erythema chronicum migrans, adenopathy) • Disseminated disease	• Prematurity • Stillbirth • Rash-like neonatal illness	Avoid tick bites (long trousers, sprays, remove all ticks)	Erythromycin

Obstetrics and Gynecology at a Glance, Fourth Edition. Errol R. Norwitz and John O. Schorge.

Viral infections (Figure 43.1)

Rubella

- *Incidence.* Rare in developed countries.
- *Transmission.* Airborne.
- *Maternal signs/symptoms.* Rubella ("German measles") is usually a mild viral illness.
- *Diagnosis.* Serologic diagnosis requires either the presence of IgM or a significant rise in IgG antibody titer (fourfold rise over 4–6 weeks).
- *Fetal/neonatal effects.* The risk of congenital rubella syndrome is 90% if maternal infection is acquired <11 weeks, 33% if 11–12 weeks, 11% if 13–14 weeks, 4% if 15–16 weeks, 0% if >16 weeks.
- *Prevention.* Measles/mumps/rubella (MMR) immunization. MMR is a live vaccine and is not recommended in pregnancy.
- *Management.* There is no treatment.

Cytomegalovirus (CMV)

- *Incidence.* One to two percent of all births.
- *Transmission.* Contact with body fluids, sexual contact.
- *Maternal signs/symptoms.* Of women 20% have a non-specific viral syndrome (fever, pharyngitis, lymphadenopathy).
- *Diagnosis.* The high prevalence of CMV seroreactivity (>50%) and multiple CMV serotypes limits the value of serologic screening.
- *Fetal/neonatal effects.* Of infected newborns 90% are asymptomatic at birth, but many later demonstrate deafness, learning disability, and/or delayed psychomotor development.
- *Prevention.* There is no vaccine.
- *Management.* There is no treatment.

Human immunodeficiency virus

- *Incidence.* Rare in developed countries, but very high prevalence in developing countries (eg, almost one in three pregnant women in South Africa is HIV positive).
- *Transmission.* Sexual contact, intravenous drug use, vertical transmission.
- *Maternal signs/symptoms.* Variable.
- *Diagnosis.* Serum enzyme-linked immunosorbent assay (ELISA) and confirmatory western blot.
- *Fetal/neonatal effects.* HIV-positive infants may develop AIDS with high perinatal mortality rate.
- *Prevention.* Safe sexual practices, avoidance of high-risk drug behavior, serial serum viral load measurements, and antiviral therapy, if indicated.
- *Management.* Prenatal HIV testing. Zidovudine (AZT) therapy reduces the risk of vertical transmission from 25–33% to 8%, with a further reduction to 0–2% if the viral load is <1,000 copies/mL. Elective cesarean delivery may reduce vertical transmission if viral load is ≥1,000 copies/mL. Continue highly active antiretroviral therapy (HAART) if the patient is already on it or consider initiating such treatment in pregnancy.

Varicella-zoster virus

- *Incidence.* One in 7,500 pregnancies.
- *Transmission.* Airborne (highly infectious).
- *Maternal signs/symptoms.* "Chickenpox." The maternal mortality rate approaches 50% for adults with pneumonitis or encephalitis.
- *Diagnosis.* Clinical suspicion. Confirmatory serologic tests.
- *Fetal/neonatal effects.* First trimester varicella-zoster virus (VZV) has a 2–3% risk of congenital varicella syndrome. Near-term infections resemble benign childhood infection.

- *Prevention.* Only 5% of adults are not immune to VZV. Consider VZIG (varicella-zoster immune globulin) or acyclovir if a susceptible woman is exposed in pregnancy.
- *Management.* Delivery should be avoided at the time of acute maternal infection. At-risk neonates should receive VZIG. Acyclovir may also be helpful.

Herpes simplex virus (see Chapter 7)

- *Incidence.* Neonatal herpes simplex virus (HSV) infection occurs in 2–4 per 10,000 births.
- *Transmission.* Direct contact.
- *Maternal signs/symptoms.* First-episode primary genital HSV may be associated with systemic symptoms. Both primary and recurrent HSV are characterized by painful, vesicular lesions.
- *Fetal/neonatal effects.* Neonatal herpes is acquired from passage through an infected birth canal. The risk of vertical transmission is 50% for primary HSV infection and 0–4% in women with recurrent disease.
- *Prevention.* Cesarean section delivery is recommended for all pregnancies complicated by primary genital HSV in labor. The management of women with a recurrent genital HSV outbreak (either lesion and/or symptoms) in labor is less clear. In the UK, such women are allowed to deliver vaginally. US practice favors cesarean section delivery for such women.
- *Management.* Prophylactic acyclovir from 35 weeks to 36 weeks may be useful in preventing active lesions in labor in some high-risk women.

Hepatitis B and C

- *Incidence.* One to two percent of pregnancies.
- *Transmission.* Sexual contact, intravenous drug use, vertical transmission.
- *Maternal signs/symptoms.* Usually mild/moderate viral illness.
- *Diagnosis.* Serologic testing.
- *Fetal/neonatal effects.* Hepatitis B and C are not teratogenic, but affected infants may become carriers. Vertical transmission rates of hepatitis B range from 15% (in women who are e-antigen negative) to 80% (e-antigen positive), and of hepatitis C from 0–5% (HIV-negative women) to 35–50% (HIV-positive women).
- *Prevention.* Safe sexual practices, avoidance of high-risk drug behavior. Breastfeeding is controversial, but is best avoided. Hepatitis B has an effective vaccine.
- *Management.* Infants born to women with detectable hepatitis B surface antigen (HBsAg) should receive hepatitis B immunoglobulin (HBIg) and hepatitis B vaccine within 12 hours of birth. There is no effective treatment for hepatitis C.

Spirochete infections (Figure 43.1)

Syphilis (see Chapter 7)

- *Incidence.* Rare in developed countries.
- *Transmission.* Sexual contact.
- *Maternal signs/symptoms.* Patients may exhibit primary, secondary, or tertiary syphilis.
- *Diagnosis.* Serum *r*apid *p*lasma *r*eagin (RPR) or *V*enereal *D*isease *R*esearch *L*aboratory (VDRL) test. Confirmatory tests are required before instituting treatment.
- *Fetal/neonatal effects.* Affected infants may be stillborn or exhibit signs of early or late congenital syphilis.
- *Prevention.* Safe sexual practices. Congenital syphilis is unusual if the mother is treated.
- *Management.* Penicillin.

Figure 44.1 RISK FACTORS FOR PRE-ECLAMPSIA

Nulliparity
African-American/African race
Prior history of pre-eclampsia
Extremes of maternal age (<15 or >35 years)
Family history of pre-eclampsia
Multiple gestation
Chronic hypertension
Chronic renal disease
Antiphospholipid antibody syndrome
Collagen vascular disease
Angiotensinogen gene T235 mutation

Figure 44.2 DIAGNOSIS OF PRE-ECLAMPSIA

Hypertension

Clinical triad

Proteinuria   ± Non-dependent edema

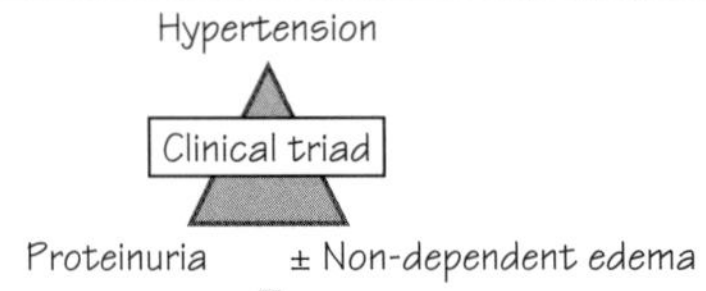

Figure 44.3 CLASSIFICATION OF PRE-ECLAMPSIA

'Severe' pre-eclampsia

Note: only one of the features listed below is required for diagnosis

'Mild' pre-eclampsia

- Includes all women with a diagnosis of pre-eclampsia, but without features of 'severe' pre-eclampsia

Symptoms	Signs	Laboratory findings
• Symptoms of central nervous system dysfunction (severe headache, blurred vision, scotomas) • Symptoms of liver capsule distention (right upper quadrant and/or epigastric pain)	• Severe elevations in BP (defined as BP ≥160/110 on two occasions at least 6 hours apart) • Pulmonary edema • Eclampsia (generalized seizures or unexplained coma) • Cerebrovascular accident • IUGR	• Proteinuria (>5 g/24 h) • Renal failure or oliguria (<500 mL/24 h) • Hepatocellular injury (serum transaminase levels >2x normal) • Thrombocytopenia (<100,000 platelets/mm^3) • Coagulopathy • HELLP (hemolysis, elevated liver enzymes, low platelets)

Figure 44.4 SHORT-TERM COMPLICATIONS

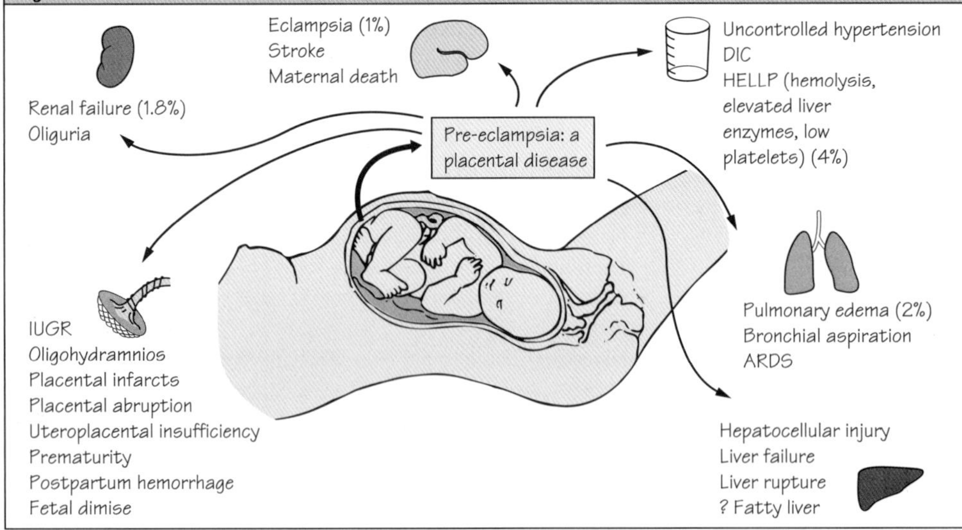

Eclampsia (1%)
Stroke
Maternal death

Renal failure (1.8%)
Oliguria

Pre-eclampsia: a placental disease

Uncontrolled hypertension
DIC
HELLP (hemolysis, elevated liver enzymes, low platelets) (4%)

IUGR
Oligohydramnios
Placental infarcts
Placental abruption
Uteroplacental insufficiency
Prematurity
Postpartum hemorrhage
Fetal dimise

Pulmonary edema (2%)
Bronchial aspiration
ARDS

Hepatocellular injury
Liver failure
Liver rupture
? Fatty liver

LONG-TERM EFFECTS

- Complications of pre-eclampsia almost always resolve completely (with the exception of cerebrovascular accident)
- ↑Risk of chronic hypertension
- Does not preclude use of OCPs (if BP returns to normal)
- ↑Risk of pre-eclampsia/eclampsia in a subsequent pregnancy (+ 25%); depends on severity, gestational age, and pressure of underlying medical conditions
- Recurrence rate for eclampsia is 10%
- ↑Risk of other obstetric complications in a subsequent pregnancy (placental abruption, IUGR, preterm labor, ↑perinatal mortality)

Hypertensive disorders of pregnancy are the second most common cause of maternal death in developed countries (after embolism), accounting for 15% of all maternal deaths.

Effects of pregnancy on maternal cardiovascular system

- Blood volume increases 800 mL by 12 weeks (1.5 L in twins).
- Blood pressure (BP) decreases in early pregnancy (due primarily to a decrease in systemic vascular resistance secondary to progesterone), nadirs in mid-pregnancy, and returns to baseline by term.

Classification

1 Chronic hypertension

- *Definition.* Hypertension before pregnancy. The diagnosis should also be entertained in women with BP ≥140/90 mmHg before 20 weeks' gestation.
- *Complications.* Such pregnancies are at increased risk of superimposed pre-eclampsia, intrauterine fetal growth restriction (IUGR), placental abruption, and stillbirth.
- *Management.* Continue antihypertensive medications with the exception of angiotensin-converting enzyme (ACE) inhibitors. These drugs have been associated with progressive and irreversible renal injury and possibly other structural anomalies in the fetus. Diuretic therapy is generally discouraged.
- Fetal testing (serial ultrasound examinations for fetal growth with or without fetal non-stress testing) should be initiated after 32 weeks' gestation. Delivery should be achieved by 40 weeks.

2 Chronic hypertension with superimposed pre-eclampsia (see Preeclampsia below)

3 Gestational hypertension

- Also known as gestational non-proteinuric hypertension.
- *Diagnosis.* Persistent elevation of BP ≥140/90 mmHg in the third trimester without evidence of pre-eclampsia. It is a diagnosis of exclusion that is best made retrospectively.
- *Etiology.* It probably represents an exaggerated physiologic response of the maternal cardiovascular system to pregnancy.
- Rarely associated with adverse maternal or fetal outcome.

4 Preeclampsia

- Also known as gestational proteinuric hypertension, preeclamptic toxemia (PET).
- *Definition.* A multisystem disorder specific to pregnancy and the puerperium. More precisely, it is a disease of the placenta because it occurs in pregnancies where there is trophoblast but no fetal tissue (complete molar pregnancies).
- *Incidence.* Six to eight percent of all pregnancies.
- *Risk factors* (Figure 44.1).
- *Diagnosis* (Figure 44.2). A clinical diagnosis with two elements:

  1 *New-onset hypertension* defined as a sustained sitting BP ≥140/90 mmHg in a previously normotensive woman (a prior definition included an elevation in systolic BP ≥30 or diastolic BP ≥15 mmHg over first trimester BP, but these criteria have now been dropped).

  2 *New-onset significant proteinuria* defined as >300 mg/24 h or ≥1+ on a clean-catch urine in the absence of urinary tract infection.

Note. A definitive diagnosis of preeclampsia should only be made after 20 weeks' gestation. Evidence of gestational proteinuric hypertension before 20 weeks should raise the possibility of an underlying molar pregnancy, drug withdrawal, or (rarely) chromosomal abnormality in the fetus.

- *Classification* (Figure 44.3). Preeclampsia is classified as "mild" or "severe." There is no category of "moderate" pre-eclampsia.
- *Etiology.* The cause of preeclampsia is not known. Theories include an abnormal maternal immunologic response to the fetal allograft, an underlying genetic abnormality, an imbalance in the prostanoid cascade, and the presence of circulating toxins and/or endogenous vasoconstrictors. What is known is that the blueprint for the development of preeclampsia is laid down early in pregnancy. The primary event is a failure of the second wave of trophoblast invasion from 8 weeks to 18 weeks, which is responsible for remodeling of the spiral arterioles in the myometrium adjacent to the developing placenta, and establishment of the definitive uteroplacental circulation. As pregnancy progresses and the metabolic demand of the fetoplacental unit increases, the spiral arterioles are therefore unable to accommodate the necessary increase in blood flow. This then leads to the development of "placental dysfunction" which manifests clinically as preeclampsia. Although attractive, this hypothesis remains to be validated. Whatever the placental abnormality, the end-result is widespread vasospasm and endothelial injury.
- *Complications* (Figure 44.4). Eclampsia – defined as one or more generalized convulsions or coma in the setting of preeclampsia and in the absence of other neurologic conditions – was thought to be the end stage of preeclampsia, hence the nomenclature. It is now clear, however, that seizures are but one clinical manifestation of "severe" pre-eclampsia; 50% of eclampsia occurs preterm. Of those at term, 75% occur either intrapartum or within 48 hours of delivery.
- *Management.* Delivery is the only effective treatment for pre-eclampsia, and is recommended:

  1 in women with "mild" preeclampsia once a favorable gestational age has been reached (>36–37 weeks).

  2 in all women with "severe" preeclampsia regardless of gestational age (with the exception of "severe" preeclampsia due to proteinuria alone or intrauterine growth restriction [IUGR] remote from term with good fetal testing). There has also been a recent trend toward expectant management of "severe" preeclampsia by BP criteria alone at <32 weeks' gestation.

- There is no proven benefit to routine delivery by cesarean section. However, the probability of vaginal delivery in a patient with preeclampsia remote from term with an unfavorable cervix is only 15–20%.
- BP control is important to prevent cerebrovascular accident (usually associated with BP ≥170/120 mmHg), but does not affect the natural course of preeclampsia.
- Intravenous magnesium sulfate should be given intrapartum and for at least 24 hours postpartum to prevent eclampsia.
- *Prevention.* Despite promising early studies, low-dose aspirin (acetylsalicylic acid or ASA) and/or supplemental calcium does not prevent preeclampsia in either high- or low-risk women.
- *Prognosis.* Preeclampsia and its complications always resolve after delivery (with the exception of cerebrovascular accident). Diuresis (>4 L/day) is the most accurate clinical indicator of resolution. Fetal prognosis is dependent largely on gestational age at delivery and problems related to prematurity.

Figure 45.1 MATERNAL COMPLICATIONS OF PREGESTATIONAL DIABETES

- Pre-eclampsia (12%)
- Chronic hypertension (10%)
- Diabetic ketoacidosis (8%)
- Polyhydramnios (18%)
- Preterm labor (8%)
- Cesarean section delivery (20–60%)
- Other obstetric emergencies (hypoglycemia, coma)
- Genetic transmission (infants of mothers with type 1 diabetes have a 4–5% risk of acquiring diabetes; infants of mothers with type 2 diabetes have a 25–50% risk of diabetes)

Figure 45.2 FETAL COMPLICATIONS OF PREGESTATIONAL DIABETES

Complications

- Congenital abnormalities
- Spontaneous abortion (↑ 2–3 x)
- Diabetic ketoacidosis (50–90% fetal mortality)
- Intrauterine growth restriction
- Late intrauterine fetal demise
- Fetal macrosomia (with or without birth injury)
- Delayed organ maturation
  - respiratory distress syndrome (RDS)
  - neonatal hypoglycemia
  - neonatal hypocalcemia
  - neonatal hypomagnesemia
  - polycythemia/hyperviscosity
  - neonatal hyperbilirubinemia (40%)

- Incidence of major anomalies is 5–10% (↑ 2–3 x) compared with controls
- Accounts for 50% of all perinatal deaths
- Incidence is related to HbA1c (if <8.5%, 3% anomalies; if ≥8.5%, 22% anomalies)

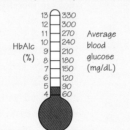

HbA1c (%) | Average blood glucose (mg/dL)
13 — 330
12 — 300
11 — 270
10 — 240
9 — 210
8 — 180
7 — 150
6 — 120
5 — 90
4 — 60

Congenital anomalies in infants of diabetic mothers

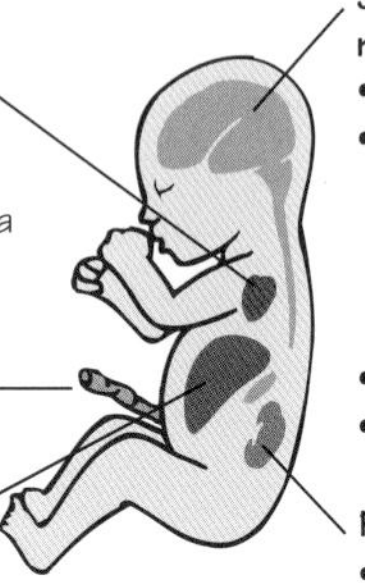

Cardiac
- Atrial septal defect
- Ventricular septal defect
- Coarctation of aorta
- Transposition of great vessels

Other
- Single umbilical artery

Gastrointestinal
- Anorectal atresia
- Duodenal atresia
- Tracheo-esophageal fistula

Skeletal and central nervous system
- Anencephaly
- Caudal regression syndrome (very rare, but highly specific for diabetes mellitus)
- Microcephaly
- Neural tube defect

Renal
- Hydronephrosis
- Renal agenesis
- Ureteral duplication
- Polycystic kidneys

Figure 45.3 RECOMMENDATIONS FOR ANTEPARTUM MANAGEMENT OF PREGESTATIONAL DIABETES

Strict glucose control using:
- Diabetic diet (36 kcal/kg or 15 kcal/lb of ideal body weight + 100 kcal per trimester given as 40–50% carbohydrate, 20% protein, 30–40% fat to avoid protein catabolism)
- Insulin (insulin therapy should be individualized, but a common regimen is 0.7–1.0 units/kg/day given 2/3 in AM (2/3 NPH, 1/3 rapid/short acting) and 1/3 in PM (50% NPH, 50% rapid/short acting))
- Goal: fasting blood glucose <95 mg/dL; 1 h postprandial blood glucose <140 mg/dL
- Home monitoring of blood sugar at least 4 x per day

Ophthalmological examination every trimester
Detailed sonographic fetal structural survey at 18–22 weeks' gestation (including fetal echocardiogram)
Consider checking thyroid functions (6% have co-existing thyroid disease), baseline preeclampsia blood tests, 24-hour urinary protein and creatinine clearance
HbA1c (above)
Fetal testing (NST, ultrasound for growth) after 32 weeks given risk of intrauterine growth restriction and fetal demise

Extent and duration of action of various types of insulin

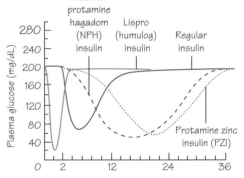

Neutral protamine hagadom (NPH) insulin

Lispro (humulog) insulin

Regular insulin

Protamine zinc insulin (PZI)

Plasma glucose (mg/dL): 280, 240, 200, 160, 120, 80, 40
(x-axis): 0, 2, 12, 24, 36

Gestational diabetes

Physiology

Pregnancy is a "diabetogenic state" with increased insulin resistance and reduced peripheral uptake of glucose (due to placental hormones with anti-insulin activity). In this way, the fetus has a continuous supply of glucose.

Incidence

Three to five percent of pregnancies.

Maternal complications

• Gestational diabetes poses little risk to the mother. Such women are not at risk of diabetic ketoacidosis (DKA), which is a disease resulting from an absolute deficiency of insulin.
• Care should be taken to avoid iatrogenic hypoglycemia due to excessive insulin administration.
• Gestational diabetes is a good screening test for insulin resistance; 50% will develop gestational diabetes in a subsequent pregnancy, and 40–60% will develop diabetes later in life.

Fetal complications

Fetuses of women with poorly controlled gestational diabetes are exposed to high concentrations of glucose and, as a result, grow large. Fetal macrosomia (see Chapter 51) is associated with an increased risk of cesarean section delivery and birth injury (see Chapter 63).

Screening

• *Glucose load test* (GLT) is used to screen for gestational diabetes. In the UK, screening is recommended only for high-risk women at approximately 28 weeks. Risk factors include women with a family history of diabetes, sustained glycosuria, obesity, or a history of gestational diabetes, fetus macrosomia, or unexplained fetal demise. US practice favors screening all pregnant women at 24–28 weeks, and high-risk women in the first trimester at 16–20 weeks and again at 24–28 weeks.
• GLT is a non-fasting test, but women should not eat after their 50-g glucose load until a venous blood sample is drawn 1 hour later. A positive test should be followed by a *glucose tolerance test* (GTT). A GLT cut-off of ≥7.8 mmol/L (≥140 mg/dL) will detect 80% of women with gestational diabetes with a false-positive rate of 14–18%; a cut-off of ≥7.2 mmol/L (≥130 mg/dL) will detect 90% with a false-positive rate of 20–25%.
• A definitive diagnosis of gestational diabetes requires a GTT; there is no GLT cut-off that is diagnostic. In the UK, a 2-hour 75-g GTT is used. Fasting glucose >5.5 mmol/L (>100 mg/dL) and at 2 hours >7.9 mmol/L (>140 mg/dL) will confirm the diagnosis. In the USA, a GTT involves a 100-g glucose load administered after an overnight fast. Venous plasma glucose is measured fasting and at 1, 2, and 3 hours. Gestational diabetes requires two or more abnormal values, defined by the NDDG as ≥105 (≥5.8), ≥190 (≥10.5), ≥165 (≥9.1), and ≥145 mg/dL (≥8.0 mmol/L), respectively. Other cutoffs exist (such as the Carpenter and Coustan criteria).

Antepartum management

• The primary aim is to prevent fetal macrosomia and its complications by maintaining blood glucose at desirable levels (defined as fasting, <95 mg/dL [<5.2 mmol/L] and 1 hour postprandial, <140 mg/dL [<7.8 mmol/L]).
• A diabetic diet is recommended for all such women.
• Treatment may be required. If fasting glucose levels are >95 mg/dL (>5.2 mmol/L), therapy can be initiated right away because "you cannot diet more than fasting." Although insulin remains the "gold standard" for the treatment of gestational diabetes in pregnancy, the use of oral hypoglycemic agents is becoming more common.

Intrapartum management

• Cesarean section delivery may be appropriate if the estimated fetal weight is excessive because of the risk of birth injury (see Chapter 63).
• As the primary source of anti-insulin hormones is the placenta, no further management is required in the immediate postpartum period.
• All women with gestational diabetes should have a standard (non-pregnant) 75-g GTT 6–8 weeks postpartum, because such women are at increased risk of developing diabetes in later life.

Pregestational diabetes

Pathophysiology

Results from either an absolute deficiency of insulin (type 1 or insulin-dependent diabetes mellitus) or increased peripheral resistance to insulin (type 2 or non-insulin-dependent diabetes mellitus).

Incidence

Less than 1% of women of childbearing age.

Classification

• The age of onset and duration of diabetes (White classification) does not correlate with pregnancy outcome.
• Poor prognostic features include DKA, poor compliance, hypertension, pyelonephritis, and vasculopathy.

Complications

In contrast with gestational diabetes, pregestational diabetes is associated with significant maternal and perinatal mortality and morbidity (Figures 45.1 and 45.2).

Antepartum management (Figure 45.3)

• Diabetic women should ideally be seen before conception. Pregnancy complications such as fetal congenital anomalies and spontaneous abortion correlate directly with the degree of diabetic control at conception.
• Intense antepartum management can reduce the perinatal mortality rate from 20% to 3–5%.
• Approximately 5% of maternal hemoglobin is glycated (bound to glucose), known as hemoglobin A1 (HbA1). HbA1c refers to the 80–85% of HbA1 that is irreversibly glycated. As red blood cells have a lifespan of 120 days, HbA1c measurements reflect the degree of glycemic control over the previous 3–4 months. HbA1c measurements should be checked before conception, at first prenatal visit, and every 4–6 weeks throughout pregnancy.

Intrapartum and postpartum management

• If metabolic control is good, spontaneous labor at term can be awaited. As a result of the risk of unexplained fetal demise, women with pregestational diabetes should be delivered by 39–40 weeks.
• If the estimated fetal weight is excessive (likely ≥4,500 g), elective cesarean section may be appropriate to avoid birth injury.
• Women may not eat during labor. As such, intravenous glucose should be administered (5% dextrose at 75–100 mL/h) and blood glucose levels checked every 1–2 hours. Regular insulin should be given by subcutaneous injection or intravenous infusion to maintain blood glucose levels at 100–120 mg/dL (5.5–6.6 mmol/L).
• During the first 48 hours postpartum, women may have a "honeymoon period" during which their insulin requirement is decreased. Blood glucose levels of 150–200 mg/dL (8.2–11.0 mmol/L) can be tolerated during this period. Once a woman is able to eat, she can be placed back on her usual regular insulin regimen.

Figure 46.1 MANAGEMENT OF SPECIFIC CARDIAC LESIONS IN PREGNANCY

Septal defects

- If lesions are small, patients are usually asymptomatic and require no specific treatment.
- Large ventricular septal defects (VSD) are associated with aortic insufficiency, congestive cardiac failure, arrhythmias, pulmonary hypertension.
- Air filters on all IV lines to prevent paradoxical air embolism

Right-to-left shunts

- Due to pulmonary hypertension with shunting of blood away from lungs
- In pregnancy, decreased systemic vascular resistance worsens shunt with increased hypoxia
- Management: avoid hypotension, maintain preload, oxygen, air filters on IV lines

Mitral/aortic valve stenosis

- Such lesions are particularly dangerous in pregnancy because of the fixed cardiac output and left atrial dilatation (which can result in arrhythmias and/or thrombus formation)
- Management: maintain preload, avoid tachycardia. Consider β-blockers for persistent heart rate >90–100 bpm. Adequate pain relief in labor to minimize tachycardia
- Autotransfusion immediately postpartum can precipitate pulmonary edema

Mitral valve prolapse

- Patients are generally asymptomatic
- Treat symptomatic prolapse with β-blocker

Prosthetic valves

- Risks include embolization, valvular dysfunction, and infection (bacterial endocarditis)
- Management: therapeutic anticoagulation for any mechanical valve, antibiotic prophylaxis against endocarditis

Prophylaxis against bacterial endocarditis

- Vaginal delivery is associated with 2–3% risk of bacteraemia
- AHA recommends endocarditis prophylaxis only for:
  (i) prosthetic heart valve/patch, (ii) prior infectious endocarditis, (iii) heart transplant, or (iv) unrepaired/partially repaired congenital heart disease

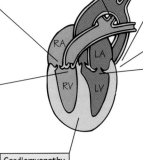

Cardiomyopathy

- Presents with left ventricular dysfunction and global dilatation
- Increased cardiac output in pregnancy may lead to decompensation
- Management: avoid hypotension, careful volume replacement, inotropic support to maximize cardiac output if needed

Regimens for endocarditis prophylaxis during labor and delivery	
Low risk regimen	Amoxicillin, 3 g p.o. 1 h before procedure or at onset of labor Repeat 1.5 g p.o q.6 h until after delivery
Standard regime	Ampicillin, 2 g i.v. plus gentamicin, 1.5 mg/kg i.v. (do not exceed 80 mg) 30 min before procedure or at onset of labor. Repeat above q.8 h until after delivery
Penicillin-allergic	Substitute vancomycin, 1 g i.v. over 1 h q.12 h

Figure 46.2 DIAGNOSIS OF DEEP VEIN THROMBOSIS

Pregnancy predisposes to thromboembolism

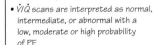

Virchow's triad describes the underlying principles of clot formation

Venous stasis — Vessel wall damage
Hypercoagulable state

CLINICAL FEATURES OF DEEP VEIN THROMBOSIS	
History:	unilateral swelling and/or pain in the calf or thigh
Examination:	may confirm unilateral swelling with or without calf tenderness or a tender 'cord' of thrombus. Homan's sign (ipsilateral calf pain on passive dorsiflexion of the foot) is only 30–40% predictive of DVT

RADIOLOGICAL STUDIES TO CONFIRM DEEP VEIN THROMBOSIS

Study	Accuracy	Comment
Doppler ultrasound*		Non-invasive, cheap, but
Proximal veins	85–95%	poor for the detection of
Calf veins	≤50%	distal thrombosis
Impedance plethysmography		Non-invasive, cheap, but
Proximal veins	90–95%	poor for the detection of
Calf veins	<30%	distal thrombosis
Venography		Accurate, but invasive with
Proximal veins	95–99%	a risk of hemorrhage
[^{125}I] Fibrinogen		Accurate, contraindicated
Distal to mid-thigh	80–90%	in pregnancy

*also known as lower extremity non-invasive (LENI) test

Figure 46.3 DIAGNOSIS OF PULMONARY EMBOLISM

Clinical features

History:	tachycardia, shortness of breath, tachypnea, pleuritic chest pain, cough, and/or hemoptysis
Examination:	may show cyanosis, pulmonary rales, and/or a friction rub. The most sensitive sign of PE is unexplained tachycardia
Labs:	EKG may show right-heart strain (S_1, Q_3, T_3 with right axis deviation). Although useful to evaluate response to treatment, arterial blood gas (ABG) is not useful in the diagnosis of PE. 70% of women with PE will have evidence of DVT on LENI.

Ventilation-perfusion ($\dot{V}/\dot{Q}$) scan

- $\dot{V}/\dot{Q}$ scans are interpreted as normal, intermediate, or abnormal with a low, moderate or high probability of PE
- If the perfusion scan is normal, PE can be reliably excluded
- Data from the 'prospective investigation of pulmonary embolism diagnosis' (PIOPED) study show that overall abnormal studies are sensitive (96%), but not specific (10%)
- A high-probability scan (one showing mismatched perfusion defects) is highly specific (97%)

Pulmonary angiography

- The most accurate test for PE, but is invasive with a number of potentially serious side-effects (hemorrhage, acute renal failure, pneumothorax)

Assessing need for pulmonary angiography			
$\dot{V}/\dot{Q}$ scan category	Clinical suspicion		
	High	Intermediate	Low
High	96%	88%	56%*
Intermediate	66%*	28%*	16%
Low	40%*	16%	4%

* pulmonary angiography indicated

Obstetrics and Gynecology at a Glance, Fourth Edition. Errol R. Norwitz and John O. Schorge.

100 © 2013 John Wiley & Sons, Ltd. Published 2013 by John Wiley & Sons, Ltd.

Maternal heart disease in pregnancy

Incidence

One percent of pregnancies.

Etiology

• Congenital lesions account for >50% of heart disease in pregnancy.
• Other common causes include coronary artery disease, hypertension, and thyroid dysfunction. Rare causes include myocarditis, cor pulmonale, cardiomyopathy, constrictive pericarditis, and cardiac dysrhythmias. Historically, rheumatic fever accounted for 90% of heart disease in pregnancy, but is now rare.

Prognosis

Prognosis depends on four factors:

1 *Cardiac function.* A clinical classification was developed by the New York Heart Association (NYHA) in 1928 (*see table below*):
2 *Clinical conditions* that may further increase cardiac output (multiple gestation, anemia, thyroid disease).
3 *Medications.*
4 The specific nature of the *cardiac lesion.*

Management (Figure 46.1)

• Allow spontaneous labor at term. Scheduled induction is indicated for women requiring invasive cardiac monitoring.
• Adequate pain relief (regional analgesia is preferred).
• Left lateral positioning with supplemental oxygen.
• Maternal pulse oximetry and ECG monitoring.
• Fluid intake and output monitoring.
• Consider invasive hemodynamic monitoring for women with NYHA class III and IV disease.
• Consider elective shortening of the second stage of labor.

Table 46.1 Maternal mortality associated with specific heart lesions

Group 1 (mortality rate <%)		Atrial septal defect
		Ventricular septal defect
		Patent ductus arteriosus
		Tetralogy of Fallot (surgically corrected)
		Bioprosthetic valve
		Pulmonary/tricuspid valve disease
		Mitral stenosis (NYHA class I and II)
Group 2 (mortality rate 5–10%)	2A	Aortic stenosis
		Mitral stenosis (NYHA class III and IV)
		Coarctation of aorta (no valvular involvement)
		Tetralogy of Fallot (uncorrected)
		Previous myocardial infarction
		Marfan syndrome with normal aorta
	2B	Mitral stenosis with atrial fibrillation
		Artificial valve
		Pulmonary hypertension
Group 3 (mortality rate 25–50%)		Coarctation of aorta (with valvular involvement)
		Marfan syndrome with aortic involvement

Table 46.2 New York Heart Association (NYHA) clinical classification of maternal heart disease

Class		
I	Uncompromised	No limitation of normal physical activity
II	Slightly compromised	Slight limitation of normal physical activity
III	Markedly compromised	Symptoms with normal activity
IV	Severely compromised	Symptoms at rest

Thromboembolic disease in pregnancy

Incidence

• The leading obstetric cause of maternal mortality.
• Deep vein thrombosis (DVT) complicates 0.05–0.3% of all pregnancies (Figure 46.2). It is three- to fivefold more common in the puerperium, and three- to fifteenfold more common after cesarean section delivery. If untreated, 15–25% of patients with DVT will have a pulmonary embolus (PE) compared with 4–5% of treated patients (Figure 46.3).

Etiology

Pregnancy is a thrombogenic state. Thromboembolic events are fivefold more common in pregnancy than in non-pregnant women. Other predisposing factors include trauma (surgery), infection, obesity, advanced maternal age, and underlying thrombophilia (*below*).

Treatment

• *Unfractionated heparin* is the treatment of choice for acute thromboembolism. It must be given intravenously or subcutaneously to keep the PTT (partial thromboplastin time) at 1.5–2.0 times normal. Heparin does not cross the placenta and, as such, is not teratogenic. Adverse effects include hemorrhage (5–10%), thrombocytopenia (2%), and osteoporosis (dose related). In the setting of acute hemorrhage, protamine sulfate can be given to reverse heparin action.
• *Low-molecular-weight heparin* (LMWH) is replacing unfractionated heparin in non-pregnant women. Although safe, its efficacy in pregnancy is not well validated. As a result of its long half-life and resistance to reversal by protamine sulfate, most authorities recommend converting LMWH to unfractionated heparin at 35–36 weeks.
• Treatment should be continued for the duration of pregnancy and for 6–12 weeks postpartum. After delivery, anticoagulation with oral warfarin (which is teratogenic and should therefore be avoided in pregnancy) can be used. Women on warfarin can breastfeed.
• Alternative therapies (fibrinolytic agents, surgical intervention) are best avoided.

Prophylaxis

• Women with prior unexplained DVT have a 5–10% incidence of recurrence in a subsequent pregnancy. In women with a documented thrombophilic disorder (*see below*), antepartum *prophylactic* heparin is indicated (5,000–1,0000 U subcutaneously twice daily). PTT will not increase. Anti-factor Xa activity should be 0.1–0.3 U/mL. The management of women with a prior DVT but no thrombophilic disorder is controversial. In the UK, such women are generally given prophylactic anticoagulation in the postpartum period only for at least 6 weeks. US practice favors *prophylactic* anticoagulation throughout pregnancy and postpartum.
• In women with a prior PE, *therapeutic* anticoagulation is indicated throughout pregnancy. Maintain PTT at 60–80 s (2.0–2.5 times control) or anti-factor Xa activity at 0.6–1.0 U/mL. Postpartum anticoagulation is indicated for at least 6 weeks.

Table 46.3 Thrombophilic disorders predisposing to thromboembolism

Condition	Is test reliable in pregnancy?
Factor V Leiden deficiency	Yes (genetic test)
Prothrombin gene defect	Yes (genetic test)
Protein C deficiency	No (levels may increase in pregnancy)
Protein S deficiency	No (levels decrease in pregnancy)
Antithrombin III deficiency	No (levels may increase in pregnancy)
Lupus anticoagulant	Yes (test for circulating antibodies)
Anticardiolipin antibodies	Yes (test for circulating antibodies)

Figure 47.1 THYROID PHYSIOLOGY

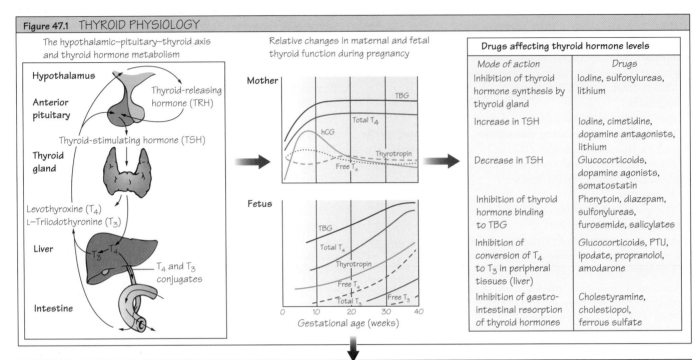

The hypothalamic–pituitary–thyroid axis and thyroid hormone metabolism

Relative changes in maternal and fetal thyroid function during pregnancy

Drugs affecting thyroid hormone levels	
Mode of action	Drugs
Inhibition of thyroid hormone synthesis by thyroid gland	Iodine, sulfonylureas, lithium
Increase in TSH	Iodine, cimetidine, dopamine antagonists, lithium
Decrease in TSH	Glucocorticoids, dopamine agonists, somatostatin
Inhibition of thyroid hormone binding to TBG	Phenytoin, diazepam, sulfonylureas, furosemide, salicylates
Inhibition of conversion of T_4 to T_3 in peripheral tissues (liver)	Glucocorticoids, PTU, ipodate, propranolol, amodarone
Inhibition of gastro-intestinal resorption of thyroid hormones	Cholestyramine, cholestiopol, ferrous sulfate

Figure 47.2 DIAGNOSIS OF MATERNAL THYROID DYSFUNCTION IN PREGNANCY

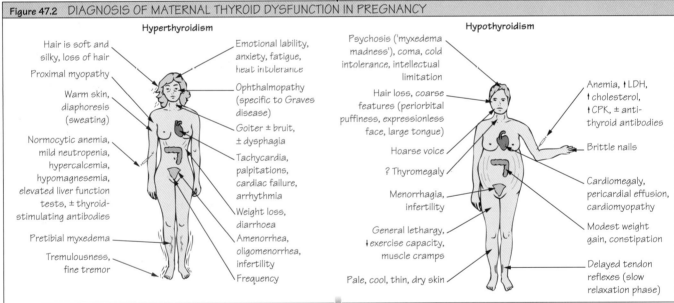

Figure 47.3 SYMPTOMS/SIGNS MAY SUGGEST THYROID DYSFUNCTION, BUT DEFINITIVE DIAGNOSIS REQUIRES THYROID FUNCTION TESTING

Thyroid function test	Units	Normal non-pregnant values (range)	Normal pregnant values (range)		Hyperthyroidism	Hypothyroidism
Thyroid-stimulating hormone (TSH)	mU/L	0.2–4.0	0.8–1.3	No change	Markedly decreased	Markedly decreased
Thyroid-binding globulin (TBG)	mg/L	11–21	23–25	Increased	No change	No change
Total levothyroxine (T_4)	μg/dL	3.9–11.6	10.7–11.5	Increased	Increased	Decreased
Free levothyroxine (T_4)	ng/dL	0.8–2.0	1.0–1.4	No change	Increased	Decreased
Total L-triiodothyronine (T_3)	ng/dL	91–208	205–233	Increased	Markedly increased	Normal to decreased
Free L-triiodothyronine (T_3)	pg/dL	190–710	250–330	No change	Increased	Decreased

Obstetrics and Gynecology at a Glance, Fourth Edition. Errol R. Norwitz and John O. Schorge.

Thyroid physiology (Figure 47.1)

- Circulating thyroxine (levothyroxine, T_4) and L-triiodothyronine (T_3) are bound primarily to thyroxine-binding globulin (TBG) with <1% circulating as free (biologically active) hormone.
- Iodine is required for thyroid hormone production and fetal thyroid function is dependent on iodine from the mother.
- Non-thyroid medical illnesses and select drugs can affect thyroid function.

Thyroid function during pregnancy

- Estrogen has two effects on thyroid function in pregnancy:
  1 It increases circulating TBG concentrations resulting in elevated levels of total T_4 and T_3
  2 It increases TBG sialylation which reduces hepatic clearance of T_4 and T_3.
  Despite these changes, circulating levels of free T_4 and T_3 remain unchanged.
- Less than 0.1% of thyroid hormone crosses the placenta. As such, tests of fetal thyroid function (although rarely, if ever, indicated) are reliable and independent of maternal thyroid status.
- Thyroid hormone can be measured in fetal blood as early as 12 weeks' gestation.

Maternal hyperthyroidism (thyrotoxicosis)
Incidence
This is 0.05–0.2% of pregnancies.

Diagnosis
A definitive diagnosis requires thyroid function testing (Figures 47.2 and 47.3).

Etiology
- *Graves disease* is the most common cause of maternal hyperthyroidism in pregnancy (95%). It results from the presence of circulating thyroid-stimulating antibodies. Eye signs (ophthalmopathy) are specific to Graves disease. As IgG antibodies cross the placenta, the fetus is at risk of thyroid dysfunction.
- *Toxic multinodular goiter* is characterized by hyperthyroidism and the presence of a large, palpable thyroid gland.
- *Hyperemesis gravidarum* is often associated with elevated human chorionic gonadotropin (hCG) levels; 50–70% of women will have biochemical studies suggestive of hyperthyroidism, but no symptoms or signs.
- Hyperthyroidism in the setting of *gestational trophoblastic neoplasia* is probably secondary to elevated levels of hCG.
- Metastatic *follicular cell carcinoma* of the thyroid (rare).
- *Exogenous* T_3 or T_3.
- *De Quervain thyroiditis* (rare) is acute and painful.

Complications
- *Maternal complications.* Infertility, recurrent pregnancy loss, cardiac failure (10–20%), thyroid storm (<0.1%).
- *Fetal complications.* Preterm delivery, intrauterine growth restriction (IUGR), increased perinatal mortality.

Management
- The goal during pregnancy is to control thyrotoxicosis while avoiding fetal and/or transient neonatal hypothyroidism.
- *Antithyroid drugs* are the treatment of choice during pregnancy. Propylthiouracil (PTU) is preferred because it blocks the release of hormone from the thyroid gland and – unlike carbimazole – also blocks peripheral conversion of T_4 to T_3. Carbimazole has also been associated with a rare congenital abnormality (aplasia cutis congenita). PTU treatment is initiated at 100–150 mg three times daily, but it takes 3–4 weeks before a clinical response is seen. Thyroid-stimulating hormone (TSH) levels should be checked every 4–6 weeks and treatment adjusted accordingly.
- Radioactive iodine to ablate the thyroid gland is absolutely contraindicated in pregnancy.
- Surgery is best avoided during pregnancy but, if indicated for failed medical therapy, is best performed in the second trimester.
- Regular fetal testing is recommended after 32 weeks to look for evidence of fetal thyroid dysfunction. Fetal tachycardia (>160 beats/min) is a sensitive index of fetal hyperthyroidism.

Maternal hypothyroidism
Incidence
This is 0.6% of all pregnancies.

Diagnosis (Figures 47.2 and 47.3)
- Thyroid function testing is required for a definitive diagnosis.
- Subclinical maternal hypothyroidism during pregnancy may be associated with long-term cognitive deficits in the offspring. However, routine TSH screening of all pregnant women is not as yet recommended.

Etiology
- *Hashimoto thyroiditis* (chronic lymphocytic thyroiditis) is characterized by hypothyroidism, a firm goiter, and the presence of circulating anti-thyroglobulin or anti-microsomal antibodies. In women with existing Hashimoto disease, pregnancy may result in a transient improvement of symptoms.
- Women *previously treated* for hyperthyroidism may manifest with hypothyroidism and require thyroid hormone replacement.
- *Infectious (suppurative) thyroiditis* is characterized by fever and a painful, swollen thyroid gland.
- *Subacute thyroiditis* is similar to suppurative thyroiditis with a painful, swollen thyroid with or without fever. It is usually the result of a viral infection, and is self-limiting.
- *Iodine deficiency* (rare).

Management
- Early diagnosis is essential to avoid antepartum complications (placental abruption, IUGR, stillbirth) and impaired neonatal and childhood development (cretinism).
- Levothyroxine (thyroxine) treatment should be initiated at 100–150 μg daily. TSH levels should be measured every 4–6 weeks, and the dose adjusted accordingly.
- Women on thyroxine before conception should have their TSH levels monitored every 4–6 weeks. Most women will need to increase their dose by 30–50% during pregnancy.

Postpartum thyroiditis
- *Incidence.* Four to ten percent of all postpartum women.
- *Etiology.* Unknown, but may be an autoimmune phenomenon.
- *Clinical features.* characterized by a transient hyperthyroid state occurring 2–3 months postpartum (with dizziness, fatigue, weight loss, palpitations) or a transient hypothyroid state 4–8 months postpartum (with fatigue, weight gain, and depression).
- *Treatment.* Therapy may be indicated to control symptoms, and can usually be tapered within 1 year.

48 Other medical and surgical conditions in pregnancy

Neurologic diseases in pregnancy
Headache
- A common complaint during pregnancy.
- *Causes.* Migraine, tension headache, depression. Less common causes include sinusitis, pseudotumor cerebri, cerebrovascular disease, cerebral tumors, temporal arteritis, infection (meningitis, encephalitis), preeclampsia, and "spinal" headache (seen in up to 30% of women within the first week after spinal analgesia, usually mild and self-limiting).
- The majority of headaches represent benign conditions. Headaches that disturb sleep are exertional in nature, or those associated with focal neurologic findings are suggestive of an underlying structural lesion.

Seizure disorders
- *Incidence.* This is 0.3–0.6% of pregnancies. The most frequently encountered major neurologic condition in pregnancy.
- *Classification.* Primary (idiopathic, epilepsy) or secondary (to trauma, infection, tumors, cerebrovascular disease, drug withdrawal, or metabolic disorders). Seizures in pregnancy should be regarded as pre-eclampsia/eclampsia until proven otherwise.
- *Effect of seizure disorder on pregnancy.* Obstetric complications include an increased risk of hyperemesis gravidarum, preterm delivery, pre-eclampsia, cesarean section delivery, placental abruption, and perinatal mortality. However, most women with seizure disorders will have an uneventful pregnancy.
- *Effect of pregnancy on seizure disorder* is variable. Estrogen lowers the seizure threshold, whereas progesterone raises it. Seizure frequency is increased in 45% of pregnant women, reduced in 5%, and unchanged in 50%. If seizures are well controlled before pregnancy, there is little risk of deterioration. However, if poorly controlled, an increase in seizure frequency can be expected. Due to a number of factors (delayed gastric emptying, increase in plasma volume, altered protein binding, accelerated hepatic metabolism), the pharmacokinetics of anticonvulsant drugs change during pregnancy.
- *Effects on fetus and neonates.* Women with epilepsy have a two- to threefold increased incidence of fetal anomalies even off treatment. Moreover, anticonvulsant drugs are teratogenic (see Chapter 49). The incidence of fetal anomalies increases with the number of anticonvulsant drugs: 3–4% with one, 5–6% with two, 10% with three, and 25% with four. Monotherapy is thus recommended. *Valproic acid* is associated with neural tube defects (NTDs) in 1% of cases. Risk is greatest from day 17 to day 30 postconception (days 31–44 from last menstrual period). Folic acid (4 mg daily) may decrease the incidence of NTDs. Of women on *phenytoin* 10–30% will have infants with one or more of the following features: craniofacial abnormalities (cleft lip, epicanthic folds, hypertelorism), cardiac anomalies, limb defects (hypoplasia of distal phalanges, nail hypoplasia), or intrauterine growth restriction (IUGR). "Fetal hydantoin syndrome" is characterized by all of the above features, and is rare. Exposure to other antiepileptic drugs (trimethadione, phenobarbital, carbamazepine) can produce similar anomalies.
- *Management of seizure disorder during pregnancy.* Discontinuation of medication before conception should be considered in women who have been seizure free for ≥2 years, although 25–40% will have recurrence of their seizures in pregnancy.

- Seizures may cause maternal hypoxemia with resultant fetal injury. The aim of therapy is to control convulsions with a single agent using the lowest possible dose.
- Labor and delivery are usually uneventful. Benzodiazepines should be used with caution in labor, because they may cause maternal and neonatal depression.
- All anticonvulsant medications cross into breast milk to some degree. The amount of transmission varies with the drug (2% for valproic acid; 30–45% for phenytoin, phenobarbital, and carbamazepine; 90% for ethosuximide). However, the use of such medications is not a contraindication to breastfeeding.

Neurologic emergencies in pregnancy
Status epilepticus
- *Definition.* Repeated convulsions with no intervals of consciousness.
- A medical emergency for both mother and fetus.
- *Management.* As for non-pregnant women. Maintain maternal vital functions, control convulsions, prevent subsequent seizures. Transient fetal bradycardia is common. Resuscitate the fetus *in utero* before making a decision about delivery. Prolonged seizure activity may be associated with placental abruption.

Disorders of consciousness
- Disorders of *content* (confusion) and *level* of consciousness (coma).
- *Differential diagnosis.* Similar to that in non-pregnant women, but also includes eclampsia.
- *Management.* Treat underlying etiology. Supportive care.

Psychiatric disorders in pregnancy
- Psychiatric medications should be continued in pregnancy. In general, the risk of a clinical relapse poses a greater threat to pregnancy than continued medication.
- Guidelines for drug treatment:
  1 Use the lowest effective dose
  2 Consider delaying treatment until after the first trimester to minimize the risk of teratogenicity (see Chapter 49)
  3 Avoid sedating agents immediately before delivery to minimize neonatal sedation
  4 Electroconvulsant therapy (ECT) is generally avoided in pregnancy, but is considered safe for the fetus.

Postpartum depression
- *Incidence.* This is 8–15% of all postpartum women.
- *Risk factors.* Prior depression (30% risk), prior postpartum depression (70–85%).
- Peak onset of symptoms is 2–3 months postpartum, and usually resolves spontaneously within 6–12 months.
- Supportive care and monthly follow-up are necessary. Medications can be started if needed.

Postpartum psychosis
- *Incidence.* This is 1–2 per 1,000 live births.
- *Risk factors.* Primiparity, personal or family history of mental illness, prior postpartum psychosis (25–30% risk).

Obstetrics and Gynecology at a Glance, Fourth Edition. Errol R. Norwitz and John O. Schorge.

- Peak onset of symptoms is 10–14 days postpartum.
- Hospitalization, pharmacologic therapy, ECT as needed.

Pulmonary disease in pregnancy
Asthma
- *Incidence.* This is 1–4% of all pregnancies.
- Pregnancy has a variable effect on asthma (25% improve, 25% worsen, 50% are unchanged). In general, women with mild, well-controlled asthma tolerate pregnancy well. Women with severe asthma are at risk of symptomatic deterioration.
- *Management.* As for non-pregnant women. Hospitalization, steroids, and/or intubation may be required.
- *Complications.* IUGR, stillbirth, maternal death.

Amniotic fluid embolism
- An obstetric emergency with 80–90% maternal mortality rate.
- *Risk factors.* Multiparity, prolonged labor, fetal demise, "excessive" oxytocin augmentation, placental abruption, cesarean section delivery.
- Characterized by acute onset of dyspnea, hypotension, coagulopathy, and hypoxemia. Therapy is primarily supportive.

Pulmonary edema
- Classified as cardiogenic or non-cardiogenic.
- *Risk factors.* Fluid overload, infection, pre-eclampsia, tocolytic therapy.
- *Management.* As for non-pregnant women. LMNOP: *l*asix (diuresis), *m*orphine, Na^{2+} and water restriction, *o*xygen, and *p*osition upright. Consider antibiotics.

Renal disease in pregnancy
Asymptomatic bacteriuria
- *Incidence.* This is 4–7% of all pregnancies, which is similar to that in non-pregnant women.
- In pregnancy, asymptomatic bacteriuria is more likely to progress to pyelonephritis (20–30%).
- *Escherichia coli* is the most common causative organism.

Chronic renal failure
- *Complications.* Infertility (usually due to chronic anovulation), spontaneous abortion, pre-eclampsia, IUGR, fetal death, and preterm birth.
- Pregnancy outcome is dependent on baseline renal function (below), and presence and severity of hypertension. The degree of proteinuria does not correlate with pregnancy outcome.
- In women with end-stage renal disease, renal transplantation offers the best chance of a successful pregnancy (especially if renal function is stable for 1–2 years and there is no hypertension). Triple-agent immunosuppression (cyclosporin, azathioprine, prednisone) should be continued in pregnancy.

Autoimmune diseases in pregnancy
Systemic lupus erythematosus
- Systemic lupus erythematosus (SLE) does not generally worsen in pregnancy. Pregnancy outcome is related primarily to the severity of underlying renal disease.
- *Complications.* Pre-eclampsia, IUGR, preterm birth.

Maternal anti-Ro and anti-La antibodies
Associated with complete fetal heart block in 5–10% of cases.

Immune (idiopathic) thrombocytopenic purpura
- Immune thrombocytopenic purpura (ITP) is a maternal disease characterized by the presence of circulating antiplatelet antibodies. It should be distinguished from *alloimmune thrombocytopenia (ATP)* in which maternal platelet counts are normal, but antiplatelet antibodies (usually anti-PLA1/2) cross the placenta to cause fetal thrombocytopenia and possibly intraventricular hemorrhage. ATP is analogous to rhesus (Rh) disease of platelets.
- *Differential diagnosis.* Pre-eclampsia, coagulopathy, drugs, gestational thrombocytopenia.
- *Complications.* IgG can cross the placenta and cause fetal thrombocytopenia. However, the correlation between maternal and fetal platelet counts is poor. Fetal intraventricular hemorrhage in the setting of ITP is rare.
- *Management.* Corticosteroids may be necessary if maternal thrombocytopenia is severe. Intravenous Ig, plasmapharesis, and splenectomy are rarely necessary in pregnancy. Cesarean section delivery has not been shown to improve perinatal outcome.

Rheumatoid arthritis
- Improves in 75% of pregnancies, but >90% of women will relapse within 6 months of delivery.
- Corticosteroids are safe in pregnancy. Gold salts, cytotoxic agents, penicillamine, and antimalarials may have adverse fetal effects, but may be used if indicated.

Surgical conditions in pregnancy
- *Incidence.* This is 2–3 per 1,000 pregnancies.
- *Indications.* Appendicitis, biliary disease, ovarian disease.
- *Complications.* Hemorrhage, anesthetic complications, infection, preterm delivery. Complications can be minimized if surgery is performed in the second trimester.
- Technical considerations:
  1 Left lateral tilt if ≥20 weeks to improve venous return
  2 Continuous fetal monitoring ≥24 weeks' gestation
  3 Avoidance of teratogenic agents (see Chapter 49)
  4 Specific anesthetic considerations (see Chapter 64).

Appendicitis
- *Incidence.* The incidence of appendicitis is not increased (1 in 1,500 pregnancies), but an infected appendix is more likely to rupture in pregnancy.
- *Diagnosis.* Symptoms and signs are similar to those in non-pregnant women, except that the appendix moves up in pregnancy.
- *Management.* Surgical removal through a right paramedian incision is generally recommended (which can be extended if the appendix cannot be located or if cesarean section delivery is indicated).

Table 48.1 Pregnancy outcome in women with chronic renal disease

	Category of chronic renal disease		
	Mild	Moderate	Severe
Serum creatinine (mmol/L)	120–150	150–250	>250
Serum creatinine (mg/dL)	<1.4	1.4–2.5	>2.5
Complications (%)	20	40	85
Viable delivery (%)	95	90	50
Long-term sequelae (%)	<5	25	55

Figure 49.1 UNITED STATES FOOD AND DRUG ADMINISTRATION (FDA) RISK CATEGORIES FOR DRUGS IN PREGNANCY

Category	Definition	Examples
A	– Controlled studies in women fail to demonstrate a risk to the fetus and the possibility of fetal harm appears remote	– Vitamin C, folate, L-thyroxine
B	– Either animal studies have not demonstrated a fetal risk but there are no controlled studies in pregnant women, or animal studies have shown an adverse effect that was not confirmed in controlled studies in women	– Hydrochlorothiazide, α-methyldopa, ampicillin
C	– Either studies in animals have revealed adverse effects on the fetus and there are no controlled studies in women, or there are no controlled studies in animals or women. Only use if potential benefit justifies risk to fetus	– Theophylline, nifedipine, digoxin, β-blockers, verapamil, zidovudine (AZT), acyclovir
D	– Positive evidence of human fetal risk, but the benefits from use in pregnant women may be acceptable despite the risk	– Cytoxan, spironolactone, ACE inhibitors, methotrexate, phenytoin
X	– Positive evidence of animal or human fetal abnormalities, or the risk of the use of the drug in pregnant women clearly outweighs any possible benefit. Contraindicated in women who are or may become pregnant	– Aminopterin, isotretinoin (vitamin A), radioisotopes, oral contraceptives

Figure 49.2 DRUGS NOT CONSIDERED TERATOGENS

- Acetaminophen
- Aciclovir
- Antiemetics (e.g. phenothiazines)
- Antihistamines (e.g. doxylamine)
- Aspirin
- Caffeine
- Hairspray
- Metronidazole
- Minor tranquilizers (e.g. fluoxetine)
- Occupational chemical agents
- Oral contraceptives
- Pesticides
- Trimethoprim/sulfamethoxazole
- Vaginal spermicides
- Zidovudine (AZT)

Figure 49.3 DRUGS WITH PROVEN BENEFIT IN PREGNANCY

- Folic acid (folate)—4 mg/day (10 x RDA) begun 4 weeks prior to conception will reduce the incidence of neural tube defects by 70–80%
- Zidovudine (AZT)—decreases vertical transmission of HIV from 25% to 8%
- Acyclovir—200 mg p.o. t.i.d. after 36 weeks' gestation to women with frequent recurrent genital herpes infection or first episode primary herpes infection in pregnancy will reduce the need for cesarean delivery for active herpes in labor
- Iron supplementation—prevents anemia
- Anesthetic agents—pain relief in labor

Figure 49.4 DRUGS WITH PROVEN TERATOGENIC EFFECTS IN HUMANS

Androgens	Virilization of female, advanced genital development in males	Effects are dose dependent. Given before 9 weeks, labio-scrotal fusion can occur. Cliteromegaly can occur any time
Angiotensin-converting enzyme (ACE) inhibitors	Fetal renal tubular dysgenesis, oligohydramnios, neonatal renal failure, lack of cranial ossification, IUGR	Incidence of fetal morbidity ~ 30%, especially with second and third trimester exposure
Anticholinergic drugs	Neonatal meconium ileus	–
Antithyroid drugs	Fetal and neonatal goitre, hypothyroidism	Propylthiouracil (PTU) is preferred over methimazole because of the association with aplasia cutis
Coumarin derivatives (e.g. warfarin)	Warfarin embryopathy (nasal hypoplasia, stippled bone epiphysis, shortened phalanges, optic atrophy, mental retardation, microcephaly), IUGR, developmental delay	15–25% of fetuses exposed to warfarin prior to 9 weeks will have some anomalies, although the embryopathy syndrome only occurs in 5–8% of cases. Later exposure is associated with optic atrophy, developmental delay, placental abruption, fetal hemorrhage
Carbamazepine (tegretol)	Neural tube defects (NTD), microcephaly, IUGR, fetal hydantoin-like syndrome	0.5% risk of NTD
Cyclophosphamide	CNS malformations	–
Folic acid antagonists (aminopterin, methotrexate)	CNS and limb malformations	All cytotoxic drugs are potentially teratogenic. Associated with increased rate of abortion. Of fetuses who survive after first trimester exposure, ~ 30% will have some anomaly
Diethylstilbestrol (DES)	Clear-cell adenocarcinoma of vagina or cervix, abnormalities of cervix and uterus, possibly infertility in males	Vaginal adenosis is seen in 50% of women whose mothers took DES before 9 weeks' gestation. Risk for vaginal adenocarcinoma is low
Lithium	Congenital heart disease (?Ebstein anomaly)	Risk of cardiac anomaly is low. Exposure in last month of gestation may be toxic to thyroid, kidneys, CNS
Phenytoin	IUGR, learning disability, microcephaly, dysmorphic craniofacial features, cardiac defects, nail and distal phalangeal hypoplasia	The full fetal hydantoin syndrome is seen in <10% of fetuses exposed in the first trimester, but ~ 30% of fetuses will have some manifestations. The effect may depend on whether the fetus inherits a mutant gene for epoxide hydrolase, an enzyme necessary to decrease the teratogenic metabolite phenytoin epoxide
Streptomycin and kanamycin	Hearing loss, eighth-nerve damage	No ototoxicity reported with gentamicin or vancomycin
Tetracycline	Hypoplasia of tooth enamel, permanent yellow-brown discoloration of deciduous teeth, ? weakening of long bones	Effects are limited to exposure in second or third trimester
Thalidomide	Bilateral limb deficiencies, microtia/anotia, cardiac and gastro-intestinal anomalies	~ 20% of fetuses have anomalies if exposed between 35 and 50 days of gestation
Trimethadione and paramethadione	Cleft palate, cardiac defects, IUGR, mental retardation, microcephaly, facial dysmorphism	~ 60–80% risk of anomaly or abortion with first trimester exposure
Valproic acid	Minor facial defects, NTD	~ 1% risk of NTD, especially open spina bifida
Vitamin A and its derivatives (e.g. isotretinoin and retinoids)	Increased spontaneous abortion, microtia, CNS defects, mental retardation, craniofacial dysmorphism, cardiac defects, cleft lip and palate, thymic agenesis	Isotretinoin is not stored, but anomalies can occur long after the drug is discontinued. Teratogenic dose >8000 µg/day (RDA = 800 µg/day). The risk of topical retin A is not known

Obstetrics and Gynecology at a Glance, Fourth Edition. Errol R. Norwitz and John O. Schorge.

106 © 2013 John Wiley & Sons, Ltd. Published 2013 by John Wiley & Sons, Ltd.

Drugs in pregnancy

Incidence
- Of women 20–25% report using medications on a regular basis throughout pregnancy.
- Major congenital anomalies occur in 3–4% of live births and 70% of such anomalies have no known cause. It is estimated that 2–3% are due to medications and 1% to environmental toxins.

Drug trials in pregnancy
- Drug trials are difficult to carry out in pregnancy because of concern over the fetus. As such, many drugs have not been validated for use or safety in human pregnancy.
- Recommendations often rely on data from animal models. The occurrence of thalidomide-associated embryopathy has led to the belief that human teratogenicity cannot be predicted by animal studies. However, every drug that has since been found to be teratogenic in humans has caused similar effects in animals.

Pharmacokinetics during pregnancy
- Pharmacokinetics is the study of how a drug moves through the body.
- Drug *absorption* is altered in pregnancy. Gastric emptying and gastric acid secretion are reduced. Intestinal motility is decreased. Pulmonary tidal volume is increased which may affect the absorption of inhaled drugs.
- The volume of *distribution* changes in pregnancy. Plasma volume rises by 40%, total body water increases 7–8 L, and body fat increases 20–40%. Despite these changes (which would be expected to decrease drug levels), albumin concentrations decline, and free fatty acid and lipoprotein values rise. As a result, protein binding of many drugs is lower in pregnancy, leading to an increase in circulating free (biologically active) drug levels.
- *Metabolism* and *elimination* are also altered in pregnancy. High steroid hormone levels affect hepatic metabolism and prolong the half-life of some drugs. Glomerular filtration rate rises 50–60%, thereby increasing the renal clearance of other drugs.

Teratogenicity
- Teratogenicity is the study of abnormal fetal development, and refers to both structural and functional abnormalities.
- With the exception of large molecules (such as heparin), all drugs given to the mother cross the placenta to some degree.
- The effect of a given drug on a fetus depends on dose, time, and duration of exposure, and as yet poorly defined genetic and environmental factors that interact to determine the susceptibility of any individual fetus for structural injury. A fetus is at highest risk for injury during embryogenesis (days 17–54 post-conception).
- Paternal exposure has never been shown to be teratogenic.

Risk categories for drugs in pregnancy (Figure 49.1)
The Food and Drug Administration (FDA) in the USA has defined five risk categories for drug use in pregnancy: A, B, C, D, X. Individual agents are assigned to a risk category according to their risk–benefit ratio (Figures 49.2, 49.3, and 49.4), eg, although oral contraceptives are not teratogenic, they are classified as category X because there is no benefit to being on the pill once you are pregnant.

Principles of drug use in pregnancy
- Use medications only if absolutely indicated.
- If possible, avoid initiating therapy during the first trimester.
- Select a safe medication (preferably an older drug with a proven track record in pregnancy).
- Use the lowest effective dose.
- Single-agent therapy is preferable.
- Discourage the use of over-the-counter drugs.

Illicit and social drug use

Cocaine
- Cocaine is associated with intrauterine fetal growth restriction (IUGR), cerebral infarction, and placental abruption. Reported congenital anomalies (limb reduction defects, porencephalic cysts, microcephaly, bowel atresias, necrotizing enterocolitis, and long-term behavioral effects) may be secondary to cocaine-induced vasospasm.
- Maternal complications include uterine rupture, hypertension, seizures, and death.

Alcohol
- Fetal alcohol syndrome is characterized by facial abnormalities (midfacial hypoplasia), central nervous system dysfunction (microcephaly, learning disability), and IUGR. Renal and cardiac defects may also occur.
- The risk of anomalies is related to the extent of alcohol use: 10% with rare use, 15% with moderate use, and 30–40% with heavy use (more than six drinks per day). There is no absolute safe level of alcohol use in pregnancy.

Marijuana
- No known teratogenic effect.
- Weak association with preterm birth, IUGR, and subsequent neurodevelopmental delay.

Cigarette smoke (nicotine and thiocyanate)
- Of pregnant women, 20–30% continue to smoke during pregnancy.
- Adverse effects include decreased fertility as well as increased spontaneous abortion, preterm birth, perinatal mortality, and low-birthweight infants (200 g decrease in birth weight for every 10 cigarettes smoked per day).
- Neonatal exposure is associated with sudden infant death syndrome, asthma, respiratory infections, and attention deficit disorder.

Caffeine
- No known teratogenic effect.
- Weak association with spontaneous abortion.

Environmental toxins

Radiation
- Associated with spontaneous abortion, learning disability, microcephaly, and (possibly) malignancy in later life.
- Fetal exposure of >5–10 rad is required for any adverse effect (estimated fetal exposure from common radiological procedures is 1–3 mrad).

Heat
- Weak association with spontaneous abortion and neural tube defects.

Electromagnetic field
- No known teratogenic effect.

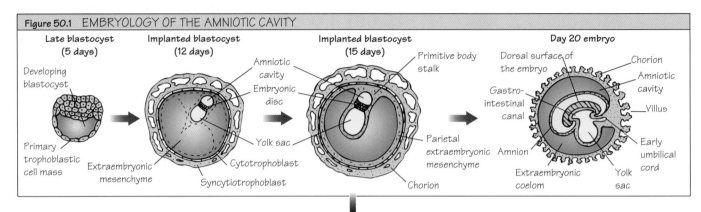

Figure 50.1 EMBRYOLOGY OF THE AMNIOTIC CAVITY

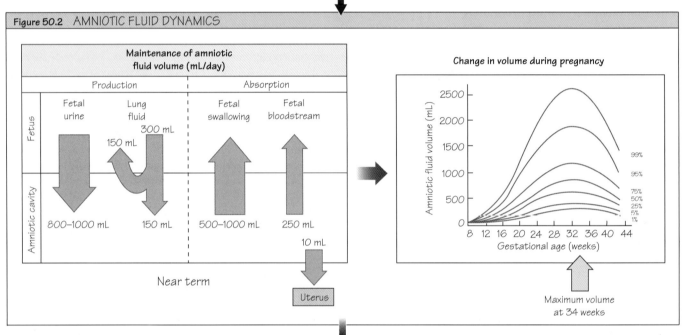

Figure 50.2 AMNIOTIC FLUID DYNAMICS

Figure 50.3 CAUSES OF OLIGOHYDRAMNIOS (LOW FLUID)

Increased absorption or loss of fluid
1 Premature rupture of membranes (PROM) accounts for 50% of cases of oligohydramnios. Perinatal outcome is dependent upon gestational age at which rupture occurs and severity of oligohydramnios

Decreased production of amniotic fluid
2 Congenital renal anomalies (renal agenesis, renal dysplasia) and exposure to ACE inhibitors will diminish fetal renal output. Bladder outlet or urethral obstruction will similarly decrease urine output
3 Uteroplacental insufficiency (caused by placental abruption, preeclampsia, postmaturity syndrome) will decrease renal perfusion and thus fetal urine output
4 Other causes include congenital infection, fetal cardiac defects, neural tube defects, twin–twin transfusion syndrome, and non-steroidal anti-inflammatory drugs

Figure 50.4 CAUSES OF POLYHYDRAMNIOS (EXCESS FLUID)

1 Idiopathic (no known cause) accounts for 50–60% of cases
2 Maternal causes include isoimmunization (leading to immune hydrops fetalis) and diabetes mellitus (volume of amniotic fluid is dependent on degree of glycemic control)
3 Fetal causes (10–15%) include non-immune hydrops fetalis (due, for example, to cardiac defect), multifetal gestation (with or without twin–twin transfusion syndrome), structural anomalies (gastrointestinal tract obstruction, cystic adenomatoid lung deformity), fetal diabetes insipidus, and defects of fetal swallowing (achalasia, esophageal obstruction, tracheoesophageal fistula, or central nervous system abnormalities)
4 Placental causes (rare) include placental chorioangioma

Embryology of the amniotic cavity (Figure 50.1)

The *amnion* is a thin fetal membrane that begins to form on the eighth post-conceptional day as a small sac covering the dorsal surface of the embryonic disc. The amnion gradually encircles the growing embryo. *Amniotic fluid* fills the amniotic cavity.

Amniotic fluid dynamics (Figure 50.2)

Maintenance of amniotic fluid volume is a dynamic process that reflects a balance between fluid production and absorption.

Fluid production

- Before 8 weeks, amniotic fluid is produced by passage of fluid across the amnion and fetal skin (transudation).
- At 8 weeks, the fetus begins to urinate into the amniotic cavity. Fetal urine quickly becomes the primary source of amniotic fluid production. Near term, 800–1000 mL of fetal urine is produced each day.
- The fetal lungs produce some fluid (300 mL per day at term), but much of it is swallowed before entering the amniotic space.

Fluid absorption

- Before 8 weeks' gestation, transudative amniotic fluid is passively reabsorbed.
- At 8 weeks' gestation, the fetus begins to *swallow*. Fetal swallowing quickly becomes the primary source of amniotic fluid absorption. Near term, 500–1000 mL of fluid are absorbed each day by fetal swallowing.
- A lesser amount of amniotic fluid is absorbed through the fetal membranes and enters the fetal bloodstream. Near term, 250 mL of amniotic fluid is absorbed by this route every day.
- Small quantities of amniotic fluid cross the amnion and enter the maternal bloodstream (10 mL per day near term).

Changes in volume during pregnancy (Figure 50.2)

Amniotic fluid volume is maximal at 34 weeks (750–800 mL) and decreases thereafter to 600 mL at 40 weeks. The amount of fluid continues to decrease beyond 40 weeks.

The role of amniotic fluid

Amniotic fluid has a number of critical functions, including:
- Cushioning the fetus from external trauma
- Protecting the umbilical cord from compression
- Allowing unrestricted fetal movement, thereby promoting the development of the fetal musculoskeletal system
- Contributing to fetal pulmonary development
- Lubricating the fetal skin
- Preventing maternal chorioamnionitis and fetal infection through its bacteriostatic properties
- Assisting in fetal temperature control.

Measurement of amniotic fluid volume

Ultrasonography is a more accurate method of estimating amniotic fluid than measurement of fundal height. Several techniques are described:
- Subjective assessment of amniotic fluid volume.
- Measurement of the single deepest pocket free of umbilical cord, known as maximal vertical pocket (MVP).
- Amniotic fluid index (AFI) is a semiquantitative method for estimating amniotic fluid volume, which minimizes inter- and intraobserver error. AFI refers to the sum of the maximum vertical pockets of amniotic fluid (in centimeters) in each of the four quadrants of the uterus. Normal AFI beyond 20 weeks' gestation ranges from 5 cm to 20 cm.

Clinical importance of amniotic fluid volume

- Amniotic fluid volume is a marker of *fetal wellbeing*.
- Normal amniotic fluid volume suggests that uteroplacental perfusion is adequate. An abnormal amount of amniotic fluid volume is associated with an unfavorable perinatal outcome.

Oligohydramnios

- *Definition.* An abnormally low amount of amniotic fluid around the fetus.
- *Incidence.* This is 5–8% of all pregnancies.
- *Diagnosis.* Oligohydramnios should be suspected if the fundal height is significantly less than expected for gestational age. It is defined sonographically as a total amniotic fluid volume <300 mL, the absence of a single 2-cm vertical pocket, or an AFI <5 cm at term or <5th percentile for gestational age.
- *Causes* (Figure 50.3).
- *Management.* Antepartum treatment options are limited, unless a structural defect (such as posterior urethral valve in a male infant) is amenable to *in utero* surgical repair. The timing of delivery depends on gestational age, etiology, and fetal wellbeing. During labor, infusion of crystalloid solution into the amniotic cavity (*amnioinfusion*) may improve abnormal fetal heart rate patterns (particularly in the setting of repetitive variable decelerations) and, possibly, decrease the cesarean delivery rate.
- *Outcome.* Oligohydramnios is associated with increased perinatal morbidity and mortality at any gestational age.
- *Complications.* Amniotic band syndrome (adhesions between the amnion and fetus causing serious deformities, including limb amputation) or musculoskeletal deformities due to uterine compression (such as clubfoot) may develop in some cases.

Polyhydramnios

- *Definition.* An abnormally large amount of amniotic fluid surrounding the fetus.
- *Incidence.* This is 0.5–1.5% of all pregnancies.
- *Diagnosis.* Polyhydramnios should be suspected if the fundal height is significantly more than expected for gestational age. It is defined sonographically as a total amniotic fluid volume >2 L, a single vertical pocket ≥10 cm, or an AFI >20 cm at term or >95th percentile for gestational age.
- *Causes* (Figure 50.4).
- *Management.* Antepartum treatment options are limited. Non-steroidal anti-inflammatory drugs (indomethacin) can decrease fetal urine production, but may cause premature closure of the fetal ductus arteriosus. Removal of fluid by amniocentesis is only transiently effective. During labor, controlled amniotomy may reduce the incidence of complications resulting from rapid decompression (placental abruption, cord prolapse).
- *Outcome.* Polyhydramnios has been associated with increased maternal morbidity as well as perinatal morbidity and mortality.
- *Complications.* Uterine overdistension may result in maternal dyspnea or refractory edema of the lower extremities and vulva. During labor, polyhydramnios can result in fetal malpresentation, dysfunctional labor, and/or postpartum hemorrhage.

51 Disorders of fetal growth

Figure 51.1 CAUSES OF INTRAUTERINE GROWTH RESTRICTION (IUGR)

Fetal causes

Genetic factors (5–15%)
- Fetal chromosomal anomalies (2–5%) including trisomies (18 >13 >21) and sex chromosome abnormalities. Most chromosomally abnormal IUGR fetuses have associated structural abnormalities, but 2% do not.
- Single gene defects (3–10%) such as phenylketonuria, dwarfism
- Confined placental mosaicism (rare)

Fetal structural anomalies (1–2%)
- Cardiovascular anomalies
- Bilateral renal agenesis

Multiple pregnancy (2–3%)
- Risk of IUGR increases with fetal number
- Worse in poly/oligo sequence (twin–twin transfusion syndrome)

Uteroplacental causes

Uteroplacental insufficiency (25–30%)
- Chronic hypertension, preeclampsia
- Antiphospholipid antibody syndrome (25% of chromosomally and structurally normal IUGR fetuses have mothers who have circulating lupus anticoagulant [LAC] or anticardiolipin antibodies [ACA])
- Unexplained chronic proteinuria (25% risk of IUGR)
- Chronic placental abruption

Velamentous insertion of umbilical cord

Maternal causes

Drug and/or toxin exposure
- Illicit drugs (cocaine)
- Heavy cigarette smoking (effect is most pronounced in older mothers)

Malnutrition (especially gestational malnutrition superimposed on poor prepregnancy nutritional status)

Maternal medical conditions
- Poorly controlled hyperthyroidism
- Hemoglobinopathies
- Chronic pulmonary disease
- Cyanotic heart disease
- Anemia

Infections (5–10%)
- Malaria (the **single greatest cause** of IUGR worldwide)
- Rubella
- Cytomegalovirus
- ? Varicella

Figure 51.2 RISK FACTORS FOR IUGR

- Hypertension (both chronic and gestational hypertension)
- Multifetal pregnancies
- Prior IUGR infant
- Poor maternal weight gain
- Severe maternal anemia
- Antiphospholipid antibody syndrome
- Diabetes with vascular disease
- Maternal drug/tobacco abuse
- Discrepancy between fundal height measurement and gestational age ≥3–4 cm

Note: maternal risk factors identify only 50% of cases of IUGR

Figure 51.3 DIAGNOSIS OF IUGR

- Suspect the diagnosis in patients at high risk
- Clinical examination will fail to identify >50% of IUGR fetuses
- Confirm the diagnosis by ultrasound:
  (i) estimated fetal weight <5th percentile (2 standard deviations from the mean) for gestational age
  OR
  (ii) estimated fetal weight <10th percentile for gestational age with evidence of fetal compromise (oligohydramnios, abnormal umbilical artery Doppler blood flow)
- Serial ultrasound examinations are more useful than a single scan to confirm the diagnosis of IUGR, to follow fetal growth, and to detect oligohydramnios or umbilical artery Doppler velocimetry abnormalities

Figure 51.5 MANAGEMENT OF IUGR

1. Attempt to determine etiology (ultrasound for fetal anomalies, check karyotype, exclude infectious etiology)
2. Regular (usually twice weekly) fetal testing
3. Consider delivery once a favorable gestational age is reached (≥34 weeks), once fetal lung maturity is documented, or for worsening fetal testing (deterioration in biophysical profile, the development of absent or reversed end-diastolic flow on umbilical artery Doppler velocimetry)
4. 50–80% of IUGR fetuses will develop 'fetal distress' in labor requiring cesarean delivery
5. Send placenta/fetal membranes to pathology after delivery to look for evidence of vasculopathy

Figure 51.4 PATHOPHYSIOLOGY OF UTEROPLACENTAL IUGR

Compromise in uteroplacental blood flow

↓

Decreased nutrients (glucose, oxygen, amino acids, ? growth factors) to fetus

↓

Fetal growth begins to diminish in a fixed sequence (subcutaneous tissue → axial skeleton → vital organs such as brain, heart, liver, kidney)

↓

Nutrient, oxygen and energy demands of the growing fetoplacental unit begin to exceed supply leading to hypoxia, acidosis, and death

↓

Changes in antepartum fetal testing reflect the pathophysiological changes (in sequence):

1. Umbilical systolic/diastolic ratio increases as placental vascular resistance increases
2. Fetal growth on ultrasound slows or stops
3. Oligohydramnios develops due to diminished perfusion of fetal kidneys
4. Loss of fetal heart rate variability with subsequent decelerations
5. Intrauterine fetal demise (IUFD)

Obstetrics and Gynecology at a Glance, Fourth Edition. Errol R. Norwitz and John O. Schorge.

110 © 2013 John Wiley & Sons, Ltd. Published 2013 by John Wiley & Sons, Ltd.

Definitions

• *Low birthweight* (LBW) refers to infants with an absolute birth weight <2500 g regardless of gestational age.
• *Small-for-gestational-age* (SGA) fetuses are <10th percentile for gestational age. Fetuses >90th percentile are termed "*large for gestational age*" (LGA). Fetuses between the 10th and 90th percentiles are referred to as "appropriate for gestational age" (AGA). Correct assignment of fetal weight category is dependent on accurate dating of the pregnancy because birthweight is a function of both gestational age and rate of fetal growth.

Intrauterine growth restriction

• *Definition.* Intrauterine growth restriction (IUGR) refers to any fetus that fails to reach its full growth potential.
• *Incidence.* Of fetuses 4–8% are diagnosed with IUGR.
• *Classification.* IUGR can be classified as *symmetric* (in which the fetus is proportionally small, suggesting long-term compromise) or *asymmetric* (in which the fetal head is proportionally larger than the body, suggesting short-term compromise with "sparing" of the brain). This distinction is, however, of little clinical value.
• *Causes.* IUGR represents the clinical end-point of many different fetal, uteroplacental, and maternal conditions. An attempt should be made to determine the cause before delivery in order to provide counseling, perform ultrasonographic evaluation for fetal growth and delineation of anatomy, and obtain neonatal consultation. Frequently, the cause is readily apparent (Figure 51.1).
• *Risk factors.* Numerous pre-existing and acquired conditions predispose the fetus to IUGR (Figure 51.2).
• *Diagnosis.* The clinical diagnosis of IUGR is unreliable, but a fundal height measurement significantly less than expected (3–4 cm) for gestational age may suggest the diagnosis. IUGR is confirmed by sonographic measurements (Figure 51.3).
• *Pathophysiology.* IUGR most commonly results from compromise of uteroplacental blood flow (Figure 51.4).
• *Prevention.* Bed rest and low-dose aspirin have been used to prevent IUGR in women at high risk, but with little or no benefit.
• *Management* (Figure 51.5). Principles of management include:
  1 the identification of women at high risk for IUGR
  2 early antepartum diagnosis
  3 determination of etiology
  4 regular (usually weekly) fetal testing with non-stress test (NST) or cardiotocography (see Chapter 52)
  5 appropriate timing of delivery.
• *Complications.* IUGR infants have higher rates of perinatal morbidity and mortality at any given gestational age, but have a better prognosis than infants with the same birthweight delivered at earlier gestational ages. Unfortunately, neonatal morbidity (meconium aspiration syndrome, hypoglycemia, polycythemia, pulmonary hemorrhage) will be present in 50% of IUGR neonates. Long-term studies show a 38-fold increase in the incidence of cerebral dysfunction (ranging from minor learning disabilities to cerebral palsy) in term IUGR infants and even more so if the infant was born preterm.

Fetal macrosomia

• *Definition.* Fetal macrosomia is defined as an estimated weight (not birthweight) of ≥4500 g.

• *Incidence.* In developing countries, 5% of infants weigh >4000 g at delivery and 0.5% weigh >4500 g.
• *Risk factors.* Although a number of factors have been associated with macrosomia, most women with risk factors have normal weight babies:
  1 *Maternal diabetes* (35–40% of all macrosomic infants) is the most common risk factor.
  2 *Post-term pregnancy* (10–20%) is another common risk factor. Of all infants born at or beyond 42 weeks, 2.5% weigh >4500 g.
  3 *Maternal obesity* (10–20%), defined as a pre-pregnancy body mass index (BMI) >30 kg/m², predisposes to fetal macrosomia. Moreover, clinical and ultrasound estimates of fetal weight in obese women are technically more difficult and may be less accurate.
  4 *Other risk factors* include multiparity, a prior macrosomic infant, a male infant, increased maternal height, advanced maternal age, and Beckwith–Wiedemann syndrome.
• *Diagnosis.* Clinical estimates of fetal weight based on the Leopold maneuvers or fundal height measurements are often unreliable. Ultrasound is generally used to estimate fetal weight (see Chapter 40). However, currently available ultrasonographic techniques are accurate only to within 15–20% of actual fetal weight.
• *Prevention.* Meticulous control of maternal diabetes throughout pregnancy reduces the incidence of fetal macrosomia.
• *Management:*
  1 *Antepartum.* Women at high risk for having a macrosomic infant or who have a known LGA fetus should be followed with serial ultrasound examinations at 3–4 weeks to chart fetal growth.
  2 *Induction of labor.* Despite the association between fetal macrosomia, and both birth trauma and cesarean section delivery, early induction of labor is not often recommended in patients with suspected fetal macrosomia at term. Induction of labor in this setting doubles the risk of cesarean section delivery without reducing shoulder dystocia or neonatal morbidity. However, induction of labor for "impending macrosomia" does not decrease the cesarean section rate. As such, this approach should not be encouraged.
  3 To prevent birth trauma, *elective (prophylactic) cesarean section delivery* should be offered to diabetic women with an estimated fetal weight >4500 g and non-diabetic women with estimated fetal weight >5000 g.
  4 *Vaginal delivery* of a macrosomic infant should take place in a controlled fashion, with immediate access to anesthesia staff and a neonatal resuscitation team. It is prudent to avoid assisted vaginal delivery in this setting.
• *Fetal morbidity and mortality.* Macrosomic fetuses have an increased risk of intrauterine and neonatal death (see Chapter 54) and birth trauma, especially shoulder dystocia and brachial plexus palsy (see Chapter 63). Other neonatal complications include hypoglycemia, polycythemia, hypocalcemia, and jaundice.
• *Maternal morbidity.* The increased maternal morbidity associated with the birth of a macrosomic infant is due primarily to a higher incidence of cesarean section delivery. Other maternal complications include postpartum hemorrhage, perineal trauma, and puerperal infection.

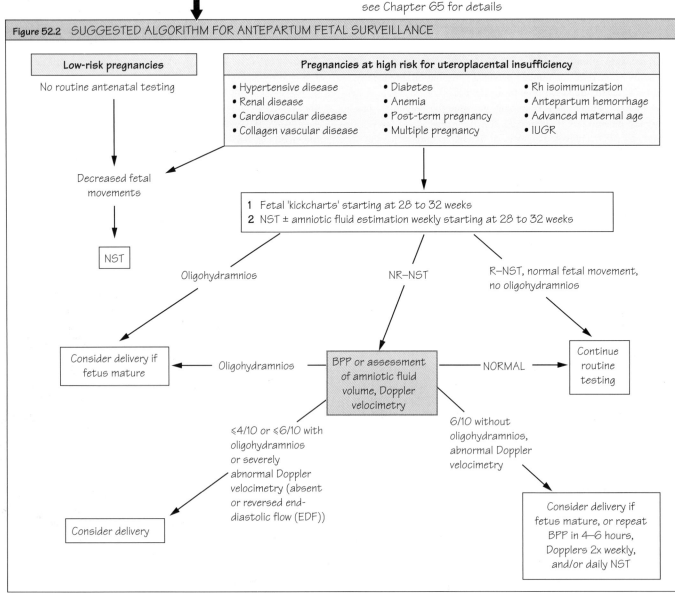

Figure 52.1 ASSESSMENT OF FETAL WELL-BEING

Antepartum	Intrapartum	Postpartum
Non-stress test (NST) • External monitor (Doppler) only Biophysical profile Fetal movement charts ('kickcharts') Umbilical artery Doppler velocimetry Vibroacoustic stimulation Contraction stress test	Non-stress test (NST) • External monitor (Doppler) • Internal (scalp electrode) Fetal scalp stimulation Fetal pulse oximetry (?)	Clinical response (seizures, poor feeding, abnormal movements) Apgar score Umbilical cord pH

see Chapter 65 for details

Figure 52.2 SUGGESTED ALGORITHM FOR ANTEPARTUM FETAL SURVEILLANCE

Low-risk pregnancies	Pregnancies at high risk for uteroplacental insufficiency
No routine antenatal testing	• Hypertensive disease • Diabetes • Rh isoimmunization • Renal disease • Anemia • Antepartum hemorrhage • Cardiovascular disease • Post-term pregnancy • Advanced maternal age • Collagen vascular disease • Multiple pregnancy • IUGR

Decreased fetal movements

NST

1 Fetal 'kickcharts' starting at 28 to 32 weeks
2 NST ± amniotic fluid estimation weekly starting at 28 to 32 weeks

Oligohydramnios

NR–NST

R–NST, normal fetal movement, no oligohydramnios

Consider delivery if fetus mature

Oligohydramnios

BPP or assessment of amniotic fluid volume, Doppler velocimetry

NORMAL

Continue routine testing

≤4/10 or ≤6/10 with oligohydramnios or severely abnormal Doppler velocimetry (absent or reversed end-diastolic flow (EDF))

6/10 without oligohydramnios, abnormal Doppler velocimetry

Consider delivery

Consider delivery if fetus mature, or repeat BPP in 4–6 hours, Dopplers 2x weekly, and/or daily NST

Introduction

Obstetric care providers have two patients: the mother and the fetus. Assessment of maternal wellbeing is relatively easy, but fetal wellbeing is far more difficult to assess. Several tests have been developed to confirm fetal wellbeing before labor and delivery (Figure 52.1).

Goal

• There are many causes of irreversible neonatal cerebral injury, including congenital abnormalities, intracerebral hemorrhage, hypoxia, infection, drugs, trauma, hypotension, and metabolic derangements (hypoglycemia, thyroid dysfunction).

• Antenatal fetal testing cannot predict or reliably detect all of these causes. The goal of antepartum fetal surveillance (Figure 52.2) is early identification of a fetus at risk for preventable morbidity or mortality due specifically to uteroplacental insufficiency.

• Antenatal fetal tests make the following assumptions:

1 that pregnancies may be complicated by progressive fetal asphyxia which can lead to fetal death or permanent handicap

2 that current antenatal tests can adequately discriminate between asphyxiated and non-asphyxiated fetuses

3 that detection of asphyxia at an early stage can lead to an intervention, which is capable of reducing the likelihood of an adverse perinatal outcome.

It is not clear whether any of these assumptions are true. At most, 15% of cerebral palsy is due to birth asphyxia.

Note. All antepartum fetal tests should be interpreted in light of the gestational age, the presence or absence of congenital anomalies, and underlying clinical risk factors.

Antepartum fetal tests

Non-stress test (NST)

• Also known as cardiotocography (CTG).

• NST refers to changes in the fetal heart rate pattern with time (see Chapter 65). It reflects maturity of the fetal autonomic nervous system. NST is non-invasive, simple to perform, readily available, and inexpensive. However, interpretation is largely subjective.

• *Is a "reactive" NST (R-NST) reassuring?* R-NST is defined as an NST with normal baseline heart rate (110–160 beats/min), moderate variability, and at least two accelerations in 20 minutes each lasting ≥15 s and peaking at ≥15 beats/min above baseline (≥10 beats/min for ≥10 s if <32 weeks). Weekly R-NST after 32 weeks' gestation has been shown to decrease perinatal mortality. R-NST is therefore reassuring.

• *Is a non-reactive NST (NR-NST) worrisome?* NR-NST should be interpreted in light of gestational age: 65% of fetuses will have R-NST by 28 weeks, 95% by 32 weeks. Once R-NST has been documented in a given pregnancy, it should remain so throughout delivery. NR-NST at term is associated with poor perinatal outcome in only 20% of cases. The significance of NR-NST depends on the clinical end-point. If the end-point is a 5-min Apgar score <7, NR-NST at term has a sensitivity of 57%, positive predictive value of 13%, and negative predictive value of 98% (assuming a prevalence of 4%). If the end-point is permanent cerebral injury, then NR-NST at term has a 99.8% false-positive rate.

• *Is there a place for vibroacoustic stimulation?* Refers to the response of the fetal heart rate to a vibroacoustic stimulus. Acceleration on NST (≥15 beats/min for ≥15 s) is a positive result. It is a useful adjunct to decrease the time to achieve R-NST and to decrease the proportion of NR-NST at term, thereby precluding the need for further testing.

Biophysical profile

• Biophysical profile (BPP) refers to a sonographic scoring system designed to assess fetal wellbeing.

• The five variables described in the original BPP were: NST, fetal movement, fetal tone, amniotic fluid volume, and fetal breathing. Two points are awarded if the variable is present or normal, 0 points if absent or abnormal. Amniotic fluid volume is the most important variable. More recently, BPP is interpreted without the NST.

• Recommended management based on the original BPP:

Score	Interpretation	Recommended management
8–10	Normal	No intervention
6	Suspect asphyxia	Repeat in 4–6 hours. Consider delivery for oligohydramnios
4	Suspect asphyxia	≥36 weeks or mature pulmonary indices, deliver
		<36 weeks, repeat in 4–6 hours versus delivery with mature pulmonary indices. If persistently ≤4, deliver
0–2	High suspicion of asphyxia	Evaluate for immediate delivery

Fetal movement charts ("kickcharts")

• Maternal appreciation of fetal movement is reliable.

• Fetal movement decreases with advancing gestational age, oligohydramnios, smoking, and antenatal corticosteroid therapy.

• "Kickcharts" involve either counting all fetal movements in 1 hour or counting the time that it takes the fetus to kick 10 times ("count-to-ten"). Measurements should be repeated at least twice daily.

• Use of "kickcharts" in high-risk pregnancies can decrease perinatal mortality fourfold.

Doppler velocimetry

• Umbilical artery Doppler velocimetry measurements reflect resistance to blood flow from the fetus to the placenta.

• Absent or reversed diastolic flow is associated with poor perinatal outcome in the setting of intrauterine growth restriction (IUGR), and urgent delivery should be considered. It is unclear how to interpret these data in the setting of a normally grown fetus.

• Abnormal flow in the middle cerebral artery (MCA) and ductus venosus may help in the timing of delivery of IUGR fetuses.

Contraction stress test (CST)

• CST refers to the response of the fetal heart rate to artificially induced uterine contractions. A minimum of three contractions in 10 minutes are required to interpret the test. A negative CST (no decelerations with contractions) is reassuring. A positive CST (severe variable or late decelerations with ≥50% of contractions) is associated with adverse perinatal outcome in 35–40% of cases. However, the false-positive rate exceeds 50%. An equivocal CST should be repeated in 24–72 hours. More than 80% of repeat tests will be negative.

• As this test is time-consuming, requires skilled nursing care, and may precipitate "fetal distress" needing emergency cesarean section delivery, it is not routinely used in clinical practice.

53 Hydrops fetalis

Figure 53.1 CLASSIFICATION OF SEVERITY OF HYDROPS FETALIS

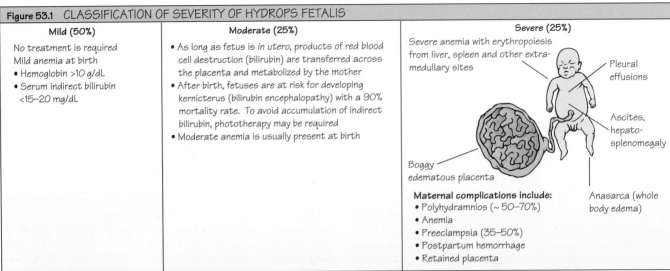

Mild (50%)

No treatment is required
Mild anemia at birth
- Hemoglobin >10 g/dL
- Serum indirect bilirubin <15–20 mg/dL

Moderate (25%)

- As long as fetus is *in utero*, products of red blood cell destruction (bilirubin) are transferred across the placenta and metabolized by the mother
- After birth, fetuses are at risk for developing kernicterus (bilirubin encephalopathy) with a 90% mortality rate. To avoid accumulation of indirect bilirubin, phototherapy may be required
- Moderate anemia is usually present at birth

Severe (25%)

Severe anemia with erythropoiesis from liver, spleen and other extra-medullary sites

Pleural effusions

Ascites, hepato-splenomegaly

Boggy edematous placenta

Anasarca (whole body edema)

Maternal complications include:
- Polyhydramnios (~ 50–70%)
- Anemia
- Preeclampsia (35–50%)
- Postpartum hemorrhage
- Retained placenta

Figure 53.2 EVALUATION AND MANAGEMENT OF Rh ISOIMMUNIZATION IN PREGNANCY

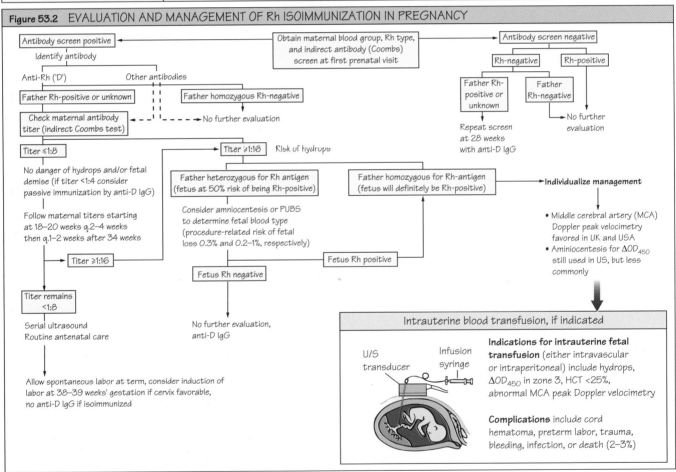

Obtain maternal blood group, Rh type, and indirect antibody (Coombs) screen at first prenatal visit

Antibody screen positive

Identify antibody

Anti-Rh ('D')   Other antibodies

Father Rh-positive or unknown   Father homozygous Rh-negative

Check maternal antibody titer (indirect Coombs test) ---- → No further evaluation

Titer <1:8

No danger of hydrops and/or fetal demise (if titer <1:4 consider passive immunization by anti-D IgG)

Follow maternal titers starting at 18–20 weeks q.2–4 weeks then q.1–2 weeks after 34 weeks

Titer ≥1:16

Titer remains <1:8

Serial ultrasound
Routine antenatal care

Allow spontaneous labor at term, consider induction of labor at 38–39 weeks' gestation if cervix favorable, no anti-D IgG if isoimmunized

Titer ≥1:18   Risk of hydrops

Father heterozygous for Rh antigen (fetus at 50% risk of being Rh-positive)

Consider amniocentesis or PUBS to determine fetal blood type (procedure-related risk of fetal loss 0.3% and 0.2–1%, respectively)

Fetus Rh negative

No further evaluation, anti-D IgG

Father homozygous for Rh-antigen (fetus will definitely be Rh-positive)

Fetus Rh positive

Antibody screen negative

Rh-negative   Rh-positive

Father Rh-positive or unknown   Father Rh-negative

Repeat screen at 28 weeks with anti-D IgG

No further evaluation

→ Individualize management

- Middle cerebral artery (MCA) Doppler peak velocimetry favored in UK and USA
- Aminiocentesis for ΔOD_{450} still used in US, but less commonly

Intrauterine blood transfusion, if indicated

U/S transducer   Infusion syringe

Indications for intrauterine fetal transfusion (either intravascular or intraperitoneal) include hydrops, ΔOD_{450} in zone 3, HCT <25%, abnormal MCA peak Doppler velocimetry

Complications include cord hematoma, preterm labor, trauma, bleeding, infection, or death (2–3%)

Definition
- Latin for "edema of the fetus."
- Refers to an abnormal accumulation of fluid in more than one fetal extravascular compartment.

Incidence
Less than 1% of pregnancies.

Diagnosis
- Hydrops fetalis is a sonographic diagnosis requiring the presence of an abnormal accumulation of fluid in more than one fetal extravascular compartment, including subcutaneous edema, ascites, pericardial effusions, and, pleural effusions. Subcutaneous edema, or placental edema. Polyhydramnios is seen in 50–75% of cases.
- A search for the underlying cause should include:
  1 a detailed history (eg, of recent maternal infection)
  2 serologic screening (blood type and antibody screen, antibody screen for **t**oxoplasmosis, **r**ubella, **c**ytomegalovirus, **h**erpes ["TORCH titers"])
  3 Kleihauer–Betke test (an acid elution test to estimate the total volume of fetal–maternal hemorrhage)
  4 ultrasound survey with or without fetal karyotype.

Prognosis
- Depends on gestational age, severity, and etiology.
- Overall perinatal mortality rate exceeds 50%.

Classification

Non-immune fetal hydrops (90%)
- *Definition.* Hydrops fetalis without an immune etiology.
- *Incidence.* This is 1 in 2000 live births. Since the introduction of anti-D immunoglobin G (IgG), non-immune hydrops is the most common cause of hydrops fetalis.
- *Etiology.* The major causes of non-immune hydrops include:
  1 idiopathic (no known cause) (50–60%)
  2 cardiac abnormalities (20–35%) including congenital dysrhythmias and structural anomalies
  3 chromosomal anomalies (15%) such as Turner syndrome
  4 hematologic aberrations (10%) such as α-thalassemia, fetal anemia
  5 other causes (fetal structural anomalies, infection, twin–twin transfusion syndrome, vascular malformations, placental anomalies, congenital metabolic disorders).
- *Management.* Depends on gestational age, severity, and etiology. Pregnancy termination is an option before fetal viability. Ultrasound may be useful to confirm diagnosis, determine severity (Figure 53.1), and monitor progression. Moderate or severe hydrops may be an indication for immediate delivery regardless of gestational age.

Immune fetal hydrops (10%)
- Also known as erythroblastosis fetalis or hemolytic disease.
- *Etiology.* Immune hydrops occurs when fetal erythrocytes express a protein(s) that is not present on maternal erythrocytes. The maternal immune system can become sensitized and produce antibodies against these "foreign" proteins. IgG antibodies can cross the placenta and destroy fetal erythrocytes, leading to fetal anemia and high-output cardiac failure. Immune fetal hydrops is usually associated with a fetal hematocrit <15% (normal 50%). The most antigenic protein on the surface of erythrocytes is D, also known as rhesus (Rh) D. Other antigens that can cause severe immune hydrops include Kell ("Kell kills"), RhE, Rhc, and Duffy ("Duffy dies"). Antigens causing less severe hydrops include ABO, Rhe, RhC, Fy^a, Ce, k, and s. Lewis incompatibility can cause mild anemia but not hydrops because they are primarily IgM antibodies, which do not cross the placenta ("Lewis lives"); 60% of immune hydrops is currently due to ABO incompatibility.
- *Screening.* Blood type and antibody screening is recommended for all women at their first prenatal visit.
- *Rh isoimmunization* (Figure 53.2). RhD antigen is expressed only on primate erythrocytes. It is evident by 38 days of intrauterine life. Mutation in the D gene on chromosome 1 results in lack of expression of D antigen on circulating erythrocytes. Such individuals are regarded as Rh negative. This mutation arose first in the Basque region of Spain, and the difference in prevalence of Rh-negative individuals between the races may reflect the amount of Spanish blood in their ancestry (white 15%, African–Americans 8%, African 4%, Native American 1%, Asian <<1%).
- If the fetus of an Rh-negative woman is itself Rh negative, Rh sensitization will not occur. However, 60% of Rh-negative women will have an Rh-positive fetus.
- Exposure of Rh-negative women to as little as 0.25 mL of Rh-positive blood may induce an antibody response (*opposite*). As the initial immune response is IgM (which does not cross the placenta), the index pregnancy is rarely affected. However, immunization in subsequent pregnancies will trigger an IgG response that will cross the placenta and cause hemolysis.
- *Risk factors* for Rh sensitization include:
  1 mismatched blood transfusion (95% sensitization rate)
  2 ectopic pregnancy (<1%)
  3 abortion (3–6%)
  4 amniocentesis (1–3%)
  5 pregnancy (16–18% sensitization rate following normal pregnancy without anti-D IgG, 1.3% with anti-D IgG at delivery, 0.13% with anti-D IgG at delivery and at 28 weeks).
- *Prevention.* Passive immunization with anti-D IgG can destroy fetal erythrocytes before they evoke a maternal immune response. Anti-D IgG should be given within 72 hours of potential exposure; 300 μg (USA) or 500 IU (UK) given intramuscularly will cover up to 30 mL fetal whole blood or 15 mL fetal red cells.
- *Management.* Immune-mediated fetal hemolysis results in release of bile pigment into amniotic fluid that can be measured as the change in optical density at wavelength 450 nm (ΔOD_{450}). Traditionally, the degree of hemolysis was measured by serial amniocentesis. Amniotic fluid ΔOD_{450} measurements were plotted against gestational age (Liley curve) in an attempt to predict fetal outcome. If the ΔOD_{450} rose into the upper 80% of zone 2 or into zone 3 of the Liley curve, prompt intervention was indicated. More recently, measurements of peak velocity in the middle cerebral artery of the fetus using non-invasive Doppler ultrasound has been shown to accurately identify fetuses with severe anemia requiring intervention. Depending on gestational age, this may include immediate delivery or fetal blood transfusion via percutaneous umbilical cord blood sampling (PUBS).

Transfusion volume (mL)	Incidence at delivery (%)	Risk of isoimmunization (%)[a]
Unmeasurable	50	Minimal
<0.1	45–50	3
>5	1	20–40
>30	0.25	60–80

[a]Without anti-D IgG.

Figure 54.1 COMPLICATIONS OF INTRAUTERINE FETAL DEMISE

Consumptive coagulopathy

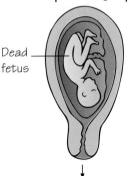

Dead fetus

↓

Transplacental leakage of thromboplastin and thromboplastin-like material into the maternal circulation

↓

Consumption of coagulation factors including factors V and VIII, prothrombin, and platelets

↓

Clinical manifestations of disseminated intravascular coagulopathy (DIC)

Multicystic encephalomalacia

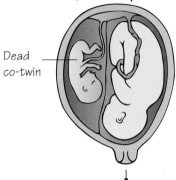

Dead co-twin

↓

Embolization of thromboplastic material from the dead fetus via placental vascular communications to the surviving fetus with or without dramatic hemodynamic changes (hypotension) at the time of fetal demise

↓

Infarction and cellular injury in the brain (known as multicystic encephalomalacia, diagnosis confirmed by electroencephalography (EEG)), bowel, kidney, lung

Figure 54.2 IDENTIFICATION OF THE CAUSE OF INTRAUTERINE FETAL DEMISE

Maternal conditions
- Random glucose or hemoglobin A1c (HbA1c)
- Maternal complete blood count
- Urine toxicology
- Thyroid function testing
- Rh antibody status

Placenta/fetal membrane complications
- Pathological examination of the placenta, fetal membranes, umbilical cord
- Histological examination

Infections
- VDRL or RPR
- CMV titers
- Bacterial/viral cultures
- Histological examination of placenta/fetal membranes

Tests which should be sent to help determine the etiology of the fetal death

Antiphospholipid antibody syndrome
- Lupus anticoagulant
- Anticardiolipin antibody ('positive' high titers IgG)
- Anti-B2-glycoprotein I

Chromosomal anomalies
- Fetal karyotype
- Fetal autopsy (including X-rays)

Fetal-maternal hemorrhage
- Kleihauer–Betke test (the only test which must be sent immediately after delivery as fetal cells will rapidly disappear from the maternal circulation)

Definition

Intrauterine fetal demise (IUFD) or stillbirth refers to fetal demise before delivery.

Incidence

In developing countries, the stillbirth rate has decreased from 15–16 per 1,000 total births in the 1960s to 7–8 per 1,000 births in the 1990s.

Risk factors

These include extremes of maternal age, multifetal pregnancy, post-term pregnancy, male fetus, and fetal macrosomia (defined as estimated fetal weight ≥4,500 g).

Diagnosis

• *Symptoms.* If fetal demise occurs early in pregnancy, there may be no symptoms aside from cessation of the usual symptoms of pregnancy (nausea, frequency, breast tenderness). Later in pregnancy, fetal demise should be suspected if there is a prolonged period without fetal movement.

• *Signs.* The inability to identify fetal heart tones at a prenatal visit beyond 12 weeks' gestation and/or the absence of uterine growth may suggest the diagnosis.

• *Laboratory tests.* Declining levels of human chorionic gonadotropin (hCG) may aid in the diagnosis early in pregnancy.

• *Radiological studies.* Historically, an abdominal radiograph was used to confirm IUFD. The three radiologic findings suggestive of fetal death include overlapping of the fetal skull bones (Spalding sign), an exaggerated curvature of the fetal spine, and gas within the fetus. However, radiographs are no longer used. Ultrasound is now the gold standard to confirm IUFD by documenting the absence of fetal cardiac activity beyond 6 weeks' gestation. Other sonographic findings include scalp edema and fetal maceration.

Singleton IUFD

Natural history

Latency (the period from fetal demise to delivery) varies depending on the underlying cause and gestational age. The earlier the gestational age, the longer the latency period. Overall, >90% of women will go into spontaneous labor within 2 weeks of fetal death.

Complications (Figure 54.1)

About 20–25% of women who retain a dead fetus for longer than 3 weeks will develop *disseminated intravascular coagulopathy* (DIC) due to excessive consumption of clotting factors.

Management

• Every effort should be made to avoid cesarean section delivery. As such, expectant management is often recommended. However, many women find the prospect of carrying a dead fetus distressing and want the pregnancy terminated as soon as possible.

• Early pregnancies can be terminated surgically by dilation and evacuation. After 20 weeks, the safest method of pregnancy termination is induction of labor. Cervical ripening may be necessary.

• Parents should be allowed to grieve for their lost child. Individualization of patient care is important, but parents should be encouraged to hold their child, give him or her a name, and be involved in the decision about disposal of remains.

• Identification of a cause for the fetal demise (Figure 54.2) may help in the grieving process and in future counseling. An autopsy is the single most useful step in identifying the cause of fetal death.

Etiology

• Of fetal deaths 50% are *idiopathic* (have no known cause).

• *Maternal medical conditions* (hypertension, pre-eclampsia, diabetes mellitus) are associated with an increased incidence of fetal death. Early detection and appropriate management will reduce the risk of IUFD.

• *Placental complications* (placenta previa, abruption) may cause fetal death. Cord accident is impossible to predict, but is most commonly seen in monochorionic/monoamniotic twin pregnancies before 32 weeks' gestation.

• Fetal karyotyping should be considered in all cases of fetal death to identify *chromosomal abnormalities*, particularly in cases with documented fetal structural abnormalities. The success of cytogenetic analysis decreases as latency increases. On occasion, amniocentesis is performed to salvage viable amniocytes for cytogenetic analysis.

• *Fetal–maternal hemorrhage* (transplacental passage of red blood cells from fetus to mother) can cause fetal death. It occurs in all pregnancies, but is usually minimal (<0.1 mL). In rare instances, fetal–maternal hemorrhage may be massive. The Kleihauer–Betke (acid elution) test allows an estimate of the volume of fetal blood in the maternal circulation.

• *Antiphospholipid antibody syndrome.* The diagnosis requires the correct clinical setting (three or more first trimester or one or more second trimester unexplained pregnancy losses, unexplained thromboembolic event, autoimmune thrombocytopenia) and one or more confirmatory laboratory tests.

• *Intra-amniotic infection* resulting in fetal death is usually evident on clinical examination. Placental culture and histologic examination of the fetus, placenta/fetal membranes, and umbilical cord may be useful.

IUFD of one twin

Prognosis

• The prognosis for the surviving twin after demise of its co-twin is dependent on the cause of death, gestational age, degree of shared fetal circulation (chorionicity), and time interval between death of the first twin and delivery of the second.

• Dizygous twin pregnancies do not share circulation (see Chapter 55). As such, death of one twin has little impact on the surviving twin. The dead twin may be resorbed completely or become compressed and incorporated into the membranes (*fetus papyraceus*). DIC in the mother is exceptionally rare.

• Some degree of shared circulation can be demonstrated in 99% of monozygous twin pregnancies. In this setting, death of one fetus often results in immediate death of the other. If, by chance, the second fetus survives, it is at high risk of developing *multicystic encephalomalacia*.

Management

• Management of a surviving co-twin depends on chorionicity and gestational age.

• Fetal wellbeing (kickcharts, non-stress testing, biophysical profile) should be assessed on a regular basis. In the setting of "fetal distress"/non-reassuring fetal testing, immediate delivery is indicated.

• Delivery should be considered once pulmonary maturity is documented or a favorable gestational age is reached.

Figure 55.1 MULTIPLE PREGANCY FLOWCHART

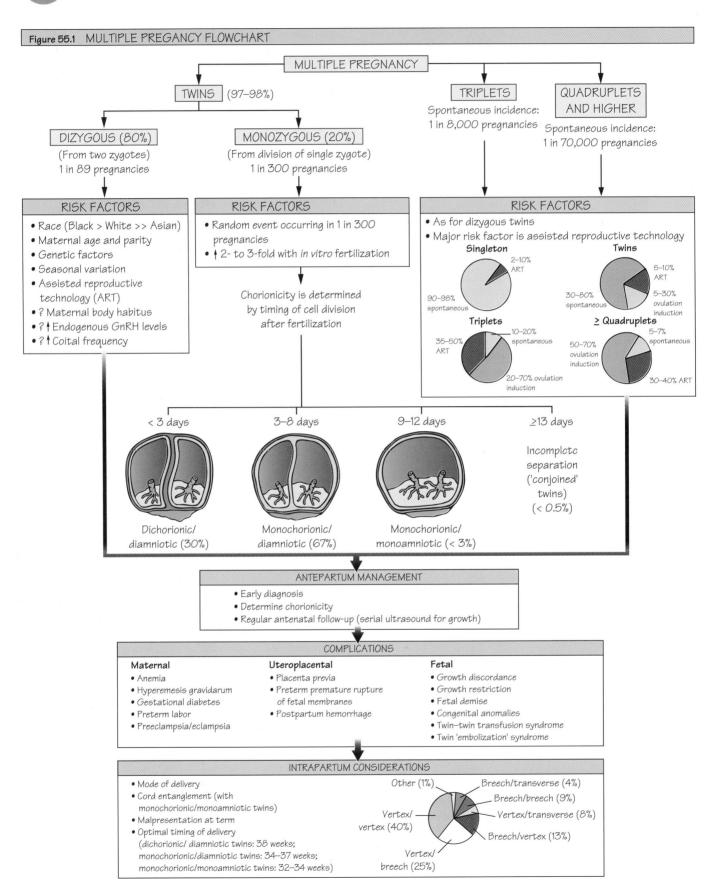

MULTIPLE PREGNANCY

TWINS (97–98%)

TRIPLETS
Spontaneous incidence:
1 in 8,000 pregnancies

QUADRUPLETS
AND HIGHER
Spontaneous incidence:
1 in 70,000 pregnancies

DIZYGOUS (80%)
(From two zygotes)
1 in 89 pregnancies

MONOZYGOUS (20%)
(From division of single zygote)
1 in 300 pregnancies

RISK FACTORS
- Race (Black > White >> Asian)
- Maternal age and parity
- Genetic factors
- Seasonal variation
- Assisted reproductive technology (ART)
- ? Maternal body habitus
- ? ↑ Endogenous GnRH levels
- ? ↑ Coital frequency

RISK FACTORS
- Random event occurring in 1 in 300 pregnancies
- ↑ 2- to 3-fold with *in vitro* fertilization

Chorionicity is determined by timing of cell division after fertilization

RISK FACTORS
- As for dizygous twins
- Major risk factor is assisted reproductive technology

Singleton
2–10% ART
90–98% spontaneous

Twins
5–10% ART
5–30% ovulation induction
30–80% spontaneous

Triplets
10–20% spontaneous
35–50% ART
20–70% ovulation induction

≥ Quadruplets
5–7% spontaneous
50–70% ovulation induction
30–40% ART

< 3 days — Dichorionic/diamniotic (30%)

3–8 days — Monochorionic/diamniotic (67%)

9–12 days — Monochorionic/monoamniotic (< 3%)

≥13 days — Incomplcte separation ('conjoined' twins) (< 0.5%)

ANTEPARTUM MANAGEMENT
- Early diagnosis
- Determine chorionicity
- Regular antenatal follow-up (serial ultrasound for growth)

COMPLICATIONS

Maternal
- Anemia
- Hyperemesis gravidarum
- Gestational diabetes
- Preterm labor
- Preeclampsia/eclampsia

Uteroplacental
- Placenta previa
- Preterm premature rupture of fetal membranes
- Postpartum hemorrhage

Fetal
- Growth discordance
- Growth restriction
- Fetal demise
- Congenital anomalies
- Twin–twin transfusion syndrome
- Twin 'embolization' syndrome

INTRAPARTUM CONSIDERATIONS
- Mode of delivery
- Cord entanglement (with monochorionic/monoamniotic twins)
- Malpresentation at term
- Optimal timing of delivery (dichorionic/diamniotic twins: 38 weeks; monochorionic/diamniotic twins: 34–37 weeks; monochorionic/monoamniotic twins: 32–34 weeks)

Other (1%)
Breech/transverse (4%)
Breech/breech (9%)
Vertex/vertex (40%)
Vertex/transverse (8%)
Breech/vertex (13%)
Vertex/breech (25%)

Obstetrics and Gynecology at a Glance, Fourth Edition. Errol R. Norwitz and John O. Schorge.

Incidence
- This is 1–2% of all deliveries.
- The majority (97–98%) are twin pregnancies; 80% of twin pregnancies are dizygous (derived from two separate embryos).
- Multiple pregnancies are becoming increasingly common, primarily as a result of assisted reproductive technology (ART). This is especially true of higher-order multiple pregnancies (triplets and up) which now constitute 0.1–0.3% of all births.

Diagnosis
- Multiple pregnancy should be suspected in women with risk factors (Figure 55.1), excessive symptoms of pregnancy, or uterine size greater than expected.
- Ultrasound will confirm the diagnosis.

Chorionicity (Figure 55.1)
- Chorionicity refers to the arrangement of membranes in multiple pregnancies. It has important prognostic implications.
- Perinatal mortality rate is higher with monozygous (30–50%) than with dizygous twins (10–20%), and is especially high with monochorionic/monoamniotic twins (65–70%).
- Chorionicity is determined most accurately by examination of the membranes after delivery. Antenatal diagnosis is more difficult. Identification of separate sex fetuses or two separate placentas confirm dichorionic/diamniotic placentation.

Complications
Antepartum complications develop in 80% of multiple pregnancies compared with 30% of singleton pregnancies.

1 Multiple pregnancies account for 10% of all *perinatal deaths.*

2 *Preterm delivery* increases as fetal number increases: the average length of gestation is 40 weeks in singletons, 37 weeks in twins, 33 weeks in triplets, and 29 weeks in quadruplets.

3 *Preterm premature rupture of membranes* occurs in 10–20% of multiple pregnancies (see Chapter 59).

4 *Fetal growth discordance* (defined as a ≥20% difference in estimated fetal weight between fetuses) occurs in 5–15% of twins and 30% of triplets. Perinatal mortality is increased sixfold.

5 *Intrauterine demise* of one twin (see Chapter 54).

6 *Twin polyhydramnios/oligohydramnios sequence* results from an imbalance in blood flow from the "donor" twin to the "recipient." Both twins are at risk for adverse events. Twin–twin transfusion syndrome is a subset of polyhydramnios/oligohydramnios sequence seen in 15% of monochorionic pregnancies, and is due to vascular communications between the fetal circulations. After delivery, a difference in birth weight of ≥20% or a difference in hematocrit ≥5 g/dL confirms the diagnosis. Prognosis depends on gestational age, severity, and underlying etiology. Overall perinatal mortality rate is 40–80%. Treatment options include expectant management, serial amniocentesis, indomethacin (to decrease fetal urine output), laser obliteration of the placental vascular communications, or selective fetal reduction.

7 *"Stuck-twin" syndrome* is an ultrasound diagnosis with severe oligohydramnios of the affected fetus which appears "vacuum packed" in its membranes. In 40% of cases, this represents severe polyhydramnios/oligohydramnios sequence. Perinatal mortality is very high.

8 *Twin reversed arterial perfusion (TRAP) sequence* is a rare complication of monozygotic twinning (1 in 35,000 deliveries) in which vascular communications within the umbilical cord or placenta cause blood to flow from one twin retrograde up the umbilical arteries to its co-twin before returning to the placenta. As a result, the co-twin (known as the "acardiac" twin) develops multiple congenital anomalies, including absent head and trunk regions, absent cardiac structures, and reduction anomalies in other organ systems. Prognosis for the normal twin may be improved if the acardiac twin is removed.

9 *Cord entanglement* is rare (1 in 25,000 births), but may occur in up to 70% of monochorionic/monoamniotic pregnancies and account for >50% of perinatal mortality in this subgroup. As such, delivery is usually by cesarean section. The risk of death due to cord entanglement appears to decrease after 32 weeks, although there is an overall increase in perinatal mortality in the third trimester. For this reason, monochorionic/monoamniotic twin pregnancies are usually delivered at 32–34 weeks.

Management issues specific to multiple pregnancy
Selective fetal reduction
- Of higher-order multiple pregnancies 10–15% will reduce spontaneously during the first trimester. For those that do not reduce, selective fetal reduction to twins at 13–15 weeks has been recommended.
- The procedure-related loss rate before 20 weeks is 15% (range 5–35%), which is comparable to the background risk for higher-order multiple pregnancies.
- The benefits of selective reduction include increased gestational length, increased birthweight, and reduced prematurity and perinatal mortality. For quadruplet pregnancies and upward, the benefits of selective reduction clearly outweigh the risks. In the absence of fetal anomaly, no clear benefit has been demonstrated for reduction of twins to a singleton. Whether triplet pregnancies benefit from selective reduction to twins, however, remains controversial. Overall, reduction of triplets to twins seems to result in a more satisfactory pregnancy outcome.

Screening for congenital anomalies
- Second trimester maternal serum analyte screening for aneuploidy and/or maternal serum α-fetoprotein (MS-AFP) for open neural tube defect is available for twins (not triplets), as it is for singletons at 15–20 weeks' gestation. *First trimester aneuploidy screening* (nuchal translucency + serum pregnancy-associated plasma protein A [PAPP-A] and β human chorionic gonadotropin [βhCG]) is rapidly becoming the preferred aneuploidy screening test for multiple pregnancies (see Chapter 39).
- In dizygous twin pregnancies, the risk of *aneuploidy* (genetic abnormality) is independent for each fetus. As such, the chance that one or both fetuses have a karyotypic abnormality is greater than for a singleton. US practice favors offering amniocentesis when the probability of aneuploidy is equal to or greater than the procedure-related pregnancy loss rate (quoted as 1 in 400). In singleton pregnancies, this balance is reached at a maternal age at delivery of 35 years. In twin pregnancies, this balance is reached at a maternal age at delivery of around 32 years.

Route of delivery
- Recommended route of delivery of twins depends on presentation, gestational age (or estimated fetal weight), and maternal and fetal wellbeing.
- Cesarean section delivery has traditionally been recommended for multiple pregnancies in which the presenting fetus is not vertex and for all higher-order multiple pregnancies, although vaginal delivery may be appropriate in selected patients.

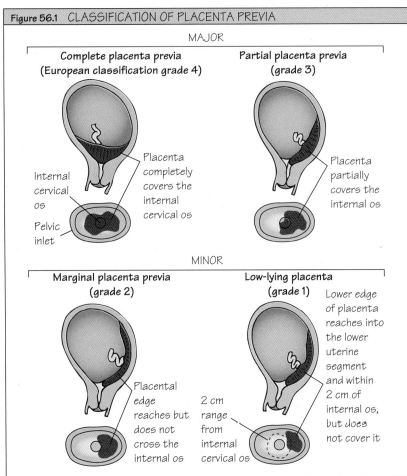

Figure 56.1 CLASSIFICATION OF PLACENTA PREVIA

MAJOR

Complete placenta previa
(European classification grade 4)

Partial placenta previa
(grade 3)

Internal cervical os

Pelvic inlet

Placenta completely covers the internal cervical os

Placenta partially covers the internal os

MINOR

Marginal placenta previa
(grade 2)

Low-lying placenta
(grade 1)

Placental edge reaches but does not cross the internal os

2 cm range from internal cervical os

Lower edge of placenta reaches into the lower uterine segment and within 2 cm of internal os, but does not cover it

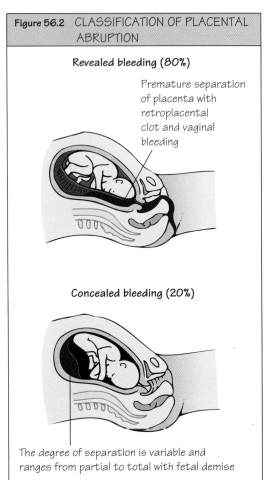

Figure 56.2 CLASSIFICATION OF PLACENTAL ABRUPTION

Revealed bleeding (80%)

Premature separation of placenta with retroplacental clot and vaginal bleeding

Concealed bleeding (20%)

The degree of separation is variable and ranges from partial to total with fetal demise

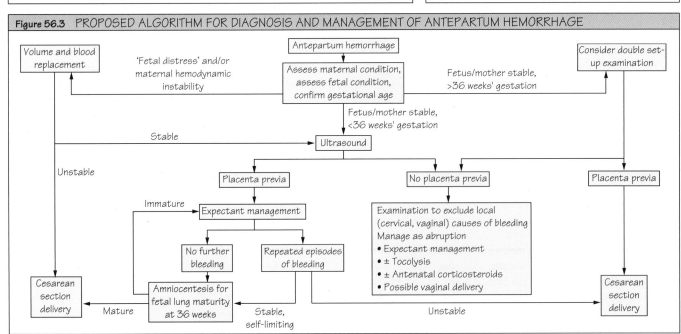

Figure 56.3 PROPOSED ALGORITHM FOR DIAGNOSIS AND MANAGEMENT OF ANTEPARTUM HEMORRHAGE

Volume and blood replacement

'Fetal distress' and/or maternal hemodynamic instability

Antepartum hemorrhage

Assess maternal condition, assess fetal condition, confirm gestational age

Fetus/mother stable, >36 weeks' gestation

Consider double set-up examination

Fetus/mother stable, <36 weeks' gestation

Stable

Ultrasound

Unstable

Placenta previa

No placenta previa

Placenta previa

Immature

Expectant management

No further bleeding

Repeated episodes of bleeding

Examination to exclude local (cervical, vaginal) causes of bleeding
Manage as abruption
• Expectant management
• ± Tocolysis
• ± Antenatal corticosteroids
• Possible vaginal delivery

Cesarean section delivery

Mature

Amniocentesis for fetal lung maturity at 36 weeks

Stable, self-limiting

Unstable

Cesarean section delivery

Obstetrics and Gynecology at a Glance, Fourth Edition. Errol R. Norwitz and John O. Schorge.

120 © 2013 John Wiley & Sons, Ltd. Published 2013 by John Wiley & Sons, Ltd.

Definition

Vaginal bleeding after 24 weeks' gestation and before labor.

Incidence

This is 4–5% of all pregnancies.

Differential diagnosis

Placenta previa (20%)

• *Definition.* Implantation of the placenta over the cervical os in advance of the fetal presenting part.

• *Incidence.* One in 200 pregnancies.

• *Risk factors.* Multiparity, advanced maternal age, prior placenta previa, prior cesarean section delivery, smoking.

• *Classification* (Figure 56.1).

• *Diagnosis.* Characterized clinically by painless, bright-red vaginal bleeding. Bleeding is of maternal origin. Fetal malpresentation is common because the placenta prevents engagement of the presenting part. May be an incidental finding on ultrasound.

Note. When a woman presents with antepartum hemorrhage, pelvic examination should be avoided until placenta previa has been excluded.

• *Ultrasound.* Ultrasound is accurate at diagnosing placenta previa. Only 5% of cases of placenta previa identified by ultrasound in the second trimester persist to term.

• *Antepartum management.* The goal is to maximize fetal maturation while minimizing risk to mother and fetus. "Fetal distress" and excessive maternal hemorrhage are contraindications to expectant management, and may necessitate immediate cesarean section irrespective of gestational age. However, most episodes of bleeding are not life threatening. With careful monitoring, delivery can be safely delayed in most cases. Outpatient management may be an option for women with a single small bleed if they can comply with restrictions on activity and maintain proximity to a hospital. Placenta previa may resolve with time, thereby permitting vaginal delivery.

• *Intrapartum management.* Elective cesarean section delivery is recommended at 36–37 weeks' gestation. Vaginal delivery is rarely appropriate, but may be indicated in the setting of intrauterine fetal demise, fetal malformation(s) incompatible with life, advanced labor with engagement of the fetal head and minimal vaginal bleeding, or an indicated delivery with a pre-viable fetus. A *double set-up examination* in labor may be appropriate when ultrasound cannot exclude placenta previa and the patient is strongly motivated for vaginal delivery. This procedure is performed in the operating room with surgical anesthesia and two surgical teams. One team is scrubbed and ready for immediate cesarean section in the event of hemorrhage or "fetal distress." The other team then performs a gentle bimanual examination, initially of the vaginal fornices and then the cervical os. If a previa is present, immediate cesarean section is indicated. If no placenta is palpated, amniotomy can be performed and labor induced.

• *Maternal complications.* Placenta accreta (abnormal attachment of placental villi to the uterine wall) is rare (1 in 2,500 pregnancies), but complicates 5% of pregnancies with placenta previa, 10–25% with placenta previa and one prior cesarean section, and >50% with placenta previa and two or more prior cesarean sections.

• *Neonatal complications.* Preterm birth, malpresentation. Placenta previa is not associated with intrauterine growth restriction (IUGR).

Placental abruption (30%)

• *Definition.* Premature separation of the placenta from the uterine side wall.

• *Incidence.* One in 120 pregnancies.

• *Risk factors.* hypertension, prior placental abruption, trauma, smoking, cocaine, uterine anomaly or fibroids, multiparity, advanced maternal age, preterm premature rupture of the membranes, bleeding diathesis, and rapid decompression of an overdistended uterus (multiple pregnancy, polyhydramnios).

• *Classification* (Figure 56.2).

• *Diagnosis* (Figure 56.3). Presents clinically with vaginal bleeding (80%), uterine contractions (35%), and abdominal tenderness (70%) with or without "fetal distress" (50%). Uterine tenderness suggests extravasation of blood into the myometrium (Couvelaire uterus). The amount of vaginal bleeding may not be a reliable indicator of the severity of the hemorrhage because bleeding may be concealed. Serial measurements of fundal height and abdominal girth are useful to monitor large retroplacental blood collections.

• *Ultrasound.* A retroplacental collection of ≥300 mL is necessary for sonographic visualization. Only 2% of abruptions can be visualized on ultrasound. Port-wine discoloration of the amniotic fluid is highly suggestive of abruption.

• *Antepartum management* (Figure 56.3) Hospitalization is indicated to evaluate maternal and fetal condition. Mode and timing of delivery depend on the condition and gestational age of the fetus, condition of the mother, and state of the cervix. In the setting of hemodynamic instability, invasive monitoring and immediate cesarean section may be necessary. If the abruption is mild and pregnancy is remote from term, expectant management may be appropriate. Placental abruption is a relative contraindication to tocolysis.

• *Maternal complications.* Maternal mortality (due to hemorrhage, cardiac failure, or renal failure) ranges from 0.5% to 5%. Aggressive volume and blood replacement should be initiated. Clinically significant coagulopathy occurs in 10% of cases.

• *Fetal complications.* Fetal demise occurs in 10–35% of cases due to fetal hypoxia, exsanguination, or complications of prematurity. Abruption is also associated with an increased rate of congenital anomalies and IUGR.

• *Recurrence.* This is 10% after one abruption, 25% after two abruptions.

Vasa previa (rare)

• *Definition.* Bleeding from fetal vessels that cross or run in close proximity to the internal cervical os umbilical vessels (fetal blood).

• *Diagnosis.* Apt test (hemoglobin alkaline elution test) involves the addition of two to three drops of an alkaline solution to 1 mL blood. Fetal erythrocytes are resistant to rupture, and the mixture will remain red. If the blood is maternal, erythrocytes will rupture and the mixture will turn brown.

• *Complications.* Bleeding is fetal in origin. As such, fetal mortality rate is >75% due primarily to fetal exsanguination.

• *Treatment.* Emergency cesarean section if the fetus is viable.

Other causes (50%)

• Early labor.

• Lesions of the lower genital tract (cervical polyps, erosion).

Figure 57.1 PHARMACOLOGICAL MANAGEMENT OF PRETERM LABOR

Tocolytic agent	Route of administration (dosage)	Efficacy†	Major maternal side-effects	Major fetal side-effects
Calcium channel blockers • Nifedipine	Oral (20–30 mg q.4–8 h)	Effective	Hypotension, reflex tachycardia, headache, nausea, flushing, potentiates the cardiac depressive effect of magnesium sulfate, hepatotoxicity	–
β-Adrenergic agonists • Terbutaline sulfate • Ritodrine hydrochloride*	IV (2 μg/min infusion, max 80 μg/min) SC (0.25 mg q.20 min) Oral maintenance (2.5–5 mg q.4–6 h) IV pump (0.02 mL/h) IV (50 mg/min infusion, max 350 μg/min IM (5–10 mg q.2–4 h) Oral maintenance (10–20 mg q.3–4 h)	Effective Effective Not effective Not effective Effective Effective Not effective	Jitteriness, anxiety, restlessness, rash, nausea, vomiting, rash, cardiac dysrythmias, chest pain, myocardial ischemia, palpitations, hypotension, tachycardia, pulmonary edema, paralytic ileus, hypokalemia, hyperglycemia, acidosis	Fetal tachycardia, hypotension, ileus, hyper-insulinemia, hypoglycemia, hyperbilirubinemia, hypocalcemia, ? hydrops fetalis
Oxytocin antagonists • Atosiban	IV (1 μmol/L per min infusion, max 32 μmol/L per min)	Effective	Nausea, headache, chest pain, arthralgia	?
Prostaglandin inhibitors • Indomethacin	Oral (25–50 mg q.4–6 h) Rectal (100 mg q.12 h)	Effective Effective	Gastrointestinal effects (nausea, heartburn), headache, rash, interstitial nephritis, increased bleeding time	Transient oliguria, oligohydramnios, premature closure of the neonatal ductus arteriosus and persistent pulmonary hypertension, ? necrotizing enterocolitis, intraventricular hemorrhage
Magnesium sulfate	IV (4–6 g bolus, 2–3 g/h infusion) Oral maintenance (100–120 mg q.4 h)	Effective Not effective	Nausea, vomiting, ileus, headache, weakness, hypotension, pulmonary edema, cardio-respiratory arrest, ? hypocalcemia (magnesium is not absorbed orally)	Decreased fetal heart rate variability, neonatal drowsiness, hypotonia, ? ileus, ? congenital ricketic syndrome (with treatment >7–10 days) ?? Increased mortality in very low birth weight infants
Others • Nitroglycerine	TD (10–50 mg q. day) IV (100 μg bolus, then 1–10 μg/kg per min)	Unproven Unproven	Hypotension, headache	Fetal tachycardia

† Efficacy is defined as proven benefit in delaying delivery by 24–48 hours as compared with placebo or standard control
IM, intramuscular; IV, intravenous; SC, subcutaneous; TD, transdermal
* the only FDH approved drug to prevent preterm birth (but no longer available in USA)

Figure 57.2 CAUSES OF PRETERM BIRTH

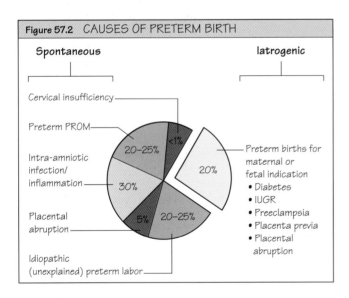

Spontaneous — Iatrogenic

- Cervical insufficiency <1%
- Preterm PROM 20–25%
- Intra-amniotic infection/inflammation 30%
- Placental abruption 5%
- Idiopathic (unexplained) preterm labor 20–25%

Preterm births for maternal or fetal indication 20%
- Diabetes
- IUGR
- Preeclampsia
- Placenta previa
- Placental abruption

Figure 57.3 FOUR MAJOR MECHANISMS RESPONSIBLE FOR PRETERM LABOR

- Intrauterine infection/inflammation
- Maternal stress (e.g., depression) and/or Fetal stress (e.g., IUGR)
- Excessive uterine stretch (e.g., mutiple pregnancy, polyhydramnios)
- Decidual hemorrhage (placental abruption)

Preterm labor

Definition

Premature (preterm) labor refers to the onset of labor before 37–0/7 weeks' gestation.

Incidence

- This is 8–12% (approximately one in eight) of all deliveries
- Accounts for 85% of all perinatal morbidity and mortality.

Pathophysiology

Preterm labor represents either a breakdown in the mechanisms responsible for maintaining uterine quiescence throughout pregnancy or a short-circuiting or overwhelming of the normal parturition cascade that triggers labor prematurely. Four discrete pathways are described, including stress, infection, stretch, and hemorrhage (Figure 57.3).

Obstetrics and Gynecology at a Glance, Fourth Edition. Errol R. Norwitz and John O. Schorge.

122 © 2013 John Wiley & Sons, Ltd. Published 2013 by John Wiley & Sons, Ltd.

Etiology

- Preterm labor represents a syndrome rather than a diagnosis because the etiologies are varied (Figure 57.2).
- Of all preterm births, 20% are iatrogenic (performed for maternal or fetal indications), 30% are associated with intra-amniotic infection/inflammation, 20–25% are associated with preterm premature rupture of membranes (PPROM), and 20–25% result from spontaneous (idiopathic) preterm labor.

Prediction of preterm birth

- *Risk factors* for preterm birth have been identified (see Table 57.1). However, reliance on historic/demographic risk factors alone will fail to identify >50% of pregnancies that deliver preterm.
- Although an increase in uterine activity is a prerequisite for preterm labor, *home uterine monitoring* has not been shown to decrease the incidence of preterm birth.
- Serial *cervical evaluation* is reassuring if the examination remains normal. However, an abnormal finding (dilation or effacement) is associated with preterm delivery in only 4% of low-risk and 20% of high-risk women.
- There is an strong inverse correlation between sonographic *cervical length* (CL) and preterm delivery in both high- and low-risk pregnancies. CL is not currently recommended in low-risk patients. In high-risk pregnancies, baseline CL is recommended at 16–20 weeks followed by serial CL every 2–4 weeks until 30–32 weeks.
- A number of *biochemical/endocrine markers* have been associated with preterm delivery, but only cervicovaginal fetal fibronectin (fFN) has been established as a screening tool. The value of fFN lies in its negative predictive value: 99% of women with a negative fFN at 22–24 weeks will still be pregnant in 1 week, 98% in 2 weeks, and 89% in 3 weeks. However, the positive predictive value is poor (only 25% of women with a positive fFN will deliver before 35 weeks).
- *Vaginal infections* (bacterial vaginosis, *Neisseria gonorrhoeae*, *Chlamydia trachomatis*, *Trichomonas vaginalis*) have been associated with preterm birth. However, routine screening and treatment of high-risk asymptomatic women does not appear to decrease this risk and is not recommended.
- *Intra-amniotic infection* is responsible for 30% of preterm labor. A positive amniotic fluid culture is necessary for a definitive diagnosis, but biomarkers of infection (high interleukin-6, low glucose, increased C-reactive protein, and high white cell count in amniotic fluid) may suggest the diagnosis.
- A number of *endocrine assays* are also being developed to predict preterm labor. Elevated maternal salivary estriol (≥2.1 ng/mL) is predictive of preterm delivery in high-risk populations. Other endocrine assays (relaxin, corticotropin-releasing hormone) are being developed.

Management

- A firm *diagnosis* of preterm labor is necessary before treatment is considered. Diagnosis requires the presence of both uterine contractions and cervical change (or an initial cervical examination ≥2 cm and/or ≥80% effacement in a nulliparous patient).
- A *cause* for preterm labor should always be sought.
- *Absolute contraindications* to tocolytic agents (drugs that inhibit uterine contractions) include intrauterine infection, "fetal distress" (non-reassuring fetal testing), vaginal bleeding, and intrauterine fetal demise. PPROM is a relative contraindication.

- Bed rest and hydration are commonly recommended, but without proven efficacy.
- Short-term *pharmacologic therapy* (Figure 57.1) remains the cornerstone of management. However, there are no reliable data to suggest that any tocolytic agent is able to delay delivery for longer than 24–48 hours. No single agent has a clear therapeutic advantage. As such, the side-effect profile of each of the drugs will often determine which to use in a given clinical setting:
  1 Calcium channel blockers (such as nifedipine) are effective, have few side effects, and are rapidly becoming the first-line tocolytic agent of choice.
  2 β-Adrenergic agonists are also commonly used, but have a higher incidence of maternal adverse effects.
  3 Atosiban (oxytocin receptor antagonist) is commonly used and nitroglycerin is used in some institutions in the UK.
  4 Magnesium sulfate (which acts as a physiologic calcium antagonist and a general inhibitor of neurotransmission) has a wide margin of safety and is still commonly used in the USA. It has the added benefit of neuroprotection in very-low-birthweight infants (<1500 g).
  5 Indometacin (a non-steroidal anti-inflammatory drug) is an effective tocolytic agent, but is associated with a number of serious neonatal complications (such as premature closure of the ductus arteriosus, persistent pulmonary hypertension, oligohydramnios). As such, it is rarely used.
- Maintenance tocolysis beyond 48 hours has not consistently been shown to delay delivery and is associated with significant adverse effects. It is therefore not generally recommended. However, recent meta-analyses suggest that maintenance tocolysis with nifedipine may be beneficial.
- The concurrent use of two or more tocolytic agents has not been shown to be more effective than a single agent alone, and the additive risk of side effects generally precludes this course of management.
- Recent data suggest that progesterone supplementation (not treatment) from 16–20 weeks through 34–36 weeks may prevent preterm delivery in some women at high risk by virtue of a prior unexplained preterm birth or short cervix (but not multiple pregnancy). Studies are under way to better define which women will benefit, and which formulation, dose, and route of administration to use.

Table 57.1 Risk factors for preterm birth

Risk factor	Relative risk
Intra-amniotic infection	50
Multiple gestation	40
Placental abruption	35
Third trimester vaginal bleeding	10
Second trimester vaginal bleeding	2
Prior preterm delivery	2–5
Uterine anomalies	5–7
Diethylstilbestrol (DES) exposure	4
Urinary tract infection	2
Smoking (≥10 cigarettes per day)	2
Illicit drug use (especially cocaine)	2
Maternal age >35 years	2–3
African–American race	2
Low socioeconomic status	1.5–2

Figure 58.1 RISK FACTORS FOR CERVICAL INSUFFICIENCY

Congenital
- Congenital cervical hypoplasia
- In utero DES exposure

Acquired
- Trauma to cervix (conization, amputation, obstetric laceration)
- ? forced cervical dilatation (may occur during elective pregnancy termination)

INDICATIONS FOR CERVICAL CERCLAGE

- History suggestive of cervical insufficiency
- ? higher-order multiple gestations
- ?? cervical shortening on ultrasound (<20mm)

ABSOLUTE CONTRAINDICATIONS TO CERVICAL CERCLAGE

Maternal
- Uterine contractions/labor
- Life-threatening maternal condition precluding anesthesia

Uteroplacental
- Rupture of fetal membranes
- Unexplained vaginal bleeding (abruption)
- Intrauterine/vaginal infection

Fetal
- Intrauterine fetal demise
- Major fetal anomaly not compatible with life
- Gestational age ≥28 weeks

— OR —

Elective (prophylactic) cerclage

- Usually performed at 13–16 weeks
- Complications rare
- Efficacy relatively well established (estimated 25 cerclages needed to salvage one pregnancy)

Expectant management

Serial clinical examinations and/or transvaginal ultrasound of the cervix every 1–2 weeks

Emergent (therapeutic) cerclage
i.e. after dilation/effacement of the cervix

- Usually performed at 18–23 weeks
- Complications more common
- Efficacy unproven

Internal os

Uterine artery

Cardinal ligament

Uterosacral ligament

TRANSABDOMINAL CERCLAGE

- No proven benefit over transvaginal cerclage
- Requires laparotomy and delivery by cesarean section
- Indicated only if transvaginal cerclage technically impossible or previously unsuccessful

TRANSVAGINAL CERCLAGE

McDonald
- Purse-string suture
- No dissection at level of
- External os

Shirodkar
- Single suture
- Dissection needed closer to
- Internal os

Obstetrics and Gynecology at a Glance, Fourth Edition. Errol R. Norwitz and John O. Schorge.

124 © 2013 John Wiley & Sons, Ltd. Published 2013 by John Wiley & Sons, Ltd.

Cervical insufficiency (also known as cervical incompetence)

Definition
Refers to an inability to support a pregnancy to term due to a *functional* defect of the cervix.

Incidence
This is 0.05–1% of all pregnancies.

Clinical features
• Cervical insufficiency is characterized by acute, painless dilation of the cervix, usually in the mid-trimester, culminating in prolapse and/or preterm premature rupture of the membranes (PPROM) with resultant preterm and often pre-viable delivery.
• Symptoms may include watery vaginal discharge, pelvic pressure, vaginal bleeding, and/or PPROM in the mid-trimester, but most women are asymptomatic.

Diagnosis
• Cervical insufficiency is a clinical diagnosis. It should be suspected when an advanced cervical dilation examination is noted at 16–24 weeks' gestation on pelvic (or sonographic) examination in the absence of uterine contractions. If uterine contractions are present, the diagnosis is more likely to be preterm labor.
• Several tests have been described in an attempt to confirm the diagnosis in non-pregnant women, but are of little clinical value.

Etiology
Cervical insufficiency is likely to be the clinical end-point of many pathologic processes. In most cases, the precise etiology is unknown.

Future pregnancies
• The probability of cervical insufficiency recurring in a subsequent pregnancy is 15–30%.
• The chance of carrying a pregnancy to term with a history of two consecutive mid-trimester pregnancy losses is 60–70%.

Cervical cerclage

Indications
• *Elective (prophylactic)* cerclage should be distinguished from emergency (therapeutic) cerclage (Figure 58.1).
• A prior history of cervical insufficiency is the only clear indication for prophylactic cerclage.
• Prophylactic cerclage in women with a history of *in utero* diethylstilbestrol (DES) exposure or multiple pregnancy (in the absence of prior pregnancy loss) is controversial.

Contraindications
• *Absolute contraindications* are listed in Figure 58.1.
• *Relative contraindications* include:
  1 fetal membranes prolapsing through the cervical os (because of the high incidence of PPROM)
  2 elevated markers of inflammation in amniotic fluid (failure rate ≥90%)
  3 placenta previa
  4 intrauterine fetal growth restriction
  5 ≥24 weeks' gestation (the limit of fetal viability).

Complications
• Complications increase with increasing gestational age and increasing cervical dilation.
• *Short-term (<48 hours) complications*: excessive blood loss, PPROM, spontaneous pregnancy loss (3–20%).
• *Long-term complications*: cervical lacerations (3–4%), chorioamnionitis (4%), cervical stenosis (1%), other (placental abruption, migration of the suture, bladder discomfort).
• *Puerperal infection* occurs in 5–6% of patients with cerclage, twice as common as in women with no cerclage.

Types of cerclage
Transvaginal cervical cerclage (Figure 58.1)
Transvaginal cerclage remains the mainstay for the management of cervical insufficiency. Shirodkar and McDonald cerclage are probably equally efficacious:
1 **Shirodkar cerclage** is a single suture placed around the cervix at the level of the internal os after surgically reflecting the bladder anteriorly and the rectum posteriorly. The suture is secured either anteriorly or posteriorly.
2 **McDonald cerclage** is one or more purse-string sutures placed around the cervix without dissection of the bladder or rectum.

Transabdominal cerclage (Figure 58.1)
Transabdominal cerclage has not been shown to be superior to transvaginal cerclage, and is a far more morbid procedure requiring a laparotomy and subsequent delivery by cesarean section. It should therefore be reserved for women in whom cerclage is indicated, but who have either failed previous transvaginal cerclages or in whom transvaginal cerclage is technically impossible to place.

Technical considerations
• An ultrasound examination should be performed before cerclage placement to exclude gross structural anomalies (such as anencephaly) and/or fetal demise.
• Confirmation of fetal viability both immediately before and after the procedure (by either auscultation or ultrasound).
• Regional anesthesia is preferred.
• Prophylactic tocolysis may be used to inhibit transient uterine contractions associated with placement, but there is no objective evidence that this improves outcome.
• Prophylactic antibiotics are recommended in emergency cerclage because of the risk of chorioamnionitis. The routine use of antibiotics for elective cerclage is, however, controversial.
• If the fetal membranes are prolapsing through the external os, the risk of iatrogenic rupture of the membranes may be as high as 40–50%. Trendelenburg position, filling the bladder, and/or amnioreduction can be used to reduce the fetal membranes before cerclage placement.

Postoperative care
• Frequent (weekly or bi-weekly) visits for cervical checks.
• Bed rest and "pelvic rest" (no coitus, tampons, or douching) until a favorable gestational age is reached.
• Remove cerclage electively at 37–38 weeks or with the onset of premature uterine contractions (to avoid cervical lacerations or uterine rupture).

59 Premature rupture of the membranes

Figure 59.1 PROPOSED MANAGEMENT ALGORITHM FOR PREMATURE RUPTURE OF MEMBRANES

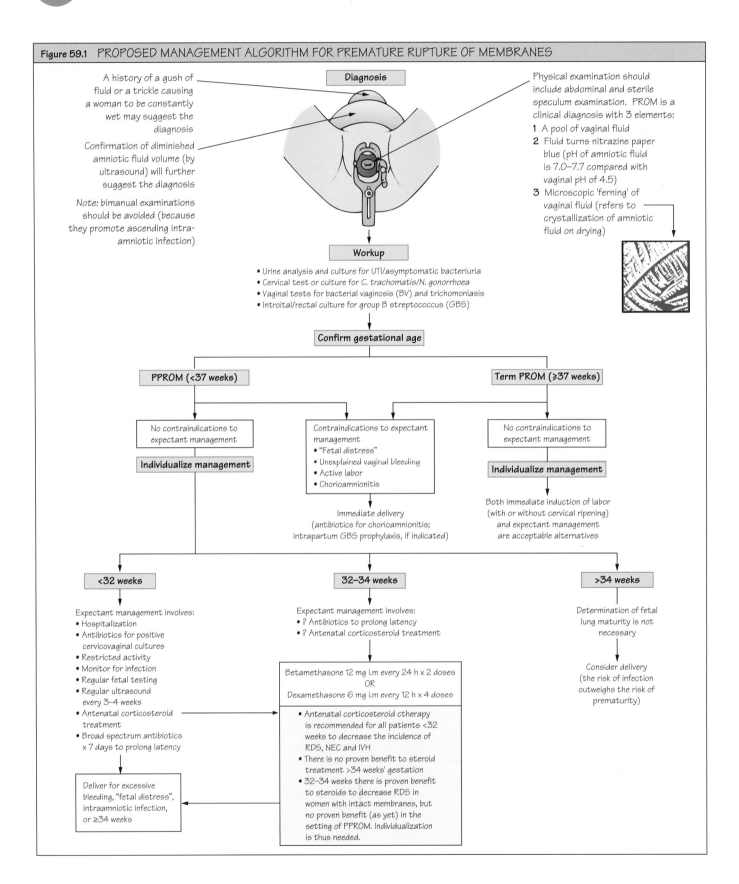

Diagnosis

A history of a gush of fluid or a trickle causing a woman to be constantly wet may suggest the diagnosis

Confirmation of diminished amniotic fluid volume (by ultrasound) will further suggest the diagnosis

Note: bimanual examinations should be avoided (because they promote ascending intra-amniotic infection)

Physical examination should include abdominal and sterile speculum examination. PROM is a clinical diagnosis with 3 elements:
1 A pool of vaginal fluid
2 Fluid turns nitrazine paper blue (pH of amniotic fluid is 7.0–7.7 compared with vaginal pH of 4.5)
3 Microscopic 'ferning' of vaginal fluid (refers to crystallization of amniotic fluid on drying)

Workup

- Urine analysis and culture for UTI/asymptomatic bacteriuria
- Cervical test or culture for *C. trachomatis/N. gonorrhoea*
- Vaginal tests for bacterial vaginosis (BV) and trichomoniasis
- Introital/rectal culture for group B streptococcus (GBS)

Confirm gestational age

PPROM (<37 weeks) | **Term PROM (≥37 weeks)**

No contraindications to expectant management
Individualize management

Contraindications to expectant management
- "Fetal distress"
- Unexplained vaginal bleeding
- Active labor
- Chorioamnionitis

Immediate delivery (antibiotics for chorioamnionitis; intrapartum GBS prophylaxis, if indicated)

No contraindications to expectant management
Individualize management

Both immediate induction of labor (with or without cervical ripening) and expectant management are acceptable alternatives

<32 weeks

Expectant management involves:
- Hospitalization
- Antibiotics for positive cervicovaginal cultures
- Restricted activity
- Monitor for infection
- Regular fetal testing
- Regular ultrasound every 3–4 weeks
- Antenatal corticosteroid treatment
- Broad spectrum antibiotics x 7 days to prolong latency

Deliver for excessive bleeding, "fetal distress", intraamniotic infection, or ≥34 weeks

32–34 weeks

Expectant management involves:
- ? Antibiotics to prolong latency
- ? Antenatal corticosteroid treatment

Betamethasone 12 mg i.m every 24 h x 2 doses
OR
Dexamethasone 6 mg i.m every 12 h x 4 doses

- Antenatal corticosteroid ctherapy is recommended for all patients <32 weeks to decrease the incidence of RDS, NEC and IVH
- There is no proven benefit to steroid treatment >34 weeks' gestation
- 32–34 weeks there is proven benefit to steroids to decrease RDS in women with intact membranes, but no proven benefit (as yet) in the setting of PPROM. Individualization is thus needed.

>34 weeks

Determination of fetal lung maturity is not necessary

Consider delivery (the risk of infection outweighs the risk of prematurity)

Obstetrics and Gynecology at a Glance, Fourth Edition. Errol R. Norwitz and John O. Schorge.

Definitions
• *Premature rupture of the membranes (PROM)* refers to rupture of the fetal membranes before the onset of labor.
• *Preterm PROM (PPROM)* refers to PROM at <37 weeks.
• *Prolonged PROM* refers to PROM >24 hours and is associated with an increased risk of intra-amniotic infection.

Diagnosis
• PROM is a clinical diagnosis (Figure 59.1).
• If clinical examination is equivocal and the pregnancy is remote from term, US practice favors an amnio-dye test ("tampon test") in which indigo carmine dye (not methylene blue because of an association with fetal methemoglobinemia) is instilled into the amniotic cavity, and leakage into the vagina confirmed by staining of a tampon within 20–30 min.
• *Differential diagnosis.* Leakage of urine, vaginal discharge.

Latency
• Latency refers to the interval between PROM and delivery.
• Of women with PROM at term 50% will go into labor within 12 hours, 70% within 24 hours, 85% within 48 hours, and 95% within 72 hours.
• Latency is influenced by gestational age (50% of women with PPROM will go into labor within 24–48 hours and 70–90% within 7 days), severity of oligohydramnios (severe oligohydramnios is associated with shortened latency), and multiple pregnancy (twins have a shorter latency period than singletons).

Etiology
• Near term, a focal weakness develops in the fetal membranes over the internal cervical os which predisposes to rupture at this site.
• Several pathologic processes (including bleeding, infection) may predispose to PPROM.

Term premature rupture of the membranes
Incidence
This is 8–10% of term pregnancies.

Management (Figure 59.1)
• In the absence of contraindications to expectant management (intra-amniotic infection, "fetal distress"/non-reassuring fetal testing, vaginal bleeding, and active labor), both expectant management and immediate augmentation of labor are acceptable options.
• If the cervix is unfavorable, cervical ripening may be required (see Chapter 60).
• Severe oligohydramnios may be associated with umbilical cord compression in labor, leading to non-reassuring fetal testing and cesarean section delivery. It is not clear whether intrapartum amnio-infusion can improve fetal testing and decrease the cesarean section delivery rate.

Preterm premature rupture of the membranes
Incidence
• This is 2–4% of singleton and 7–10% of twin pregnancies.
• PPROM is associated with 20–25% of preterm births and 10% of all perinatal mortality.

Risk factors
• Risk factors include prior PPROM (recurrence risk 20–30%), unexplained vaginal bleeding, placental abruption (seen in 10–15% of women with PPROM, but may be a result rather than a cause), cervical insufficiency, vaginal or intra-amniotic infection, amniocentesis, smoking, multiple pregnancy, polyhydramnios, chronic steroid treatment, connective tissue diseases, anemia, low socioeconomic status, and single women.
• Factors not associated with PPROM include coitus, cervical examinations, maternal exercise, and parity.

Complications
• *Neonatal complications* are related primarily to prematurity, including respiratory distress syndrome (RDS), intraventricular hemorrhage (IVH), sepsis, pulmonary hypoplasia (especially with PPROM <22 weeks), and skeletal deformities (related to severity and duration of PPROM). Overall, PPROM is associated with a fourfold increase in perinatal mortality.
• *Maternal complications* include increased cesarean section delivery (due to malpresentation, cord prolapse), intra-amniotic infection (15–30%), and postpartum endometritis.

Management (Figure 59.1)
• Management of PPROM should be individualized and depends in large part on gestational age. The risk of prematurity should be weighed against the risk of expectant management, primarily intra-amniotic infection.
• Areas of controversy in the management of PPROM:
  1 *Antibiotics.* Empiric, prophylactic, broad-spectrum antibiotics prolong latency in women with PPROM <34 weeks and are therefore recommended for 7 days. There is currently no evidence to recommend one antibiotic regimen over another.
  2 *Tocolysis.* PPROM is a relative contraindication to the use of tocolytic agents (drugs that inhibit uterine contractions).
  3 *Steroids.* Antepartum glucocorticoid administration decreases the incidence of RDS by 50%. Maximal benefit is achieved 24–48 hours after the initial dose. This effect lasts for 7 days, but it is unclear what happens thereafter. Steroids also decrease the incidence of necrotizing enterocolitis (NEC) and IVH. Intramuscular dexamethasone can also be used, but not prednisone (as it does not cross the placenta) or oral dexamethasone (because of a 10-fold increase in neonatal infection and IVH). Of note, multiple (three or more) courses of steroids may be associated with intrauterine growth restriction (IUGR), smaller head circumference, and (possibly) an increased risk of cerebral palsy. As such, repeat courses of steroids are not routinely recommended. However, a single repeat ("rescue") course before 34 weeks may provide additional benefit if the first course was given >2 weeks previously.
  4 *Fetal surveillance.* After PPROM, fetuses are at risk for ascending infection, cord accident, placental abruption, and (possibly) uteroplacental insufficiency. It is generally accepted that some form of fetal monitoring is necessary, but the type and frequency of monitoring are controversial. Options include non-stress testing and/or biophysical profile (see Chapter 52), but none has been shown to be superior to fetal kickcharts.

Figure 60.1 MYOMETRIAL CONTRACTILITY

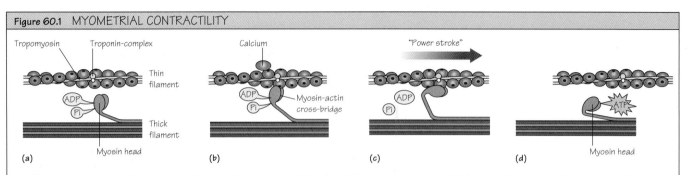

The mechanics of muscle contraction depend on the movement of thin (actin) filaments relative to thick (myosin) filaments within the contractile unit. In the resting state (**a**), myosin binding sites are obscured by tropomyosin. As intracellular calcium concentrations increase (**b**), calcium binds to the troponin-complex resulting in a conformational change that exposes these binding sites leading to the formation of actin-myosin cross-bridges. This results in hydrolysis of bound adenosine triphosphate (ATP) with release of adenosine diphosphate (ADP) and inorganic phosphate (Pi), which causes the myosin heads to bend and slide past the myosin fibers. The resultant "power stroke" results in shortening of the contractile unit and generation of force. The myosin head then releases the actin binding site, is cocked back to its furthest position, and binds to a new molecule of ATP in preparation for another contraction.

Figure 60.2 FACTORS AFFECTING THE COURSE OF LABOR (THE 3 Ps)

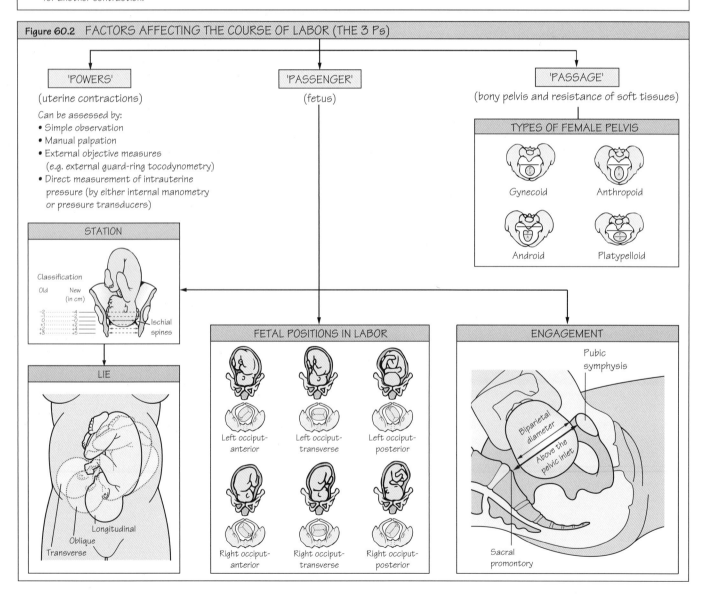

Obstetrics and Gynecology at a Glance, Fourth Edition. Errol R. Norwitz and John O. Schorge.

128 © 2013 John Wiley & Sons, Ltd. Published 2013 by John Wiley & Sons, Ltd.

Definition

Labor is the physiologic process by which a fetus is expelled from the uterus to the outside world. It is a clinical diagnosis requiring two elements: (1) regular phasic uterine contractions increasing in frequency and intensity, and (2) progressive effacement and dilation of the cervix. Normal labor occurs at term (defined as 37–0/7 to 42–0/7 weeks' gestation).

The endocrine control of labor

Labor may be regarded physiologically as a release from the inhibitory effects of pregnancy on the myometrium rather than as an active process mediated by uterine stimulants. In vivo, however, both inhibitory and stimulatory factors appear to be important. It is likely that there is a "parturition cascade" at term that removes the mechanisms maintaining uterine quiescence and recruits factors promoting uterine activity (see Chapter 37). Regardless of whether the trigger for labor begins within the fetus or outside the fetus, the final common pathway ends in the maternal tissues of the uterus, and is characterized by the development of regular phasic uterine contractions.

Myometrial contractility

As in other smooth muscles, myometrial contractions are mediated through the ATP-dependent binding of thick filaments (myosin) to thin filaments (actin) (Figure 60.1). Electrical stimuli (action potentials) must be generated and propagated in the myometrium to cause contractions, which are achieved through the rapid shift of ions (especially calcium) through membrane ion channels. The frequency of contractions correlates with the frequency of action potentials, the force of the contractions correlates with the number of spikes in the action potential and the number of cells activated together, and the duration of contractions correlates with the duration of the action potentials. The transition of the uterus from a quiescent entity to a contractile one comes in part through an increase in gap junctions leading to recruitment and improved communication between adjacent myometrial cells (Figure 60.1). In contrast to vascular smooth muscle, myometrial cells have a sparse innervation which is further reduced during pregnancy. The regulation of uterine contractility is therefore largely humoral and/or dependent on intrinsic factors within myometrial cells.

Mechanics of normal labor

The ability of the fetus to successfully negotiate the pelvis is dependent on the interaction of three variables (known as "the 3 Ps"): powers, passenger, and passage. The "powers" refers to the forces generated by the uterine musculature, the "passenger" is the fetus, and the "passage" consists of the bony pelvis and resistance provided by soft tissues, specifically the cervix and pelvic floor musculature.

Powers

• Several techniques are available to assess uterine activity (Figure 60.2). Uterine activity is characterized by frequency, intensity (amplitude), and duration of contractions.

• Despite technological advances, the definition of "adequate" uterine activity remains unclear. Classically, three to five strong contractions in 10 minutes has been used to define adequate labor. This contraction pattern is seen in 95% of women in normal labor at term. Remember that the external uterine monitor is a tonometer (it measures muscle tone). It provides an accurate measure of the timing of contractions, but not the intensity. If an intrauterine pressure catheter (IUPC) is used, 150–200 Montevideo units (strength of contractions in millimeters of mercury multiplied by the frequency per 10 minutes) are deemed adequate. The ultimate barometer of uterine activity is the rate of cervical dilation and descent of the presenting part.

Passenger

• Two main fetal variables influence the course of labor: *fetal size* and *attitude* (degree of flexion or extension of the head). When the fetal head is optimally flexed, the smallest possible diameter (suboccipito-bregmatic diameter 9.5 cm) presents at the pelvic inlet.

• The lie, presentation, position, and station of the fetus can be assessed on clinical examination. *Lie* refers to the long axis of the fetus relative to the long axis of the uterus, and can be longitudinal, transverse, or oblique (Figure 60.2). *Presentation* can be either cephalic or breech, referring to the pole of the fetus that overlies the pelvic inlet. *Position* refers to the relationship of a nominated site on the presenting part of the fetus to a nominated location on the maternal pelvis, and can be assessed most accurately on bimanual examination. In a cephalic presentation, the nominated site is usually the occiput. In the breech, the nominated site is the sacrum. *Station* refers to the leading bony edge of the presenting part relative to the maternal pelvis (specifically the ischial spines) as assessed on bimanual examination (Figure 60.2). The vertex is said to be *engaged* when the widest diameter has entered the pelvic inlet, which is best assessed on abdominal examination.

• *Fetal weight* can be estimated clinically or by ultrasound. Using birth weight as the gold standard, both techniques are equally accurate with an error of 15–20%.

Passage

• The bony pelvis is composed of the sacrum, ilium, ischium, and pubis. The shape of the pelvis can be classified into one or more four broad categories: gynecoid, android, anthropoid, and platypelloid (Figure 60.2). The gynecoid pelvis is the classic female shape.

• Clinical pelvimetry can be used to estimate the shape and adequacy of the bony pelvis, but has not been shown to accurately predict the course of labor or to change clinical management.

• Pelvic soft tissues (cervix and pelvic floor musculature) can provide resistance in labor. In the second stage, the pelvic musculature may play an important role in facilitating rotation and descent of the head. Excessive resistance may, however, contribute to failure to progress in labor.

Figure 61.1 NORMAL PROGRESS IN LABOR (FRIEDMAN, 1955)

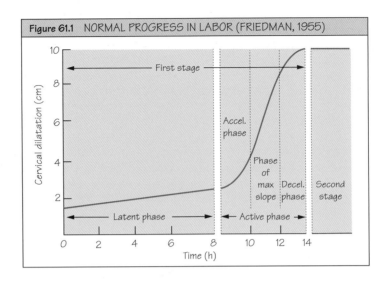

Figure 61.2 PROGRESSION OF SPONTANEOUS LABOR AT TERM

Parameter	Mean	5th percentile
Nulliparas		
Total duration of labor (hours)	10.1 hours	25.8 hours
Stage of labor		
Duration of the first stage (hours)	9.7 hours	24.7 hours
Duration of second stage (minutes)	33.0 minutes	117.5 minutes
• Duration of latent phase (hours)	6.4 hours	20.6 hours
• Rate of cervical dilation during active phase (cm/hour)	3.0 cm/hour	**1.2 cm/hour**
Duration of the third stage (minutes)	5.0 minutes	30.0 minutes
Multiparas		
Total duration of labor (hours)	6.2 hours	19.5 hours
Stage of labor		
Duration of the first stage (hours)	8.0 hours	18.8 hours
Duration of second stage (minutes)	8.5 minutes	46.5 minutes
• Duration of latent phase (hours)	4.8 hours	13.6 hours
• Rate of cervical dilation during active phase (cm/hour)	5.7 cm/hour	**1.5 cm/hour**
Duration of the third stage (minutes)	5.0 minutes	30.0 minutes

Data from Friedman EA. Labor: Clinical evaluation and management. Conneticut, Appleton-Century-Crofts, 1978

Figure 61.3 CARDINAL MOVEMENTS IN NORMAL LABOR

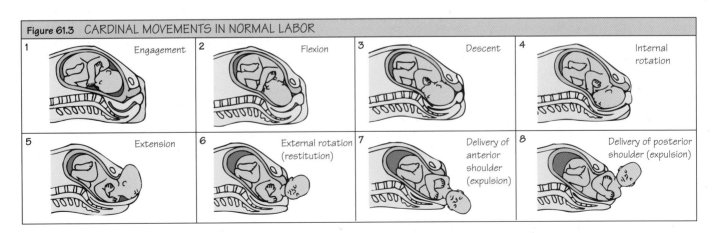

Stages of labor

Labor is a continuous process. For clinical purposes, however, it is divided into three stages:

1 The *first stage* refers to the interval between the onset of labor and full cervical dilation. It is further divided into the *latent phase* (the period between the onset of labor and a point at which a change in the slope of the rate of cervical dilation is noted) and the *active phase* (which is associated with a greater rate of cervical dilation and usually begins at around 3–4 cm dilation). The partogram (Friedman curve) is a graphic representation of the normal labor curve against which a patient's progress is plotted (Figure 61.1). Normal latent phase is <20 hours in nullipara and <14 hours in multipara. In active phase, the cervix should dilate a minimum of >1.2 cm/h in nullipara (>1.5 cm/h in multipara) (Figure 61.2). A delay in cervical dilation in the active phase of ≥2 hours over that expected suggests labor dystocia and requires further evaluation.

2 The *second stage* commences when the cervix achieves full dilation (10 cm) – not when the mother starts to push – and ends with delivery of the fetus. Prolonged second stage refers to >3 hours with or >2 hours without regional analgesia in a nullipara and >2 hours with or >1 hour without regional analgesia in a multipara.

3 The *third stage* refers to delivery of the placenta and fetal membranes and usually lasts <10 min. In the absence of excessive bleeding, up to 30 min may be allowed before intervention (see Chapter 68).

Cardinal movements in normal labor (Figure 61.3)

The cardinal movements refer to the changes in position of fetal head required for the fetus to successfully negotiate the birth canal and include the following:

1 *Engagement* refers to passage of the widest diameter of the presenting part to a level below the plane of the pelvic inlet. In a cephalic fetus with a well-flexed head, the largest transverse diameter is the biparietal diameter (9.5 cm). In nulliparas, engagement of the fetal head usually occurs by 36 weeks. Failure of the head to engage by this time may be a sign of cephalopelvic disproportion (CPD). In multipara, engagement can occur later or even during labor.

2 *Descent* refers to the downward passage of the presenting part through the pelvis.

3 *Flexion* of the fetal head on to the chest occurs passively as it descends due to the shape of the bony pelvis and the resistance of the pelvic floor. Although flexion of the head is present to some degree in most fetuses before labor, complete flexion occurs only during labor. The result of complete flexion is to present the smallest diameter of the fetal head (suboccipitobregmatic diameter) for optimal passage through the pelvis.

4 *Internal rotation* refers to rotation of the presenting part from its original position (transverse with regard to the birth canal) to the anteroposterior position as it passes through the pelvis. As with flexion, internal rotation is a passive movement resulting from the shape of the pelvis and the pelvic floor musculature. As the head descends, the occiput of the fetus rotates towards the symphysis pubis (or, less commonly, towards the hollow of the sacrum), thereby allowing the widest portion of the fetus to negotiate the pelvis at its widest dimension. Due to the angle of inclination between the maternal lumbar spine and pelvic inlet, the fetal head engages in an asynclitic fashion (ie, with one parietal eminence lower than the other). With uterine contractions, the leading parietal eminence descends and is first to engage the pelvic floor. As the uterus relaxes, the pelvic floor musculature causes the fetal head to rotate until it is no longer asynclitic.

5 *Extension* occurs once the fetus has descended to the level of the introitus. This descent brings the base of the occiput into contact with the inferior margin at the symphysis pubis. At this point, the birth canal curves upwards. The fetal head is delivered by extension and rotates around the symphysis pubis. The forces responsible for this motion are the downward force exerted on the fetus by the uterine contractions along with the upward forces exerted by the muscles of the pelvic floor.

6 *External rotation*, also known as restitution, refers to the return of the fetal head to the correct anatomic position in relation to the fetal torso. This can occur to either side depending on the orientation of the fetus. This is again a passive movement resulting from a release of the forces exerted on the fetal head by the maternal bony pelvis and its musculature, and mediated by the basal tone of the fetal musculature.

7 *Expulsion* refers to delivery of the rest of the fetus. After delivery of the head and external rotation, further descent brings the anterior shoulder to the level of the symphysis pubis. The anterior shoulder is delivered in much the same manner as the head, with rotation of the shoulder under the symphysis pubis. After the shoulder, the rest of the body is usually delivered without difficulty.

Clinical assistance at delivery

The goals of clinical assistance at delivery are to support the mother psychologically, reduce maternal trauma, prevent fetal injury, and resuscitate the newborn if required.

• As the fetal head crowns, the clinician's hand is used to control delivery and prevent precipitous expulsion (which has been associated with perineal injury in the mother and intracranial hemorrhage in the neonate).

• Mouth and pharynx can be gently suctioned, although this maneuver has largely fallen out of favor as it has not been shown to change perinatal outcome. Vigorous suctioning can cause a vagal response and fetal bradycardia, and should be avoided.

• If a nuchal cord is present, it should be reduced at this time.

• Following restitution of the fetal head, a hand is placed on each parietal eminence and the anterior shoulder delivered by gentle downward traction.

• The posterior shoulder and torso are then delivered by upward traction.

• The umbilical cord should be double clamped and cut. Delayed cord clamping has been shown to increase blood flow to the infant and thus increase its hematocrit. It may have clinical benefit in preterm infants, but has not been shown to significantly improve perinatal outcome at term.

• The infant should be supported at all times.

• The third stage of labor can be managed either passively or actively (see Chapter 68).

• The placenta and fetal membranes should be examined, and the number of blood vessels in the umbilical cord recorded. If indicated, the placenta should be sent for pathologic examination.

62 Induction and augmentation of labor

Figure 62.1 PATIENT ASSESSMENT BEFORE INDUCTION OF LABOR

Confirm indication for induction
Review for contraindications to labor and/or vaginal delivery
Confirm gestational age
Estimate fetal weight (clinically or by ultrasound)
Determine fetal presentation
Assess shape and adequacy of bony pelvis (clinical pelvimetry)
Assess cervical examination (Bishop score)
Assess need for documentation of fetal lung maturity
Review risk and benefits of induction of labor

CONTRAINDICATIONS TO INDUCTION OF LABOR

Absolute contraindications

Maternal contraindications
  Active genital herpes
  Serious chronic medical conditions
Fetal contraindications
  Malpresentation
  "Fetal distress"/non-reassuring fetal testing
Uteroplacental contraindications
  Cord prolapse
  Placenta previa
  Vasa previa
  Prior 'classic' cesarean section

Relative contraindications

Maternal contraindications
  Cervical carcinoma
  Pelvic deformities
Fetal contraindications
  Extremely large fetus
Uteroplacental contraindications
  Low-lying placenta
  Unexplained vaginal bleeding
  Cord presentation
  Myomectomy involving the uterine cavity

INDICATIONS FOR INDUCTION OF LABOR AT TERM

Absolute indications

Maternal indications
  Pre-eclampsia/eclampsia
  Maternal medical problems
  • Diabetes mellitus
  • Chronic renal disease
  • Chronic pulmonary disease

Fetal indications
  Chorioamnionitis
  Abnormal antepartum testing
  Intrauterine growth restriction
  Post-term pregnancy (>42 weeks)
  Isoimmunization

Uteroplacental indications
  Placental abruption

Relative indications

Maternal indications
  Chronic hypertension
  Gestational hypertension
  Gestational diabetes
  Logistic factors
  • History of rapid labor
  • Distance from the hospital
  • Psychosocial indications
Fetal indications
  Premature rupture of membranes
  Fetal macrosomia (?)
  Fetal demise
  Previous stillbirth
  Fetus with a major congenital anomaly
Uteroplacental indications
  Unexplained oligohydramnios

ASSESSMENT OF CERVICAL STATUS BY BISHOP SCORE

	Score			
	0	1	2	3
Dilation (cm)	0	1–2	3–4	≥5
Effacement (%)	0–30	40–50	60–70	≥80
Station	–3	–2	–1 or 0	≥1+
Consistency	Firm	Medium	Soft	–
Cervical position	Posterior	Mid-position	Anterior	–

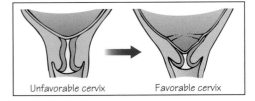

Unfavorable cervix → Favorable cervix

METHODS OF CERVICAL RIPENING AND INDUCTION OF LABOR

Preinduction cervical ripening

Hormonal techniques
  Prostaglandins
  • PGE₂ (dinoprostone)*
  • PGE₁ (misoprostol)
  Oxytocin
  Estrogen (?)
  RU486 (mifepristone) (?)
  Relaxin (?)
Amniotomy
Membrane stripping
Mechanical dilators
  Hygroscopic dilators
  • Laminaria (desiccated seaweed)
  • Dilapan (polyacrylonitrile)
  • Lamicel (magnesium sulfate in alcohol)
  Balloon catheter (alone, with traction, with infusion)

Initiation/augmentation of uterine contractility

Hormonal techniques
  Oxytocin
  Prostaglandins
  • PGE₂ (Dinoprostone)
  • PGE₁ (Misoprostol)
  • PGF₂α (Prostin) (?)
  RU486 (Mifepristone) (?)
Amniotomy

* Only PGE2 is approved by the FDA for pre-induction cervical ripening

Induction of labor

Definition

• *Induction* refers to interventions designed to initiate labor before spontaneous onset with a view to achieving vaginal delivery.
• This should be distinguished from *augmentation* which refers to enhancement of uterine contractility in women in whom labor has already begun.

Patient assessment (Figure 62.1)

• The appropriate timing for induction is the point at which benefit to mother and/or fetus is greater if pregnancy is interrupted than if pregnancy is continued, and depends on gestational age.
• Indications and contraindications are detailed in Figure 62.1.

Bishop score

• The success of induction depends in large part on the status of the cervix. In 1964, Bishop designed a cervical scoring system to prevent iatrogenic prematurity. This system has since been modified (Figure 62.1) and used to predict the success rate of induction. If the Bishop score is favorable (defined as ≥ 6), the likelihood of a successful induction and vaginal delivery is high. If unfavorable (<6), the probability of successful induction is reduced and pre-induction cervical "ripening" (maturation) may be indicated.
• Cervical ripening describes a complex series of biochemical events that alter cervical collagen and ground substance composition, resulting in a softer and more pliable cervix. A number of agents are available to facilitate this maturation (Figure 62.1). Potential benefits include fewer failed inductions, shorter hospital stay, lower fetal and maternal morbidity, lower medical costs, and possibly lower cesarean section delivery rates.

Methods (Figure 62.1)

The choice of induction regimen should be individualized. A single technique is not always rarely effective, on its own, and a combination of interventions may be required:

• *Prostaglandin E_2* (PGE$_2$) improves the rate of vaginal delivery, regardless of route of administration. Gastrointestinal side effects are lower with vaginal administration. The rate of failed induction is only 1–6%. The most commonly used local PGE$_2$ preparation is dinoprostone gel (Prepidil). PGE$_1$ analogs, such as misoprostol (Cytotec), are cheaper, can be administered orally with few side effects, and are as effective as PGE$_2$ for cervical ripening and labor induction. PGE$_2$ should be avoided in women with asthma, glaucoma, and severe renal, pulmonary, or hepatic disease. Prostaglandin induction of labor should be avoided in patients with a prior cesarean section delivery, because of a fourfold increased risk of uterine rupture.
• *Oxytocin* infusion by any protocol (low dose or high dose, continuous or pulsatile) has been shown to be effective in pre-induction cervical ripening and labor induction. Continuous low-dose infusion is as effective as other protocols, while minimizing oxytocin requirements and adverse effects (especially maternal water intoxication due to an antidiuretic hormone-like effect). Advantages of oxytocin include cost and familiarity for the clinician. Fetal monitoring is required because of the risk of uterine tachysystole and "fetal distress."
• *Progesterone receptor antagonists* (RU 486 [mifepristone], ZK98299 [onapristone]) have been shown to promote cervical ripening and lower oxytocin requirements in labor.
• *Amniotomy* (artificial rupture of the membranes – AROM) may be sufficient on its own to induce labor, but is more effective if used in combination with oxytocin. It shortens the interval from induction to delivery by 1–3 hours, but does not appear to lower the rate of cesarean section delivery. Contraindications to amniotomy include HIV, active perineal herpes infection, and viral hepatitis.
• *Sweeping (stripping) of the membranes* refers to digital separation of the fetal membranes from the lower uterine segment before labor at term. It may accelerate the onset of labor by releasing endogenous prostaglandins. However, most studies show no significant increase in the proportion of women going into labor within 7 days.
• *Mechanical dilators* (transcervical Foley catheter placement, hygroscopic dilators) significantly shorten the induction to delivery interval compared with no pre-induction ripening, and are as effective as PGE$_2$. Hygroscopic dilators rely on absorption of water to swell and forcibly dilate the cervix. A disadvantage of mechanical dilators is patient discomfort both at the time of insertion and with progressive cervical dilation.

Augmentation of labor

Indications

Augmentation of uterine activity is indicated for failure to progress in labor in the presence of inadequate contractions and in the absence of absolute cephalopelvic disproportion (see Chapter 63).

Methods

These include amniotomy and/or oxytocin. It is still unclear whether such interventions improve obstetric outcome or merely produce the same outcome in a shorter period of time.

Active management of labor

• "Active management" describes a protocol of clinical management based on the premise that enhancing uterine contractility in the first stage of labor will improve obstetric outcome. It applies only to nullipara in spontaneous labor with a cephalic presentation.
• Active management protocols rely on strict criteria for the diagnosis of labor, amniotomy within 1 hour of labor onset, and high-dose oxytocin if cervical dilation is not maintained at ≥ 1.0 cm/h. Other components include antenatal education, one-on-one nursing care, and close supervision by a senior obstetrician.
• The National Maternity Unit in Dublin, Ireland, pioneered active management in 1968. Although the aim was to shorten the duration of nulliparous labor, it has attracted much attention for its apparent (but as yet unproven) ability to lower the cesarean section delivery rate. Active management does decrease the duration of labor in nulliparas, but an improvement in obstetric outcome has yet to be conclusively demonstrated.

Figure 63.1 BREECH PRESENTATION

Definition: fetus presenting buttocks first (position of the breech is defined relative to the sacrum)

Diagnosis: by the Leopold maneuver, vaginal examination or ultrasound

Incidence: 3–4% at term

Risk factors:
- Prematurity (30% breech at 28 weeks, 15% at 30 weeks)
- Uterine anomaly
- Polyhydramnios
- Prior breech delivery
- Multiple gestation
- Placenta previa
- Fetal anomalies (anencephaly, hydrocephalus)

Associated with:
- Twofold ↑risk of congenital abnormality
- ↑Risk of cord prolapse, preterm labor, birth trauma, maternal morbidity

Types of breech

Frank breech (70%)

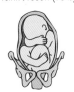
Complete breech (10%)

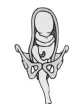
Footling or incomplete breech (20%)

External cephalic version (ECV)

- Refers to attempted conversion of breech to vertex by manual manipulation through maternal abdomen
- Performed after 36 weeks

Benefits: ↓breech at term

Risks of ECV: "fetal distress", abruption, cord accident, rupture of fetal membranes, neurological injury

Contraindications to ECV may be absolute (uterine anomaly) or relative (prior cesarean, IUGR, twins, oligohydramnios, labor)

Predictors of success: frank breech, normal amniotic fluid volume, operator experience, non-engaged breech, multiparous and thin mother, laterally located fetal spine

Techniques of ECV:
- >36 weeks, no labor, consent obtained, reactive NST
- Anti-D IgG if needed
- Under ultrasound guidance
- ± Epidural/β-mimetic tocolysis
- Check NST after ECV

Success rate: 50%

Vaginal breech delivery

- Preterm singleton breeches are best delivered by cesarean section (because of risk of head entrapment)
- Management of breech second twin is addressed in Chapter 52
- Term breech fetuses are most commonly delivered abdominally (because of the ↑risk of head entrapment, cord prolapse, asphyxia, birth trauma with vaginal breech delivery)
- Vaginal breech delivery may be a safe alternative to cesarean section under the following conditions:
  – term frank breech
  – estimated fetal weight 2,500–3,500 g by ultrasound
  – no hyperextension of fetal head
  – capacity for emergent cesarean section
  – experienced operator
  – adequate anesthesia
  – adequate progress in labor
  – absence of "fetal distress"
  – preferably multiparous woman ('proven pelvis')

Figure 63.2 SHOULDER DYSTOCIA AND BRACHIAL PLEXUS INJURIES

Definition: Impaction of the anterior shoulder of the fetus behind the pubic symphysis following delivery of the head

Risk factors:
- Fetal macrosomia (EFW ≥4,500g)
- History of prior shoulder dystocia
- Diabetes mellitus
- Midcavity operative vaginal delivery
- Labor dystocia (second stage >60 min)
- Post-term pregnancy
- Obesity

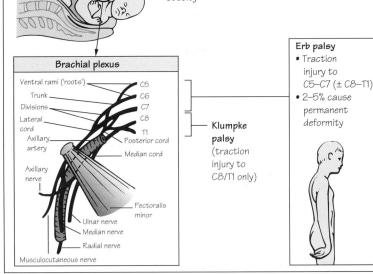

Brachial plexus

Ventral rami ('roots') — C5, C6, C7, C8, T1
Trunk
Divisions
Lateral cord
Axillary artery — Posterior cord
— Median cord
Axillary nerve
Pectoralis minor
Ulnar nerve
Median nerve
Radial nerve
Musculocutaneous nerve

Klumpke palsy (traction injury to C8/T1 only)

Erb palsy
- Traction injury to C5–C7 (± C8–T1)
- 2–5% cause permanent deformity

Management of shoulder dystocia

?? Prevention (difficult because it is almost impossible to predict)

↓

Identify problem immediately. Call for help. Note the time (you have ± 5 min to deliver the baby safely)

↓

Create space (empty bladder, consider generous episiotomy, remove the bottom of the bed)

↓

Perform the McRobert maneuver ± suprapubic pressure

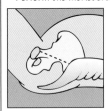 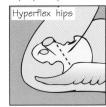
Hyperflex hips

If unsuccessful consider:
- Suprapubic (not fundal) pressure
- Wood screw or Ruben maneuver
- Cut proctoepisiotomy
- Deliver posterior arm
- ? Break clavicle (pull outwards)
- ? Zavanelli maneuvre (replace head, cesarean)
- ? Symphysiotomy
- ? Place patient in knee–chest position

Obstetrics and Gynecology at a Glance, Fourth Edition. Errol R. Norwitz and John O. Schorge.

Labor dystocia

- *Definition.* Abnormal or inadequate progress in labor (see Chapter 61).
- Also known as failure to progress, prolonged labor, failure of cervical dilation, failure of descent of the fetal head.
- *Causes.* Inadequate "power" (uterine contractions), inadequate "passage" (bony pelvis), or abnormalities of the "passenger" (fetal macrosomia, hydrocephalus, malpresentation, extreme extension or asynclitism (lateral tilting) of the fetal head).
- *Cephalopelvic disproportion* (CPD) is classified as absolute (where the disparity between the size of the bony pelvis and the fetal head precludes vaginal delivery even under optimal conditions) or relative (where fetal malposition, asynclitism, or extension of the fetal head prevents delivery). Absolute CPD is an absolute contraindication to attempted vaginal delivery.
- *Management.* Exclude absolute CPD. Confirm "adequate" uterine activity (see Chapter 60). If contractions are "adequate," one of two events will occur: dilation and effacement of the cervix with descent of the head, or worsening caput succedaneum (scalp edema) and molding (overlapping of the skull bones). Proceed with timely cesarean section delivery, if indicated.

Malpresentation

Breech (Figure 63.1)

Transverse (shoulder presentation) or oblique lie

- *Incidence.* This is 0.3% of term pregnancies.
- *Etiology.* Prematurity, placenta previa, grandmultiparity, multiple gestation, uterine anomalies (fibroids, bicornuate uterus).
- *Management.* Consider external cephalic version. Cesarean section delivery if unsuccessful.

Other malpresentations

- Malpresentations can occur in a vertex fetus. Some can be delivered vaginally (such as occiput posterior, face with mentum [chin] anterior). In others (brow, face with mentum posterior), conversion to occiput anterior is necessary for vaginal delivery.
- *Compound presentation* (<0.1% of all deliveries) refers to the presence of a fetal extremity alongside the presenting part. It is associated with prematurity, polyhydramnios, and multiple gestations. Vaginal delivery can often be affected.
- *Funic presentation* refers to presentation of the umbilical cord below the head. It is rare. If identified in labor, cesarean section delivery may be indicated because of the risk of cord prolapse.

Intrapartum complications

Cord prolapse

- An obstetric emergency characterized by prolapse of the umbilical cord into the vagina after rupture of the fetal membranes.
- *Incidence.* Less than 0.5% of term cephalic pregnancies.
- *Risk factors.* Malpresentation (breech, transverse lie), polyhydramnios, small fetus, prematurity.
- *Diagnosis.* Palpation of a pulsatile cord on vaginal examination with or without fetal bradycardia.
- *Prevention.* Perform amniotomy only once the vertex is well applied to the cervix and always with fundal pressure.
- *Management.* Replace cord manually and expedite delivery immediately (usually by emergency cesarean section).

Shoulder dystocia and brachial plexus injury
(Figure 63.2)

- *Shoulder dystocia* is an obstetric emergency associated with neonatal birth trauma (neurologic injury, fractures of the humerus, skull, clavicle) in up to 30% of cases. Immediate identification and prompt and appropriate intervention may prevent neonatal birth trauma in some cases. Shoulder dystocia complicates 0.2–2% of all vaginal deliveries. Although several risk factors are described, most cases occur in women with no risk factors.
- *Brachial plexus paralysis* is the second most common neurologic birth injury (after facial nerve palsy) complicating 0.5–3 per 1,000 deliveries. It results from "excessive" lateral traction on the head and neck at delivery with resultant injury to the brachial plexus, usually to cervical nerve roots C5–7 (Erb/Duchenne palsy). The lower brachial plexus (C8–T1) may also be involved. On examination, the arm hangs limply at the side of the body with the forearm extended and internally rotated, the classic "waiter's tip" deformity (Figure 63.2). The function of the fingers is usually retained; 95% of brachial plexus injuries resolve completely within 2 years with the help of physical therapy. Elective cesarean section delivery will prevent most (but not all) brachial plexus injuries. Given the difficulty in predicting shoulder dystocia, however, cesarean section delivery cannot be recommended for all women with identifiable risk factors.

Other congenital neurologic birth injuries

- *Facial nerve paralysis* results from pressure on the facial nerve (cranial nerve VII) as it exits the skull through the stylomastoid foramen. It is the most common neurologic birth injury (0.1–8 per 1,000 live births). It is more common after surgical vaginal (forceps) delivery. Resolution is usually complete within a few days.
- *Injuries to the neck and spinal cord* may result from excessive traction at delivery with fracture or dislocation of the vertebrae. Such injuries may prove fatal. The true incidence of spinal injuries is not known.
- *Multicystic encephalomalacia* is a pathologic condition specific to monochorionic twin multiple pregnancies in which cerebral damage develops in the surviving fetus after intrauterine demise of its co-twin (see Chapter 55). The mechanism of cerebral injury is not known. Unfortunately, immediate cesarean section delivery does not appear to prevent neurologic injury in the surviving twin.

Intracranial hemorrhage

- Bleeding into the fetal head can occur at several anatomic sites. Intraventricular hemorrhage (IVH), defined as bleeding into the germinal matrix within the ventricles, occurs most commonly.
- *Incidence.* Of term infants 4–5% will have sonographic evidence of IVH unrelated to obstetric factors.
- *Risk factors.* Prematurity, fetal bleeding diathesis, alloimmune thrombocytopenia. Birth trauma is an uncommon cause of intracranial hemorrhage.
- *Treatment.* Primarily supportive. Surgery is rarely indicated.
- *Prognosis* depends on gestational age at delivery, the presence and extent of ventriculomegaly, and the extent and location of the hemorrhage (parenchymal and subdural hemorrhages have a poor prognosis in 90% of cases because the hemorrhage is often more excessive; IVH has a poor prognosis in 45% of cases; only grade 3 and 4 IVH are associated with significant long-term neurologic sequelae).

Figure 64.1 PAIN RELIEF IN LABOR

Techniques	Efficacy
Pharmacological techniques	
General endotracheal analgesia	Very effective
Systemic analgesia	
• Opioid (narcotic) agonists (such as morphine, meperidine, fentanyl)	Effective
• Partial opioid agonist/antagonists (such as nalbuphine, butorphanol)	Effective
• 'Twilight sleep' (morphine plus scopolamine. historical interest only)	-
Regional analgesia	
• Pudendal block	Moderately effective
• Epidural block	Very effective
• Spinal block	Very effective
• Caudal block (saddle block)	Very effective
Local analgesia	
• Field block (local infiltration)	Minimally effective
• Paracervical block	Minimally effective
Inhalation analgesia	
• Ether (historical interest only)	-
• Chloroform (historical interest only)	-
• Nitrous oxide (alone, with air, with oxygen)	Moderately effective
Non-pharmacological techniques	
Acupuncture	Probably effective
Hypnosis	Probably ineffective
Aromatherapy	No data
Transcutaneous electrical nerve stimulation (TENS)	Probably ineffective
Psychoprophylaxis (pioneered by Lamaze in France)	Probably ineffective

Figure 64.2 EPIDURAL ANALGESIA

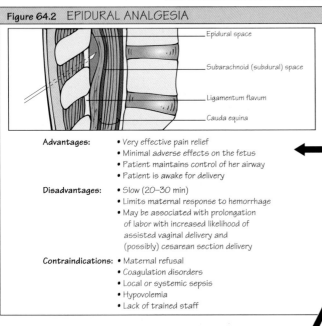

Epidural space
Subarachnoid (subdural) space
Ligamentum flavum
Cauda equina

Advantages:
• Very effective pain relief
• Minimal adverse effects on the fetus
• Patient maintains control of her airway
• Patient is awake for delivery

Disadvantages:
• Slow (20–30 min)
• Limits maternal response to hemorrhage
• May be associated with prolongation of labor with increased likelihood of assisted vaginal delivery and (possibly) cesarean section delivery

Contraindications:
• Maternal refusal
• Coagulation disorders
• Local or systemic sepsis
• Hypovolemia
• Lack of trained staff

Figure 64.3 PAIN PATHWAYS FOR LABOR AND DELIVERY

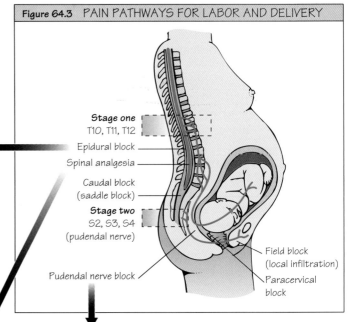

Stage one
T10, T11, T12
Epidural block
Spinal analgesia
Caudal block (saddle block)
Stage two
S2, S3, S4 (pudendal nerve)
Pudendal nerve block
Field block (local infiltration)
Paracervical block

Figure 64.4 SPINAL ANALGESIA

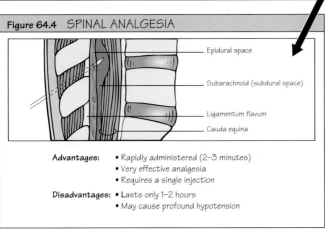

Epidural space
Subarachnoid (subdural space)
Ligamentum flavum
Cauda equina

Advantages:
• Rapidly administered (2–3 minutes)
• Very effective analgesia
• Requires a single injection

Disadvantages:
• Lasts only 1–2 hours
• May cause profound hypotension

Figure 64.5 PUDENDAL NERVE BLOCK

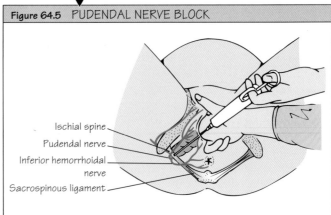

Ischial spine
Pudendal nerve
Inferior hemorrhoidal nerve
Sacrospinous ligament

Obstetrics and Gynecology at a Glance, Fourth Edition. Errol R. Norwitz and John O. Schorge.

136 © 2013 John Wiley & Sons, Ltd. Published 2013 by John Wiley & Sons, Ltd.

- Pain during labor is generally severe, with only 2–4% of women reporting minimal pain in labor.
- Pain relief (analgesia – Figure 64.1) during normal labor is not mandatory. However, all women should be aware of the options available to them. There are no contraindications for pain relief in labor.
- Analgesia is strongly recommended for certain maternal conditions (select cardiac disorders, suspected difficult intubation) and in situations where intrapartum manipulation is likely (breech, multiple pregnancy).
- Adequate analgesia is mandatory for assisted vaginal delivery, perineal repair, manual removal of placenta, and cesarean section delivery.

Pain pathways (Figure 64.3)
- During the *first stage* of labor, pain results from both cervical dilation and uterine contractions (myometrial ischemia). Pain sensation travels from the uterus via visceral afferent (sympathetic) nerves that enter the spinal cord through the posterior segments of thoracic spinal nerves, T10–12.
- Pain during the *second stage* of labor results primarily from distension of the pelvic floor, vagina, and perineum by the presenting part of the fetus, and travels via sensory fibers of sacral nerves, S2–4 (pudendal nerve). The sensation of uterine contractions also contributes, but is probably secondary.

Non-pharmacologic techniques
- Acupuncture, hypnosis, and aromatherapy may have a place in clinical practice, but their efficacy is not yet proven.
- Transcutaneous electrical nerve stimulation (TENS) is thought to act by promoting endogenous enkephalin release within the spinal cord, where it acts to inhibit the transmission of pain. Its efficacy is unproven.
- Warm baths, massage, relaxation, antenatal classes, breathing exercises, and the presence of a supportive "doula" (midwife) have all been shown to decrease analgesic requirements in labor.

Pharmacologic techniques
General endotracheal anesthesia
- *Indications.* General anesthesia should generally be avoided. It is best reserved for emergency cesarean section or instrumental vaginal delivery (because of speed of administration) and for entrapment of the after-coming head at vaginal breech delivery (because it relaxes the cervix).
- *Advantages.* Rapidly administered, low incidence of hypotension, appropriate for women with hypovolemia and women at high risk of hemorrhage.
- *Disadvantages.* Higher incidence of aspiration (because the patient is unable to protect her airway), neonatal depression, and postpartum hemorrhage (due to uterine relaxation).
- *Complications.* Aspiration of gastric contents leading to pneumonia or pneumonitis (Mendelson syndrome), maternal hypoxic cerebral injury (due to failed intubation or obstructed endotracheal tube), or injury to the upper airway. Complications can be minimized by preoperative starvation or use of a orogastric tube, intravenous fluid and antacid administration, cricoid pressure at intubation, and careful monitoring throughout the procedure.

Systemic analgesia
- *Opiate agonists* have good analgesic and sedative properties, but delay gastric emptying and can cause neonatal sedation and respiratory depression. A reversal agent (naloxone) should be available in the event of maternal or neonatal depression.
- *Partial opioid agonists/antagonists* have fewer side effects, but are less effective analgesics.
- *Advantages.* Readily available, easily administered, does not adversely affect the progress of labor.
- *Side effects.* Nausea and vomiting, respiratory depression, oversedation, and decreased fetal heart rate variability.

Regional
- Regional blockade of the spinal sensory nerves can be achieved through a number of techniques.
  1 *Epidural analgesia* (Figure 64.2) involves insertion of a cannula at L2–3 or L3–4. The cannula is left in place in the peridural fat, which allows for administration of local analgesic agents by intermittent bolus injections or continuous infusion. Advantages and disadvantages are reviewed in Figure 64.2. Epidural analgesia provides superior pain relief, but may prolong labor and limit a woman's ability to push. Moreover, epidural analgesia may be associated with an increased incidence of malpresentation (occiput posterior), instrumental vaginal delivery, severe perineal trauma, and (possibly) cesarean section delivery. Complications include hypotension (which can usually be avoided by preloading with 500 mL crystalloid), accidental dural puncture (<1%), postdural puncture headache (5–25%), drug toxicity, direct neurologic injury, and spinal hematoma (very rare). Maternal hypotension may be associated with fetal bradycardia which is usually short-lived and may be reversed by maternal ephedrine administration.
  2 *Spinal analgesia* (Figure 64.4) involves an injection of local anesthetic into the subarachnoid space. It is usually reserved for cesarean section, because its effect is limited to 1–2 hours.
  3 *Combined spinal–epidural analgesia.*
- *Pudendal nerve block* (Figure 64.5) is a regional block achieved through transvaginal infiltration of the pudendal nerves (S2–4) bilaterally as they exit the Alcock canal and circumnavigate the ischial spines. It is most useful for outlet manipulations in the second stage of labor.
- *Caudal block* (saddle block) is a localized regional block of the cauda equina administered through the sacral hiatus.

Local analgesia
- *Field block* (infiltration of the nerve endings in the vulva) is used most often to repair perineal laceration or episiotomy.
- *Paracervical block* (bilateral infiltration of the sensory nerves leaving the uterus through the cardinal ligaments) is used most often to provide analgesia for the latter part of the first stage of labor.
- Local analgesic agents include bupivacaine, lidocaine, chloroprocaine. Prilocaine is generally avoided because of the risk of methemoglobinemia.

Inhalational analgesia
Inhalational analgesia, especially Entonox (50% oxygen/50% nitrous oxide), is widely used in developing countries with good patient satisfaction.

Figure 65.1 ASSESSMENT OF FETAL WELL-BEING

Antepartum	Intrapartum	Postpartum
Non-stress test (NST) • External monitor (Doppler) only Biophysical profile Vibroacoustic stimulation Contraction stress test Fetal movement charts ('kickcharts') Doppler velocity (?)	Non-stress test (NST) • External monitor (Doppler) • Internal (scalp electrode) Vibroacoustic stimulation Contraction stress test Fetal scalp sampling Biophysical profile (?) Fetal pulse oximetry (?)	Clinical response (seizures, poor feeding, abnormal movements) Apgar score Umbilical cord pH

see Chapter 52 for details

INTERPRETATION OF NON-STRESS TESTS

Accelerations

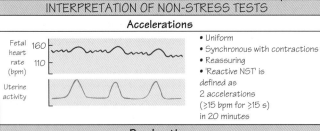

Fetal heart rate (bpm) / Uterine activity

• Uniform
• Synchronous with contractions
• Reassuring
• 'Reactive NST' is defined as 2 accelerations (≥15 bpm for ≥15 s) in 20 minutes

Decelerations

Early decelerations

Fetal heart rate (bpm) / Uterine activity

• Uniform
• Synchronous with contractions
• Rarely falls below 110 bpm
• Reflects head compression and is mediated through the parasympathetic nervous system (vagus nerve)
• Not a sign of "fetal distress"

Variable decelerations

Fetal heart rate (bpm) / Uterine activity

• Variable in appearance and timing
• May be associated with increased variability
• Reflects umbilical cord compression
• May be a sign of "fetal distress"

Late decelerations

Fetal heart rate (bpm) / Uterine activity

• Uniform
• Starts after peak of contraction
• Associated with decreased variability
• Reflects a chemoreceptor response
• May indicate fetal hypoxemia

Other fetal heart rate patterns

Moderate variability (5–25 bpm)

Marked (exaggerated) variability (>25 bpm)

Minimal variability (<5 bpm)

Sinusoidal pattern (concerning for fetal anemia)

APGAR SCORING SYSTEM

	Score		
	0	1	2
Appearance	Blue, pale	Pink body, blue extremity	Pink all over
Heart rate (bpm)	Absent	<100	≥100
Grimace	No response	Some response	Cry, cough
Activity	Limp	Some flexion	Active motion
Respiratory effort	Absent	Slow	Strong cry

NORMAL FETAL ACID–BASE VALUES AT TERM

	pH	PO₂ (mmHg)	PCO₂ (mmHg)	Bicarbonate (mmol/L)	O₂ saturation (%)
Umbilical vein	7.35 ± 0.05	29.2 ± 5.9	38.2 ± 5.6	20.4 ± 2.1	70
Umbilical artery	7.28 ± 0.05	18.0 ± 6.2	14.2 ± 8.4	22.3 ± 2.5	28
Fetal scalp blood					
• Early first stage	7.33 ± 0.03	21.8 ± 2.6	44.0 ± 4.05	20.1 ± 1.2	
• Late first stage	7.23 ± 0.02	21.3 ± 2.1	42.0 ± 5.1	19.1 ± 2.1	
• Second stage	7.29 ± 0.04	16.5 ± 1.4	46.3 ± 4.2	17.0 ± 2.0	

DRUGS AFFECTING INTRAPARTUM FETAL HEART RATE TRACING

Effect on fetus	Drug
Fetal tachycardia	Adrenalin Atropine β-Agonists (ritodrine, terbutaline)
Fetal bradycardia	Anti-thyroid agents (including propothiouracil) β-Blockers (such as propranolol) Epidural anesthesia (regardless of the agent used) Methergine (contraindicated before delivery) Oxytocin (if associated with excessive uterine activity)
Sinusoidal heart rate pattern	Opioid analgesics (especially alphaprodine butorphamol, meperidine)
Diminished variability	Atropine Anticonvulsants (but not phenytoin) β-Blockers Betamethasone Ethanol General anesthesia Hypnotics (including diazepam) Insulin (if associated with hypoglycemia) Magnesium sulfate Narcotic analgesics Promethazine (Phenergan)

Introduction

- Fetal morbidity and mortality can occur as a consequence of labor. A number of tests have been developed to assess fetus wellbeing (Figure 65.1).
- Attention has focused on *hypoxic ischemic encephalopathy* (HIE) as a marker of birth asphyxia and a predictor of long-term outcome. HIE is a clinical condition that develops within the first hours or days of life. It is characterized by abnormalities of tone and feeding, alterations in consciousness, and convulsions. In order to attribute such a state to birth asphyxia, the following four criteria must all be fulfilled:

  1 profound metabolic or mixed acidemia (pH <7.00) on an umbilical cord arterial blood sample, if obtained

  2 Apgar score of 0–3 for longer than 5 min

  3 neonatal neurologic manifestations (seizures, coma)

  4 multisystem organ dysfunction.

- At most, only 15% of cerebral palsy and learning disability can be attributed to HIE.

Intrapartum fetal monitoring

Non-stress test (NST) or fetal cardiotocography (CTG)

A fetal scalp electrode for the continuous monitoring of the fetal heart rate during labor was introduced by Hon and Lee in 1963. A year later, Doppler technology made external fetal heart analysis possible. Continuous intrapartum CTG is now recommended for all high-risk pregnancies and is commonly used in low-risk pregnancies too.

Characteristics of intrapartum fetal heart rate patterns

- *Baseline fetal heart rate* refers to the dominant reading taken over ≥10 min. Normal baseline fetal heart rate is 110–160 beats/min. Bradycardia is a baseline rate <110 beats/min. Tachycardia is a baseline rate >160 beats/min.
- *Fetal heart rate variability* is classified as moderate (which refers to peak-to-trough excursions of 5–25 beats/min around the baseline, and is a healthy sign), minimal (<5 beats/min excursions, which is concerning for hypoxia and requires further evaluation), absent (0 beats/min excursions, which is worrisome for hypoxia), or marked (>25 beats/min excursions, which suggests hypoxia without acidosis).
- *Accelerations* are periodic, transient increases in fetal heart rate of ≥15 beats/min for ≥15 s (or ≥10 beats/min for ≥10 s for fetuses <32 weeks). Accelerations are often associated with fetal activity, and are a sign of a healthy fetus (specifically the absence of metabolic acidosis).
- *Decelerations* are periodic, transient decreases in fetal heart rate usually associated with uterine contractions. They can be further classified into early, variable, or late decelerations by their shape and timing in relation to contractions. Decelerations are regarded as "repetitive" if they occur with more than 50% of contractions.

Interpretation of NST (Figure 65.1)

- Fetal heart rate patterns in labor are classified as:

  1 "reactive" (defined as two or more accelerations in 20 min), which is considered reassuring

  2 suspicious or equivocal (indeterminate)

  3 ominous or agonal (non-reassuring).

- Reassuring elements of the intrapartum fetal heart rate include normal baseline, moderate variability, and accelerations (class I). Non-reassuring elements include bradycardia, tachycardia, minimal or absent variability, and/or repetitive severe variable or late decelerations (class III). Class II refers to an intermediate pattern.

- Non-reassuring patterns are seen in up to 60% of labors, suggesting that they are not specific to fetal hypoxia. Severely abnormal fetal heart rate patterns (specifically, repetitive severe variable or late decelerations), on the other hand, occur in only 0.3% of intrapartum fetal heart rate tracings.

- NST interpretation is largely subjective and should always take into account gestational age, the presence or absence of congenital anomalies, and underlying clinical risk factors. Fetuses that are premature or growth restricted are less likely to tolerate episodes of decreased placental perfusion and, as such, may be more prone to hypoxia and acidosis. Drugs can also affect heart rate and variability (Figure 65.1).

- Only two intrapartum fetal heart rate patterns have been associated with poor perinatal outcome, namely repetitive severe variable (defined as decreasing to <70 beats/min and lasting for ≥60 s) and repetitive late decelerations.

- When compared with intermittent fetal heart rate auscultation, continuous fetal heart rate monitoring during labor is associated with a decrease in the incidence of seizures before 28 days of life, but no difference in other measures of short-term perinatal morbidity or mortality. Moreover, the increase in neonatal seizures does not translate into differences in long-term morbidity (cerebral palsy, learning disability, or seizures after 28 days of life). However, continuous fetal heart rate monitoring is associated with a significant increase in obstetric intervention, including surgical vaginal and cesarean section delivery.

- Several unusual fetal heart rate patterns have been described:

  1 A *salutatory* pattern (in which there are large oscillations in baseline) is of unclear clinical significance. It may indicate intermittent cord occlusion.

  2 A *lambda* pattern (an acceleration followed by a deceleration) is attributed to fetal movement. It is not felt to be of pathological significance.

  3 A *sinusoidal* pattern (one with normal baseline, decreased variability, and a cyclic sinusoidal pattern with a frequency of 2–5 cycles/min and amplitude of 5–15 beats/min) is associated most strongly with fetal anemia. It may also be seen in the setting of chorioamnionitis, impending fetal demise, and maternal drug administration (especially opiate analgesics).

Fetal scalp sampling

- The pH of fetal capillary blood lies between that of fetal arterial and venous blood (see table below).
- Fetal scalp blood sampling was introduced by Saling in 1962. It is most useful in labor when alternative non-invasive tests are unable to confirm fetal wellbeing.
- Suggested management based on fetal scalp pH:

Scalp pH	Suggested management
>7.25	May manage expectantly, consider repeating in 1 hour if cardiotocography still abnormal
7.20–7.25	Repeat at 30-minute intervals
<7.20	Expedite delivery immediately

Figure 66.1 PERINEAL INJURY AT DELIVERY

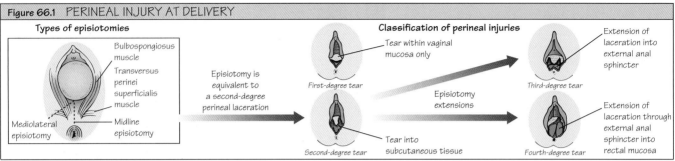

Types of episiotomies

Bulbospongiosus muscle

Transversus perinei superficialis muscle

Mediolateral episiotomy — Midline episiotomy

Episiotomy is equivalent to a second-degree perineal laceration

Classification of perineal injuries

Tear within vaginal mucosa only

First-degree tear

Tear into subcutaneous tissue

Second-degree tear

Episiotomy extensions

Extension of laceration into external anal sphincter

Third-degree tear

Extension of laceration through external anal sphincter into rectal mucosa

Fourth-degree tear

Figure 66.2 SURGICAL VAGINAL DELIVERY

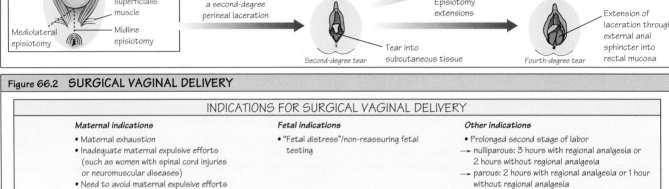

INDICATIONS FOR SURGICAL VAGINAL DELIVERY

Maternal indications
- Maternal exhaustion
- Inadequate maternal expulsive efforts (such as women with spinal cord injuries or neuromuscular diseases)
- Need to avoid maternal expulsive efforts (such as women with certain cardiac or cerebrovascular diseases)

Fetal indications
- "Fetal distress"/non-reassuring fetal testing

Other indications
- Prolonged second stage of labor
  → nulliparous: 3 hours with regional analgesia or 2 hours without regional analgesia
  → parous: 2 hours with regional analgesia or 1 hour without regional analgesia

CRITERIA WHICH NEED TO BE FULFILLED BEFORE SURGICAL VAGINAL DELIVERY

Maternal criteria
- Adequate analgesia
- Verbal and/or written consent
- Lithotomy position
- Bladder empty
- Adequate clinical pelvimetry

Fetal criteria
- Vertex presentation
- Vertex engaged (i.e. biparietal diameter of the head has passed through the pelvic inlet)
- Station (i.e. leading bony point of the head relative to the ischial spines) ≥ + 2/+ 5 cm
- Position, attitude of fetal head as well as presence of caput or moulding is known

Uteroplacental criteria
- Cervix fully dilated
- Membranes ruptured
- No placenta previa

Other criteria
- An experienced operator
- Capability to perform an emergency cesarean section delivery if required

FORCEPS

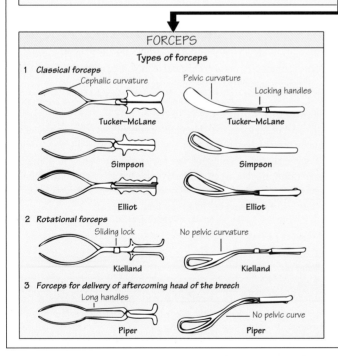

Types of forceps

1 *Classical forceps*

Cephalic curvature

Tucker–McLane

Pelvic curvature

Locking handles

Tucker–McLane

Simpson

Simpson

Elliot

Elliot

2 *Rotational forceps*

Sliding lock

Kielland

No pelvic curvature

Kielland

3 *Forceps for delivery of aftercoming head of the breech*

Long handles

Piper

No pelvic curve

Piper

VACUUM

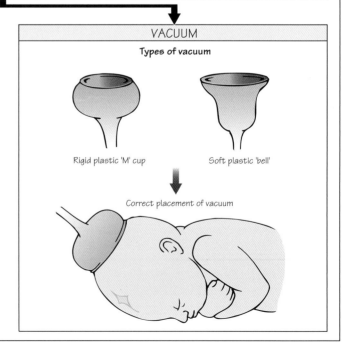

Types of vacuum

Rigid plastic 'M' cup

Soft plastic 'bell'

Correct placement of vacuum

Obstetrics and Gynecology at a Glance, Fourth Edition. Errol R. Norwitz and John O. Schorge.

140 © 2013 John Wiley & Sons, Ltd. Published 2013 by John Wiley & Sons, Ltd.

Episiotomy

- *Definition.* A surgical incision made in the perineum to facilitate delivery.
- *Incidence.* It used to be performed in >30% of vaginal deliveries, most often in nulliparous women, but there was a steep decline to <10% by 2006. It remains highly dependent on practice style and provider preference.
- *Indications.* It may be performed in isolation or in preparation for surgical vaginal delivery. It may also be used to facilitate delivery complicated by shoulder dystocia (see Chapter 63).
- *Goal.* Episiotomy was introduced to reduce complications of pelvic floor trauma at delivery, including bleeding, infection, genital prolapse, and incontinence. However, there does not appear to be any benefit to the mother of elective episiotomy.
- *Types/extensions* (Figure 66.1):
  1 *Midline episiotomy* refers to a vertical midline incision from the posterior forchette toward the rectum. It is effective in hastening delivery, but is associated with increased severe perineal trauma involving the external anal sphincter (third and fourth degree extensions). Used more commonly in the USA.
  2 *Mediolateral episiotomy* is cut at 45° to the posterior forchette on one side. Such incisions appear to protect against severe perineal trauma, but have been associated with increased blood loss, wound infection, and worsened postpartum pain (none of which has been definitively demonstrated). Used more commonly in the UK.
- *Episiotomy repair.* Primary approximation affords the best opportunity for functional repair, especially if there is rectal involvement. The external anal sphincter should be repaired by securing the cut ends using interrupted sutures.

Assisted vaginal delivery

- Assisted vaginal delivery refers to any surgical procedure designed to expedite vaginal delivery, and includes forceps delivery and vacuum extraction.
- There is no proven benefit of one instrument over another.
- The choice of which instrument to use is dependent largely on clinician preference and experience.

Forceps
Instruments
Since their introduction into obstetric practice by the Chamberlain family in the eighteenth century in Europe, the use of forceps has been controversial.

Forceps can be classified into three categories (see table below).
1 Classic forceps (such as Simpson forceps), which have a pelvic curvature, a cephalic curvature, and locking handles.
2 Rotational forceps (such as Kielland forceps), which lack a pelvic curvature and have sliding shanks.
3 Forceps designed to assist breech deliveries (such as Piper forceps), which lack a pelvic curve and have long handles on which to place the body of the breech while delivering the head.

Indications Figure 66.2 and contraindications
Relative contraindications include prematurity, fetal macrosomia, and suspected fetal coagulation disorder.

Complications
- Increased maternal perineal injury, especially with rotational forceps delivery.

- Fetal complications include facial bruising and/or laceration. Facial nerve palsy, skull fractures, cervical spine injuries, and intracranial hemorrhage are rare.

Classification of forceps deliveries

Type of procedure	Criteria
Outlet forceps	Fetal head is at or on the perineum, scalp is visible at the introitus without separating the labia, sagittal suture is in the anteroposterior diameter or right or left occiput anterior or posterior position, rotation is ≤45°
Low forceps	Leading point of the fetal skull is at ≥+2 cm but not on the pelvic floor, rotation may be: (a) ≤45° *or* (b) >45°
Mid-forceps	Station <+2 cm but head engaged
High forceps	(Not included in classification)

Vacuum
Instruments
- In 1954, Malmström developed the vacuum extractor (Ventouse) which now bears his name. The first (classic) Malmström vacuum extractor used a metal cup (the "M" cup). Current instruments are plastic, polyethylene, or silicone.
- There are two general types (Figure 66.2): (1) a firm, mushroom-shaped cup similar to the "M" cup (the rigid cup); and (2) a pliable, funnel-shaped cup (the soft cup).

Indications and contraindications
The same as for forceps delivery.

Technical considerations
- To promote flexion of the fetal head with traction, the suction cup is placed over the "median flexing point" (symmetrically astride the sagittal suture with the posterior margin of the cup 1–3 cm anterior to the posterior fontanelle).
- Low suction (100 mmHg) is applied. After ensuring that no maternal soft tissue is trapped between the cup and fetal head, suction is increased to 500–600 mmHg and sustained downward traction applied along the pelvic curve in concert with uterine contractions. Suction is released between contractions.
- Ideally, episiotomy should be avoided as pressure of the perineum on the vacuum cup will help to keep it applied to the fetal head and assist in flexion and rotation.
- The procedure should be abandoned if the cup detaches three times or if no descent of the head is achieved.

Complications
- *Failed delivery* may be more common with the soft cup.
- *Fetal complications* include cephalohematoma (bleeding into the scalp) and scalp lacerations ("cookie-cutter" injuries that result from the operator attempting to manually rotate the head with the vacuum). It remains unclear whether fetal intracerebral hemorrhage is increased with vacuum extraction.
- *Maternal* perineal injuries are not significantly increased.

Figure 67.1	INDICATIONS FOR CESAREAN SECTION DELIVERY	
	Absolute	**Relative**
Maternal	• Failed induction of labor • Failure to progress (labor dystocia) • Cephalopelvic disproportion	• Elective repeat cesarean section • Maternal disease (severe pre-eclampsia, cardiac disease, diabetes, cervical cancer)
Utero-placental	• Previous uterine surgery (classical cesarean) • Prior uterine rupture • Outlet obstruction (fibroids) • Placenta previa, large placental abruption	• Prior uterine surgery (full-thickness myomectomy) • Funic (cord) presentation in labor
Fetal	• "Fetal distress"/non-reassuring fetal testing • Cord prolapse • Fetal malpresentation (transverse lie)	• Fetal malpresentation (breech, brow, compound presentation) • Macrosomia • Fetal anomaly (hydrocephalus)

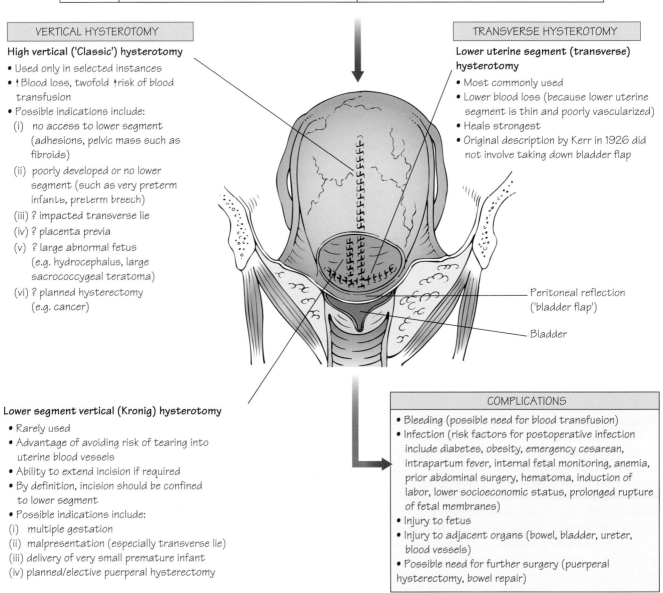

VERTICAL HYSTEROTOMY

High vertical ('Classic') hysterotomy

• Used only in selected instances
• ↑Blood loss, twofold ↑risk of blood transfusion
• Possible indications include:
  (i)   no access to lower segment (adhesions, pelvic mass such as fibroids)
  (ii) poorly developed or no lower segment (such as very preterm infants, preterm breech)
  (iii) ? impacted transverse lie
  (iv) ? placenta previa
  (v)   ? large abnormal fetus (e.g. hydrocephalus, large sacrococcygeal teratoma)
  (vi) ? planned hysterectomy (e.g. cancer)

Lower segment vertical (Kronig) hysterotomy

• Rarely used
• Advantage of avoiding risk of tearing into uterine blood vessels
• Ability to extend incision if required
• By definition, incision should be confined to lower segment
• Possible indications include:
  (i)   multiple gestation
  (ii) malpresentation (especially transverse lie)
  (iii) delivery of very small premature infant
  (iv) planned/elective puerperal hysterectomy

TRANSVERSE HYSTEROTOMY

Lower uterine segment (transverse) hysterotomy

• Most commonly used
• Lower blood loss (because lower uterine segment is thin and poorly vascularized)
• Heals strongest
• Original description by Kerr in 1926 did not involve taking down bladder flap

Peritoneal reflection ('bladder flap')

Bladder

COMPLICATIONS

• Bleeding (possible need for blood transfusion)
• Infection (risk factors for postoperative infection include diabetes, obesity, emergency cesarean, intrapartum fever, internal fetal monitoring, anemia, prior abdominal surgery, hematoma, induction of labor, lower socioeconomic status, prolonged rupture of fetal membranes)
• Injury to fetus
• Injury to adjacent organs (bowel, bladder, ureter, blood vessels)
• Possible need for further surgery (puerperal hysterectomy, bowel repair)

Definition

Delivery of a fetus via the abdominal route (laparotomy) requiring an incision into the uterus (hysterotomy).

Incidence

Cesarean section delivery is the second most common surgical procedure (behind male circumcision), accounting for around 20–25% of all deliveries in the UK and 32% in the USA.

Indications (Figure 67.1)

• Most indications for cesarean section are relative and rely on the judgment of the obstetric care provider.
• The most common indication for a primary (first) cesarean section is failure to progress in labor.
• Absolute cephalopelvic disproportion (CPD) refers to the clinical setting in which the fetus is too large relative to the bony pelvis to allow for vaginal delivery even under optimal circumstances. Relative CPD is where the fetus is too large for the bony pelvis because of malpresentation (brow, compound presentation).

Technical considerations

• Elective cesarean section can be performed after 39 weeks' gestation without documenting fetal lung maturity.
• Regional is preferred over general analgesia.
• Routine use of prophylactic antibiotics will decrease the incidence of postoperative febrile morbidity.
• Skin incision may be Pfannenstiel (low transverse incision, muscle separating, strong, but limited exposure), midline vertical (offers the best exposure, but is weak), or paramedian (vertical incision lateral to rectus muscles, rarely used). Pfannenstiel incisions may rarely be modified to improve exposure by dividing the rectus muscles horizontally (Maylard incision) or lifting the rectus off the pubic bone (Cherney incision).
• Types of hysterotomy are reviewed in Figure 67.1.
• Elective surgery (such as myomectomy) should not be performed at the time of cesarean section, because of the risk of bleeding.

Puerperal (cesarean section) hysterectomy
Incidence

Around 1 in 6,000 deliveries.

Indications

• Performed primarily as an emergency procedure when the mother's life is at risk due to uncontrolled hemorrhage (30–40%).
• Other indications include abnormal placentation (see Chapter 56), severe cervical dysplasia, and cervical cancer.
• Permanent sterilization is not an acceptable indication for puerperal hysterectomy.

Technical considerations

• A highly morbid procedure usually requiring general anesthesia. As such, it should be performed only as a last resort.
• Warming blanket, three-way Foley catheter, and blood products should be available.
• Emergency puerperal hysterectomies are associated with a fourfold increased risk of complications compared with elective procedures. Blood loss is often excessive (2–4 L) and blood transfusions are usually required (90%). Despite a high morbidity, overall maternal mortality rate is low (0.3%).

• It may be possible to leave the cervix behind (subtotal or supracervical hysterectomy), thereby minimizing complications, especially blood loss. This may not be possible if the cervix is the source of the excessive bleeding, such as with placenta previa.
• Although women will be amenorrheic and sterile, menopausal symptoms will not develop if the ovaries are left in place.

Vaginal birth after cesarean section
Background

• Of cesarean section deliveries, 30% are elective repeat procedures.
• Maternal mortality rate from cesarean section delivery is <0.1%, but is 2- to 10-fold higher than that associated with vaginal birth.
• Maternal morbidity (infection, thromboembolic events, wound dehiscence) is markedly higher with cesarean section.

Results

• Successful vaginal birth after cesarean section (VBAC) can be achieved in 65–80% of women.
• Factors associated with successful VBAC include prior vaginal delivery, estimated fetal weight <4,000 g, and a non-recurrent indication for the previous cesarean section (breech, placenta previa) rather than a potential recurrent indication (such as CPD).

Contraindications

• Absolute contraindications include a prior classic (high vertical) cesarean section, "fetal distress," transverse lie, and placenta previa.
• Relative contraindications include breech presentation, prior full-thickness uterine myomectomy, prior uterine rupture, and (possibly) multiple gestations.

Complications

• *Uterine dehiscence* (subclinical separation of the prior uterine incision) occurs in 2–3% of cases. It is often detected only by manual exploration of the scar after vaginal delivery. In the absence of vaginal bleeding, no further treatment is necessary.
• *Uterine rupture* may be life threatening. Symptoms and signs include acute onset of fetal bradycardia (70%), abdominal pain (10%), vaginal bleeding (5%), hemodynamic instability (5–10%), and/or loss of the presenting part (<5%). Epidural anesthesia may mask some of these features. Risk factors include:
  1 type of prior uterine incision (<1% for lower segment transverse incision, 2–3% for lower segment vertical, and 4–8% for high vertical);
  2 two or more prior cesarean sections (4%)
  3 prior uterine rupture
  4 "excessive" use of oxytocin (although "excessive" is poorly defined)
  5 dysfunctional labor pattern (especially prolonged second stage or arrest of dilation)
  6 induction of labor using prostaglandins.

Factors NOT associated with an increased risk for rupture include epidural anesthesia, unknown uterine scar, fetal macrosomia, and indication for prior cesarean section.

Clinical considerations

• Continuous intrapartum fetal monitoring is recommended.
• Follow labor curve carefully for evidence of labor dystocia.
• The capacity to perform an emergency cesarean section should be at hand.

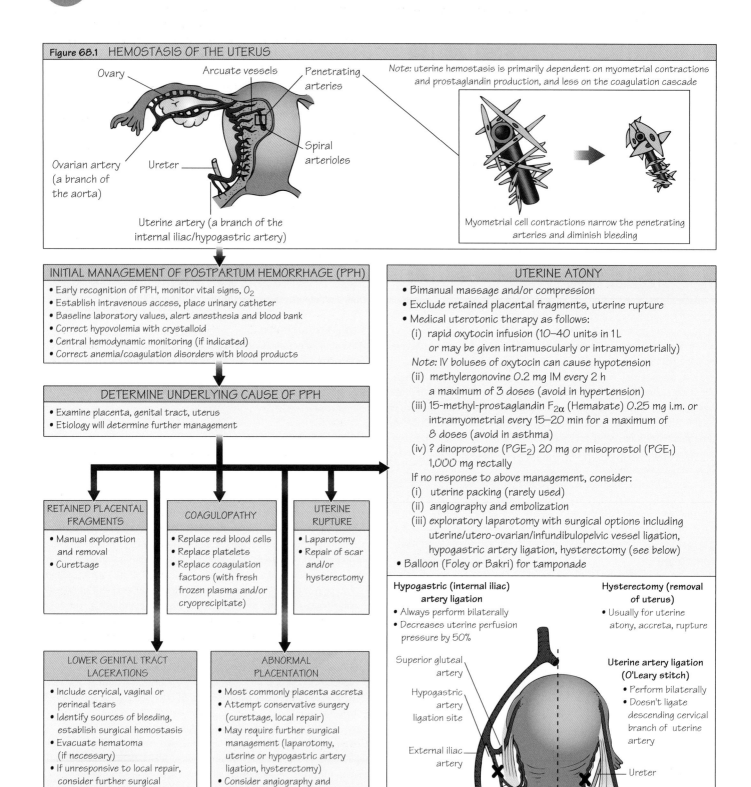

Figure 68.1 HEMOSTASIS OF THE UTERUS

Ovary
Arcuate vessels
Penetrating arteries
Spiral arterioles
Ovarian artery (a branch of the aorta)
Ureter
Uterine artery (a branch of the internal iliac/hypogastric artery)

Note: uterine hemostasis is primarily dependent on myometrial contractions and prostaglandin production, and less on the coagulation cascade

Myometrial cell contractions narrow the penetrating arteries and diminish bleeding

INITIAL MANAGEMENT OF POSTPARTUM HEMORRHAGE (PPH)
- Early recognition of PPH, monitor vital signs, O_2
- Establish intravenous access, place urinary catheter
- Baseline laboratory values, alert anesthesia and blood bank
- Correct hypovolemia with crystalloid
- Central hemodynamic monitoring (if indicated)
- Correct anemia/coagulation disorders with blood products

DETERMINE UNDERLYING CAUSE OF PPH
- Examine placenta, genital tract, uterus
- Etiology will determine further management

RETAINED PLACENTAL FRAGMENTS
- Manual exploration and removal
- Curettage

COAGULOPATHY
- Replace red blood cells
- Replace platelets
- Replace coagulation factors (with fresh frozen plasma and/or cryoprecipitate)

UTERINE RUPTURE
- Laparotomy
- Repair of scar and/or hysterectomy

LOWER GENITAL TRACT LACERATIONS
- Include cervical, vaginal or perineal tears
- Identify sources of bleeding, establish surgical hemostasis
- Evacuate hematoma (if necessary)
- If unresponsive to local repair, consider further surgical management (such as uterine packing, hypogastric artery ligation, uterine artery ligation, hysterectomy, embolization)

ABNORMAL PLACENTATION
- Most commonly placenta accreta
- Attempt conservative surgery (curettage, local repair)
- May require further surgical management (laparotomy, uterine or hypogastric artery ligation, hysterectomy)
- Consider angiography and embolization if time permits

UTERINE ATONY
- Bimanual massage and/or compression
- Exclude retained placental fragments, uterine rupture
- Medical uterotonic therapy as follows:
  (i) rapid oxytocin infusion (10–40 units in 1L or may be given intramuscularly or intramyometrially)
  Note: IV boluses of oxytocin can cause hypotension
  (ii) methylergonovine 0.2 mg IM every 2 h a maximum of 3 doses (avoid in hypertension)
  (iii) 15-methyl-prostaglandin $F_{2\alpha}$ (Hemabate) 0.25 mg i.m. or intramyometrial every 15–20 min for a maximum of 8 doses (avoid in asthma)
  (iv) ? dinoprostone (PGE_2) 20 mg or misoprostol (PGE_1) 1,000 mg rectally
  If no response to above management, consider:
  (i) uterine packing (rarely used)
  (ii) angiography and embolization
  (iii) exploratory laparotomy with surgical options including uterine/utero-ovarian/infundibulopelvic vessel ligation, hypogastric artery ligation, hysterectomy (see below)
- Balloon (Foley or Bakri) for tamponade

Hypogastric (internal iliac) artery ligation
- Always perform bilaterally
- Decreases uterine perfusion pressure by 50%

Hysterectomy (removal of uterus)
- Usually for uterine atony, accreta, rupture

Uterine artery ligation (O'Leary stitch)
- Perform bilaterally
- Doesn't ligate descending cervical branch of uterine artery

Superior gluteal artery
Hypogastric artery ligation site
External iliac artery
Uterine artery
Obturator artery
Ureter
Uterine artery
Bladder

Third stage of labor

Definition
- Begins with delivery of the fetus and ends with delivery of the placenta and fetal membranes.

Duration
- Median duration of the third stage of labor is 10 min.
- Of pregnant women 3–5% have a third stage lasting ≥30 min.

Management
- The third stage of labor is usually managed expectantly. Uterine contractions result in cleavage of the placenta between the zona basalis and zona spongiosum.
- The three clinical signs of placental separation include:
  1 a sudden gush of blood ("separation bleed")
  2 apparent lengthening of the umbilical cord
  3 elevation and contraction of the uterine fundus.
- Placental separation can be encouraged by "controlled cord traction" using either the Brandt–Andrews maneuver (where the uterus is secured and controlled traction is applied to the cord) or the Credé maneuver (where the cord is secured and the uterus elevated). Care should be taken to avoid uterine placental inversion.

Complications
- Postpartum hemorrhage (Figure 68.1).
- Retained placenta is defined as failure of the placenta to deliver within 30 min. If there is excessive bleeding, manual removal may be required earlier. Failed manual removal of the placenta suggests abnormal placentation (see Chapter 56).

Postpartum hemorrhage

Definition
- Postpartum hemorrhage (PPH) has traditionally been defined as an estimated blood loss of ≥500 mL. However, blood loss is underestimated clinically by 30–50%. The average blood loss after vaginal delivery is 500 mL, with 5% of women losing >1,000 mL. Blood loss after cesarean section averages 1,000 mL.
- More recently, PPH has been defined as a 10% drop in hematocrit from admission or bleeding requiring blood transfusion.

Incidence
Approximately 5% of all deliveries (4% after vaginal delivery, 6–8% after cesarean section delivery).

Classification
Early PPH
- Defined as PPH <24 hours after delivery.
- Causes include uterine atony, retained placental fragments, lower genital tract lacerations, uterine rupture, uterine inversion, abnormal placentation, and coagulopathy.

Late or delayed PPH
- Defined as PPH >24 hours but <6 weeks post-delivery.
- Causes include retained placental fragments, infection (endometritis), coagulopathy, and placental site subinvolution.

Etiology and management of PPH (Figure 68.1)
Uterine atony
- *Risk factors* include uterine overdistension (due to polyhydramnios, multiple pregnancy, fetal macrosomia), high parity, rapid or prolonged labor, infection, prior uterine atony, and use of uterine-relaxing agents.
- *Management* is reviewed in Figure 68.1.

Retained placental fragments
- May result from retention of a cotyledon or succenturiate lobe (seen in 3% of placentas). Examination of the placenta may identify defects suggestive of retained products.
- *Management.* Dilation and curettage, preferably under ultrasound guidance.

Lower genital tract lacerations
- *Risk factors* include assisted vaginal delivery, fetal macrosomia, precipitous delivery, and use of episiotomy.
- *Diagnosis* should be considered when vaginal bleeding continues despite adequate uterine tone.
- *Management.* Primary repair.

Uterine rupture
- *Incidence.* One in 2,000 deliveries.
- *Risk factors* include prior uterine surgery, obstructed labor, "excessive" use of oxytocin, abnormal fetal lie, grandmultiparity, and uterine manipulations in labor (forceps delivery, breech extraction, and intrauterine pressure catheter insertion).
- *Treatment.* Laparotomy with repair or hysterectomy.

Uterine inversion
- *Incidence.* One in 2,500 deliveries.
- *Risk factors* include uterine atony, excessive umbilical cord traction, manual removal of placenta, abnormal placentation, uterine anomalies, and fundal placentation.
- *Symptoms* include acute abdominal pain and shock (30%). The uterus may be visibly extruding through the vulva.
- *Treatment.* Immediate manual or hydrostatic replacement.

Abnormal placentation
- Includes abnormal attachment of placental villi to the myometrium (accreta), invasion into the myometrium (increta), or penetration through the myometrium (percreta).
- Placenta accreta is the most common type (1 in 2,500 deliveries).
- *Risk factors* include prior uterine surgery, placenta previa, smoking, and grandmultiparity. Placenta previa alone is associated with a 5% incidence of accreta, which increases to 10–25% with placenta previa and one prior cesarean section and >50% with placenta previa and two or more prior cesarean sections.
- *Management.* Dilation and curettage, or hysterectomy.

Coagulopathy
- *Congenital coagulopathy* complicates 1–2 per 10,000 pregnancies. The most common diagnoses are von Willebrand disease and idiopathic thrombocytopenic purpura (ITP).
- *Acquired* causes include anticoagulant therapy and consumptive coagulopathy resulting from obstetric complications (such as pre-eclampsia, sepsis, abruption, and amniotic fluid embolism).
- *Management.* Stop ongoing bleeding and replace blood products (including platelets, coagulation factors, and red blood cells).

Figure 69.1 PHYSIOLOGY OF LACTATION

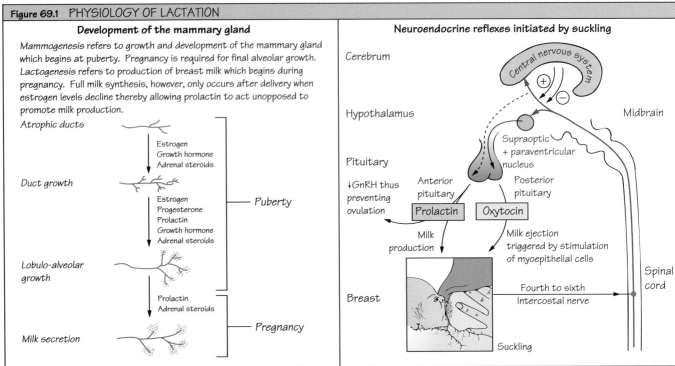

Development of the mammary gland

Mammogenesis refers to growth and development of the mammary gland which begins at puberty. Pregnancy is required for final alveolar growth. *Lactogenesis* refers to production of breast milk which begins during pregnancy. Full milk synthesis, however, only occurs after delivery when estrogen levels decline thereby allowing prolactin to act unopposed to promote milk production.

Atrophic ducts

Duct growth
- Estrogen
- Growth hormone
- Adrenal steroids

- Estrogen
- Progesterone
- Prolactin
- Growth hormone
- Adrenal steroids

} Puberty

Lobulo-alveolar growth
- Prolactin
- Adrenal steroids

Milk secretion

} Pregnancy

Neuroendocrine reflexes initiated by suckling

Cerebrum — Central nervous system (+) (−)

Hypothalamus — Midbrain

Supraoptic + paraventricular nucleus

Pituitary
↓GnRH thus preventing ovulation

Anterior pituitary — Prolactin

Posterior pituitary — Oxytocin

Milk production

Milk ejection triggered by stimulation of myoepithelial cells

Spinal cord

Breast

Fourth to sixth Intercostal nerve

Suckling

Figure 69.2 COMPLICATIONS OF THE PUERPERIUM

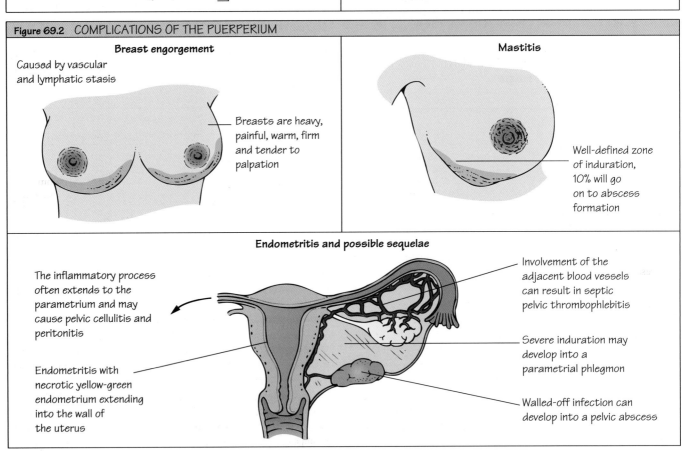

Breast engorgement

Caused by vascular and lymphatic stasis

Breasts are heavy, painful, warm, firm and tender to palpation

Mastitis

Well-defined zone of induration, 10% will go on to abscess formation

Endometritis and possible sequelae

The inflammatory process often extends to the parametrium and may cause pelvic cellulitis and peritonitis

Endometritis with necrotic yellow-green endometrium extending into the wall of the uterus

Involvement of the adjacent blood vessels can result in septic pelvic thrombophlebitis

Severe induration may develop into a parametrial phlegmon

Walled-off infection can develop into a pelvic abscess

Obstetrics and Gynecology at a Glance, Fourth Edition. Errol R. Norwitz and John O. Schorge.

Physiology

- The *puerperium* is the 6-week period after delivery when the reproductive tract returns to its non-pregnant state.
- Immediately after delivery, the uterus shrinks down to the level of the umbilicus. By 2 weeks postpartum, it is no longer palpable above the symphysis. By 6 weeks, the uterus has returned to its non-pregnant size.
- Decidual sloughing after delivery results in a physiologic vaginal discharge, known as *lochia*.
- The abdomen will resume its pre-pregnancy appearance, with the notable exception of *abdominal striae* ("stretch marks"). These fade with time.
- Most women will experience the return of menstruation by 6–8 weeks postpartum.

Postpartum care

- In the *immediate postpartum period*, maternal vital signs should be taken frequently, the uterine fundus should be palpated to ensure it is well contracted, and the amount of vaginal bleeding should be noted.
- Early ambulation is encouraged regardless of route of delivery. Adequate pain management is essential.
- Shortly after birth, neonates should receive topical ophthalmic prophylaxis (to prevent ophthalmia neonatorum) and vitamin K (to prevent hemorrhagic disease of the newborn due to a physiologic deficiency of vitamin K-dependent coagulation factors).
- Prior to discharge, skilled nursing staff should be made available to prepare the mother for care of the newborn. The mother should receive anti-D immunoglobulin (if she is rhesus [Rh] negative and her baby Rh positive) and MMR (measles, mumps, rubella) vaccine (if she is rubella non-immune).
- Coitus can be resumed 2–3 weeks after delivery depending on the patient's desire and comfort. Contraception is necessary to prevent conception.
- A *routine visit* is recommended 6 weeks postpartum. Contraceptive counseling and breastfeeding should be addressed.

Lactation and breastfeeding (Figure 69.1)

- *Advantages.* Breastfed infants have a lower incidence of allergies, gastrointestinal infections, otitis media, respiratory infections, and (possibly) higher intelligence quotient (IQ) scores. Women who breastfeed appear to have a lower incidence of breast cancer, ovarian cancer, and osteoporosis. Breastfeeding is also a bonding experience between infant and mother.
- *Contraindications.* HIV, cytomegalovirus, and possibly chronic hepatitis B or C. Most drugs given to the mother are secreted to some extent into breast milk, but the amount of drug ingested by the infant is typically small. There are some drugs, however, in which breastfeeding is contraindicated (radioisotopes, cytotoxic agents).
- *Physiology.* Prolactin is essential for lactation. Women with pituitary necrosis (Sheehan syndrome) do not lactate. Cigarette smoking, diuretics, bromocriptine, and combined oral contraceptives (not the progestin-only pill) decrease milk production.
- *Colostrum* is a lemon-colored fluid secreted by the breasts during the first 4–5 days postpartum. It contains more minerals and protein than mature milk, but less sugar and fat. *Mature milk* production is established within a few days. It contains high concentrations of lactose, vitamins (except vitamin K), immunoglobulins, and antibodies.

Complications of the puerperium (Figure 69.2)

Breast engorgement

- May occur on days 2–4 postpartum in women who are not nursing or at any time if breastfeeding is interrupted.
- Conservative measures (tight-fitting brassiere, ice packs, analgesics) are usually effective. Bromocriptine may be indicated in refractory cases.

Mastitis

- Refers to a regional infection of the breast parenchyma, usually by *Staphylococcus aureus*.
- *Incidence.* Uncommon. More than 50% of cases occur in primiparas.
- Mastitis is a *clinical diagnosis* with fever, chills, and focal unilateral breast erythema, edema, and tenderness. It usually occurs during the third or fourth week postpartum.
- *Treatment.* Overcome ductal obstruction (by continuing breastfeeding or pumping), symptomatic relief, and oral antibiotics (usually flucloxacillin). Ten percent of women will develop an abscess requiring surgical drainage.

Endometritis

- Refers to a polymicrobial infection of the endometrium that often invades the underlying myometrium.
- *Incidence.* Less than 5% after vaginal delivery, but 5- to 10-fold higher after cesarean section delivery.
- *Risk factors.* Cesarean section delivery, prolonged rupture of membranes, multiple vaginal examinations, manual removal of the placenta, and internal fetal monitoring.
- Endometritis is a *clinical diagnosis* with fever, uterine tenderness, a foul purulent vaginal discharge, and/or increased vaginal bleeding. It occurs most commonly 5–10 days after delivery.
- *Treatment.* Broad-spectrum antibiotics (until the patient is clinically improved and afebrile for 24–48 hours) and dilation and curettage (if retained products of conception are suspected).
- *Complications.* Abscess, septic pelvic thrombophlebitis.

Necrotizing fasciitis

- Refers to necrotic infection of the superficial fascia that spreads rapidly along tissue planes to the abdominal wall, buttock, and/or thigh, leading to septicemia and circulatory failure. Maternal mortality rate approaches 50%.
- *Diagnosis.* Skin edema, blue–brown discoloration, or frank gangrene with loss of sensation or hyperesthesia.
- *Treatment.* Early diagnosis, antibiotics, aggressive surgical debridement.

Psychiatric complaints (see Chapter 48)

- A mild *transient depression* ("postpartum blues") is common after delivery, occurring in >50% of women.
- *Postpartum depression* occurs in 8–15% of women. Risk factors include a history of depression (30%) or prior postpartum depression (70–85%). Symptoms develop 2–3 months postpartum and resolve slowly over the next 6–12 months. Supportive care and monthly follow-up are necessary.
- *Postpartum psychosis* is rare (1–2 per 1,000 live births). Risk factors include young age, primiparity, and a personal or family history of mental illness. Symptoms typically start 10–14 days postpartum. Hospitalization, pharmacologic and/or electroconvulsive therapy (ECT) may be necessary. Recurrence of postpartum psychosis is high (25–30%).

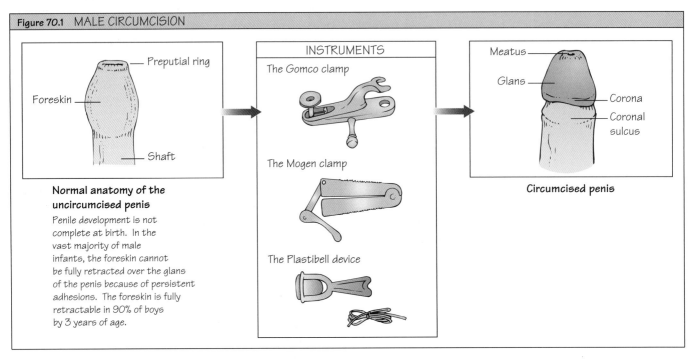

Figure 70.1 MALE CIRCUMCISION

Normal anatomy of the uncircumcised penis

Penile development is not complete at birth. In the vast majority of male infants, the foreskin cannot be fully retracted over the glans of the penis because of persistent adhesions. The foreskin is fully retractable in 90% of boys by 3 years of age.

INSTRUMENTS

The Gomco clamp

The Mogen clamp

The Plastibell device

Circumcised penis

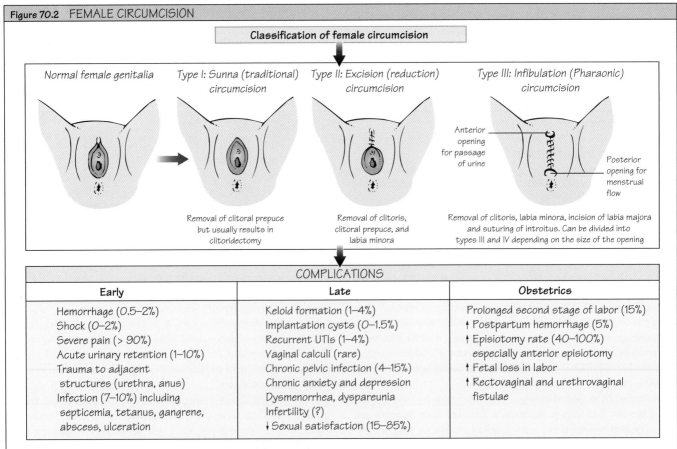

Figure 70.2 FEMALE CIRCUMCISION

Classification of female circumcision

Normal female genitalia

Type I: Sunna (traditional) circumcision — Removal of clitoral prepuce but usually results in clitoridectomy

Type II: Excision (reduction) circumcision — Removal of clitoris, clitoral prepuce, and labia minora

Type III: Infibulation (Pharaonic) circumcision — Anterior opening for passage of urine — Posterior opening for menstrual flow — Removal of clitoris, labia minora, incision of labia majora and suturing of introitus. Can be divided into types III and IV depending on the size of the opening

COMPLICATIONS

Early	Late	Obstetrics
Hemorrhage (0.5–2%)	Keloid formation (1–4%)	Prolonged second stage of labor (15%)
Shock (0–2%)	Implantation cysts (0–1.5%)	↑ Postpartum hemorrhage (5%)
Severe pain (> 90%)	Recurrent UTIs (1–4%)	↑ Episiotomy rate (40–100%)
Acute urinary retention (1–10%)	Vaginal calculi (rare)	especially anterior episiotomy
Trauma to adjacent structures (urethra, anus)	Chronic pelvic infection (4–15%)	↑ Fetal loss in labor
Infection (7–10%) including septicemia, tetanus, gangrene, abscess, ulceration	Chronic anxiety and depression	↑ Rectovaginal and urethrovaginal fistulae
	Dysmenorrhea, dyspareunia	
	Infertility (?)	
	↓ Sexual satisfaction (15–85%)	

Obstetrics and Gynecology at a Glance, Fourth Edition. Errol R. Norwitz and John O. Schorge.

148 © 2013 John Wiley & Sons, Ltd. Published 2013 by John Wiley & Sons, Ltd.

Male circumcision (Figure 70.1)

Definition

Male circumcision refers to the surgical removal of all or part of the foreskin of the male penis.

Incidence

• It is the most common surgery performed on males.
• Circumcision rates vary from country to country: 90–95% in Israel, 60–90% in the USA, 50% in Canada and the UK.

Indications

• The most common indications are religious traditions and/or social beliefs. Cultural traditions also often dictate the timing of the procedure and the person responsible for performing it.
• Newborn (male) circumcision has potential medical benefits and advantages as well as disadvantages and risks. It is generally accepted that there is no medical indication for routine circumcision of newborn males.
• Medical indications are rare. These include persistent non-retractability (especially if associated with urinary obstruction), phimosis and paraphimosis (acute onset of pain and swelling of the glans due to obstruction of venous return, resulting from a persistent retracted foreskin), and possibly recurrent urinary tract infections and/or sexually transmitted infections.

Potential benefits

• Facilitates genital cleanliness. It does not eliminate the need for proper genital hygiene; it simply makes it easier.
• May reduce the incidence of urinary tract infections from 1% in uncircumcised to 0.1% in circumcised males.
• May reduce the risk of transmission of some sexually transmitted infections (such as HIV and human papillomavirus [HPV]).
• Penile carcinoma is a disease of elderly people with an incidence of around 1 in 600 uncircumcised males. It can be almost completely prevented by circumcision. However, poor genital hygiene may be equally important in the pathogenesis of this disease.
• May prevent cervical cancer in the partners of uncircumcised males infected with HPV.
• Will avoid circumcision later in life where the procedure may be more complicated and more traumatic for the patient. Of all uncircumcised males, up to 10% will require circumcision later in life for medical indications.

Contraindications

• *Absolute contraindications* include a documented or family history of a bleeding disorder or a structural defect of the penis (such as hypospadias in which the foreskin is used as a surgical graft to repair the defect). Circumcision is an elective procedure. It should be performed only in healthy, stable infants.
• *Relative contraindications* include prematurity, infants <24 hours old, and a very small appearing penis ("micropenis") that may result from webbing or tethering of the glans to the scrotum.

Technical considerations

• Informed consent should be obtained from the parent(s).
• Examination of the external genitalia should be performed.
• The infant is temporarily restrained.
• Infants do experience pain and discomfort with the procedure. Analgesia is not universally used, but is highly recommended. The preferred method of analgesia has not been determined. Swaddling, sucrose by mouth, and acetaminophen may reduce stress. Local infiltration (dorsal penile block or ring block) is effective. Epinephrine should not be given. Topical anesthesia (5% lidocaine/prilocaine – Emla) may be effective, but should be applied 1 hour before the surgery. General anesthesia is not justified.
• Instruments available for male circumcision are detailed in Figure 70.1.

Complications

• Complications occur in 0.2–0.6% of procedures. The most common complication is excessive bleeding. Other immediate complications include postoperative infection, hematoma formation, injury to the penis, and excessive skin removal (denudation).
• The Plastibell device is left in place over a number of days until the foreskin separates by infarction and falls off. It may be associated with a higher incidence of infection.
• Long-term complications are rare and include stenosis of the urethral meatus. As regards future sexuality, Masters and Johnson found no difference in sexual experience and sensitivity between circumcised and uncircumcised men.
• More serious complications are exceptionally rare and invariably involve breach of protocol (such as complete destruction of the penis by electrocautery or ischemia after the inappropriate use of epinephrine-containing local anesthetics).

Female circumcision (genital mutilation)
(Figure 70.2)

General considerations

• Despite universal condemnation, this practice persists in many countries with prevalence rates ranging from <1% to 99%.
• It is practiced on all continents, across socioeconomic classes, and among different ethnic, religious, and cultural groups, including indigenous African and Arab cultures.
• There are at least 100 million circumcised women worldwide.

Indications

• There is no medical indication for female circumcision.
• In many cultures, female circumcision is looked upon as an initiation into womanhood.
• Reasons given for the procedure include prevention of immorality, to make a woman eligible for marriage, to make intercourse more enjoyable for the man, and to promote cleanliness. In reality, it symbolizes social control of a woman's sexual pleasure (clitoridectomy) and reproductive capacity (infibulation).

Technical considerations

• Techniques of female circumcision are detailed in Figure 70.2. Sunna (the Arabic word for "traditional") circumcision is the least mutilating procedure with removal of the clitoral prepuce alone. It is said to be analogous to male circumcision; however, it invariably results in severe clitoral damage and/or amputation.
• Circumcision is generally performed by untrained operators without anesthesia or sterilized instruments. Hemostasis is achieved by the application of cow dung or mud, by pressure with dirty clothes, or by crude suturing. A girl's legs may be tied together for weeks to facilitate healing.

Complications

The complications of female circumcision (early, late, and intrapartum) and their respective incidence are detailed in Figure 70.2.

Case studies and questions

Case 1: Ectopic pregnancy

You are called to the emergency room to evaluate a 21-year-old woman in excruciating pain. She is sexually active, her partner uses condoms for contraception, and she is 6 weeks late for her period. Her blood pressure is 90/55 mmHg and her pulse is 115.

1 *What is the quickest way to make a diagnosis based on this presentation?*
2 *What is the etiology for most maternal deaths?*
3 *Are there any consistent symptoms of ectopic pregnancy?*
4 *Why has there been a recent increase in the number of women diagnosed with ectopic pregnancy?*
5 *What are the surgical treatment options?*
6 *What are potential problems of methotrexate medical management?*

Case 2: Vaginitis

Beth is a 33-year-old single woman who has been in your practice for several years and left a message with your nurse that she has a pruritic vaginal discharge that has persisted for 2 weeks despite her attempts at using an over-the-counter yeast cream.

1 *Is it ever appropriate to treat without an examination?*
2 *What are the other disadvantages of using non-prescription antifungal agents?*
3 *What else should be considered in the differential diagnosis?*
4 *How should Beth be evaluated?*
5 *On examination the vaginal pH is high, but microscopic findings are equivocal. How should this patient be managed?*
6 *How do you confirm the diagnosis of candidiasis? What is the treatment?*

Case 3: Adnexal mass

You are asked to consult on an asymptomatic 46-year-old woman who is currently an inpatient. She had a CT scan performed of the abdomen and pelvis for an unrelated medical indication and a 5-cm adnexal mass was inadvertently seen.

1 *How commonly do adnexal masses occur?*
2 *How should this patient be evaluated?*
3 *What TVU findings suggest a benign etiology?*
4 *Is a CA-125 test warranted?*
5 *This patient has a complex cyst, a CA-125 level of 337 U/mL, no ascites, and her CT scan is otherwise normal. Her sister was diagnosed with breast cancer at age 34. Is aspiration of cyst fluid appropriate?*
6 *What type of operation should be proposed?*

Case 4: Amenorrhea

A 37-year-old G_0 presents to your office for her annual visit. For the past 5 years she has noted irregular menses, but now she has not had a period in 7 months and wonders if this is abnormal.

1 *How is amenorrhea defined?*
2 *How should this patient be evaluated?*
3 *Her TSH and prolactin are both normal. The FSH level is not in the menopausal range. What is the next step?*

4 *She has a "period" after 7 days of progestin therapy and her examination suggests PCOS. As she is not attempting to get pregnant, what is the best medical therapy to treat anovulation and amenorrhea?*
5 *Does weight loss improve ovarian function in obese women with PCOS?*

Case 5: Endometrial cancer

An obese, but otherwise healthy, 62-year-old woman presents to your office after having her "period" for the first time in over a decade.

1 *What is your differential diagnosis?*
2 *What is the initial evaluation?*
3 *The biopsy demonstrates grade 1 endometrial cancer. What is the best management?*
4 *Her final pathology demonstrates a grade 13 tumor with 70% depth of invasion into the myometrium, negative lymph nodes, no cervical extension or lymph vascular invasion, and normal pelvic washings. What is her stage and does she need postoperative therapy?*
5 *What is the appropriate follow-up for patients with endometrial cancer?*

Case 6: Preterm labor

A 28-year-old G_5P_2 is admitted to your office at 28 weeks' gestation with regular painful uterine contractions every 3 minutes. Bimanual examination shows her cervix to be long and closed.

1 *How is preterm labor defined? Is this patient in preterm labor?*
2 *What are the causes of preterm birth?*
3 *This patient has had three prior spontaneous preterm deliveries at 28–31 weeks' gestation and is very concerned that this pregnancy too will end prematurely. What tests are available to screen for preterm labor?*
4 *The patient continues to contract. A repeat cervical examination 4 hours later shows her cervix to be 4 cm dilated and 90% effaced. You make a diagnosis of preterm labor and are considering initiating tocolytic therapy. Are there any contraindications to tocolysis?*
5 *Should you recommend strict bed rest and aggressive intravenous hydration?*
6 *Is antibiotic administration recommended? If so, what is the indication and for how long should treatment be continued?*
7 *You are considering starting a tocolytic agent. What is the goal of tocolysis? What tocolytic agents are available and which are most effective?*
8 *Is there a place for progesterone to prevent preterm birth?*

Case 7: Preterm PROM

A 30-year-old G_2P_{1001} at 29 weeks' gestation presents to the obstetric triage unit with suspected leakage of clear fluid, described as a constant trickle since 2am. She has a history of systemic lupus erythematosus (SLE) and is maintained on prednisone 20 mg daily. In addition, she reports having experienced scant vaginal bleeding throughout the first trimester only. Currently, fetal wellbeing is reassuring and the patient has no contractions noted on tocometry. Her abdomen is soft, and she is afebrile.

1 *Does the patient have any specific risk factors for preterm PROM?*
2 *How do you confirm the diagnosis of preterm PROM?*

3 *What other diagnoses should be considered?*

4 *What are the complications of preterm PROM?*

5 *Is this patient a candidate for expectant management?*

6 *Is this patient a candidate for antenatal corticosteroids?*

7 *How should this patient be managed?*

Case 8: Post-term pregnancy

A nulliparous woman presents for a routine prenatal visit at 41 weeks' gestation. She is concerned that she has not yet gone into labor. Fetal wellbeing is reassuring.

1 *How is post-term pregnancy defined? How often does it occur?*

2 *What causes some pregnancies to continue post-term?*

3 *On further review, she is not certain of her LMP. Is this important and, if so, what criteria should be used to confirm gestational age?*

4 *What are the risks to the fetus of post-term pregnancy?*

5 *Does post-term pregnancy pose any increased risk to the mother?*

6 *What are the current recommendations for the management of post-term pregnancy?*

7 *After weighing the risks and benefits of induction of labor, the patient and her husband decide that they would like to go home and await the spontaneous onset of labor. How should this patient be followed?*

Case 9: Gestational diabetes

A 28-year-old G_4P_2 presents to your office for a routine prenatal visit at 24 weeks' gestation. Her physical examination is unremarkable and fetal wellbeing is reassuring. You recommend testing for gestational diabetes mellitus (GDM).

1 *What is GDM?*

2 *Should everyone be screened for GDM? If so, at what gestational age should they be screened?*

3 *Her 1-hour GLT is 182 mg/dL. Does she have GDM?*

4 *All four values of her 3-hour GTT are elevated and her fasting glucose level is 127 mg/dL. How would you manage her GDM? How long would you allow her to try dietary restriction before adding a hypoglycemic agent?*

5 *The estimated fetal weight at 38 weeks' gestation is 4,600 g (10 lb 2 oz). She has had six prior uncomplicated vaginal deliveries. How would you counsel her about delivery?*

6 *After extensive counseling, the couple decline elective cesarean section delivery. She is now 38 weeks' gestation. How should she be managed at this point in time?*

Case 10: Pre-eclampsia

A healthy 29-year-old G_2P_{0101} is admitted to labor and delivery at 28 weeks' gestation complaining of a severe headache and blurred vision. Her BP is 200/110 mmHg with 2+ proteinuria on urinalysis. Repeat BP a few hours later is 160/110 mmHg. Laboratory studies showed a normal hematocrit, platelet count, and liver transaminase levels.

1 *How is pre-eclampsia defined?*

2 *Her 24-hour urinalysis reveals 1.2 g protein. This patient meets criteria for the diagnosis of pre-eclampsia. What type of pre-eclampsia does she have?*

3 *What causes pre-eclampsia?*

4 *Are there risk factors for the development of pre-eclampsia? Can we accurately predict and prevent pre-eclampsia?*

5 *This patient has severe pre-eclampsia by symptoms and BP criteria. She is only 28 weeks' gestation. Should she be delivered or can she be managed expectantly?*

6 *The decision has been made to proceed with delivery. Bimanual examination shows her cervix to be long and closed. Does this mean that the patient has to have a cesarean section delivery?*

Answers

Case 1: Ectopic pregnancy

1 This patient is becoming hemodynamically unstable and should receive urgent attention. Based on the brief history, the first priority should be to determine if she has an ectopic pregnancy. Other less likely possibilities include a ruptured ovarian hemorrhagic cyst, appendicitis, or a septic abortion with imminent shock. A bedside sonogram should be performed to look for hemoperitoneum and/or βhCG (βhuman chorionic gonadotropin) level sent. Although ectopic pregnancies are increasingly diagnosed before rupture, in this emergency case, a high clinical suspicion should prompt an immediate call to the operating room for expeditious surgical intervention. In the presence of a ruptured tubal pregnancy, it will be positive in >90% of cases if performed correctly. It is a useful, albeit infrequently used, diagnostic tool for this urgent situation. Maternal blood in the abdomen is initially able to clot in the same way that peripheral blood does. However, when an ectopic pregnancy has continued bleeding, this blood undergoes lysis. Retrieval of non-clotting blood obtained by culdocentesis will generally have a hematocrit >15% and confirm the diagnosis.

2 More than 90% of women who die experience rapid catastrophic blood loss, hemoperitoneum, shock, and ultimately cardiovascular collapse. Rarely, infections or anesthetic complications contribute to mortality. In about half of cases, significant delays by physicians or misdiagnosis by other medical personnel is at least partially responsible.

3 Typically, early symptoms include an absence of menstrual bleeding and some description of spotting or irregular bleeding. Patients often seek medical attention at this point and are followed closely with sonograms and βhCG levels before the onset of dramatic symptoms. The pain of an ectopic pregnancy may be manifest in a variety of ways. Before rupture, it may only be a vague unilateral soreness or a colicky type of pain. After rupture, the severity of escalating pelvic pain depends on the rate of blood loss. Referred shoulder pain occurs in 25% as a result of diaphragmatic irritation from the hemoperitoneum.

4 Several factors have resulted in the steep rise in the incidence of ectopic pregnancy. First, pelvic inflammatory disease (PID – see Chapter 8) is not only much more common than it was in the 1970s, but the management has gravitated toward conservative medical therapy or fertility-sparing surgery. As a result, more women with a prior episode of PID are at risk. Second, advances in diagnostic techniques (eg, transvaginal sonogram, βhCG) have resulted in earlier, and probably more frequent, diagnoses. Historically, tubal abortions were much more common without knowledge of the ectopic pregnancy location. In fact, about half of ectopic pregnancies are believed to undergo spontaneous tubal abortion without further sequelae. Third, the dramatic increase in infertility treatment and assisted reproductive technologies (ART – see Chapter 27) has contributed.

5 When a patient is diagnosed with an *unruptured* ectopic pregnancy, the treatment options include non-surgical management. If surgery is decided upon, then, if equipment is available, laparoscopy is preferred.

• *Salpingotomy* (serosal defect in the fallopian tube is closed with sutures) and *salpingostomy* (serosal defect is left open to close by secondary intention – most common in the USA). These variations have about equal success in preserving fertility. In 5–10% of cases, postoperative methotrexate is required due to persistent trophoblast (placental) tissue at the ectopic site.

• Partial or complete *salpingectomy* may be indicated when (1) child-bearing is complete, (2) the patient has a prior history of an ectopic in the same fallopian tube, (3) there is significant damage to the inner lumen of the tube, or (4) if the health of the woman is significantly improved by more definitive management (eg, large-volume blood loss).

If the patient has a *ruptured* ectopic pregnancy and is *hemodynamically stable*, then surgery is required and laparoscopy is not necessarily contraindicated. The advantage of laparoscopy is a *quicker* postoperative recovery. The disadvantage is that in a woman with a hemoperitoneum it can take longer to clear the blood out, identify the ectopic, and treat it. The same type of surgery would be done regardless of whether a laparotomy is performed.

In the presented case of a woman with a *ruptured* ectopic pregnancy who is *hemodynamically unstable*, a laparotomy should probably be performed and usually a (partial) salpingectomy. The removal of the damaged tube allows rapid control of bleeding and the best chance for continued hemostasis throughout the postoperative period.

6 Treatment failure is the main worry with methotrexate therapy of an unruptured ectopic pregnancy. Every potential patient has a constellation of findings that factor into deciding whether it is safe to treat her medically. In general, the more advanced the gestation, the more likely it is to fail methotrexate and ultimately rupture without surgery. When evaluating a patient, at a minimum she must have an unruptured mass, be hemodynamically stable, and desire future fertility (see Chapter 5 for other relative and absolute indications and contraindications). Medical treatment is considered to have failed when the βhCG levels either increase or plateau by day 7 post-injection or when the tube ruptures. If medical therapy fails, rapid surgical intervention may be necessary. Patients treated with methotrexate *must* therefore be able to return for follow-up care.

Methotrexate side effects are usually very mild in the typical, young, otherwise healthy patient. On occasion, significant nausea, stomatitis, diarrhea, dizziness, or pneumonitis can occur. During therapy, women should discontinue folic acid supplements (eg, prenatal vitamins) and avoid non-steroidal anti-inflammatory drugs.

Treatment-related complications frequently include at least one episode of increased abdominal pain due to swelling of the tube. Typically it is a milder event than with tubal rupture, is of limited duration (1–2 days), and should not be associated with a surgical abdomen or hemodynamic instability. A sonogram can help confirm the absence of intra-abdominal blood.

See Chapters 5, 6, 8, and 27.

Case 2: Vaginitis

1 Very frequently, women will attempt to self-diagnose their vaginitis and self-treat with any number of readily available topical or oral agents. The benefits of using a non-prescription antifungal include convenience, the potential to avoid the cost of a physician visit, and, most importantly, the ability to quickly initiate effective treatment. However, the accuracy of self-diagnosis is often worse than is widely assumed. Given the non-specific nature of vulvovaginal symptoms, patients requesting treatment by telephone should be asked to come in for evaluation, particularly – as in this patient – if she has treated herself with a non-prescription antifungal without success. However, in a reasonably compliant woman with multiple confirmed episodes and similar symptoms, a short course of treatment may be initiated over the phone. In these cases, she should be asked to come in for evaluation only if symptoms persist.

2 A patient with a simple, straightforward case of vulvovaginal candidiasis who uses an over-the-counter non-prescription product should respond to therapy. Failure to respond should prompt clinical evaluation. Side effects consist primarily of localized burning and irritation in 5% of women. Mainly, it leads to a delay in accurate diagnosis and appropriate treatment. Although such delay may have minimal effect on vulvovaginal symptoms, such as pruritis, odor, or discharge, it may be of greater concern if she ends up being diagnosed with pelvic inflammatory disease (see Chapter 8), sexually transmitted infection, or a urinary tract infection.

3 Vaginitis is a general term that refers to a spectrum of conditions causing vulvovaginal burning, itching, irritation, and/or abnormal discharge. The differential diagnosis is extensive. Bacterial vaginosis is the most common cause, followed by candidiasis and trichomoniasis. Many cases will remain undiagnosed or end up attributed to atrophic vaginitis or various vulvar dystrophies.

4 The first step is to obtain a focused history to understand the extent of symptoms, including any recent changes and whether she has been experiencing associated dyspareunia and/or dysuria. Questions about the duration of symptoms, relation to menstrual cycle, prior attempts at treatment, and a sexual history also may yield important insights into the etiology.

The pertinent parts of the physical examination include careful inspection of the vulva. During speculum examination, samples should be obtained for vaginal pH, the "whiff" test, and slide preparations for a saline (wet mount) and 10% KOH microscopy. Importantly, the pH swab should be obtained from the mid-portion of the vaginal side wall to avoid false elevation from cervical mucus, blood, semen, or previous intravaginal medications.

5 Usually when the pH is elevated in a symptomatic patient, microscopic findings will quickly confirm the diagnosis (eg, trichomonads, clue cells). However, recent intercourse, menses, sampling of cervical mucus, or recent intravaginal therapy can also elevate the pH of the vagina.

Although light microscopy is a standard part of the diagnostic evaluation, it misses a large percentage of patients with symptomatic vulvovaginal candidiasis. As in this patient, self-treatment before evaluation may also make it more difficult to visualize yeast.

Vaginal cultures are not obtained routinely because of their cost, the delay in obtaining results, and the fact that many women may be asymptomatically colonized with group B streptococci or lactobacilli. However, cultures should be obtained in cases of recurrent vulvovaginal candidiasis, possible non-*albicans* candida infection (eg, persistent yeast symptoms after antifungal therapy), or symptomatic women with negative microscopic findings. Therefore, this symptomatic patient should be treated in a manner similar to other women with vaginitis where the diagnosis is unclear and cultures may be helpful.

6 The diagnosis may be suggested on the basis of history and physical examination, but confirmation requires either (1) visualization of branched and budding hyphae on KOH wet mount or (2) a positive culture in a symptomatic woman. Uncomplicated patients may be treated with either topical clotrimazole or oral fluconazole. Occasion-

ally, in more severe cases, a second dose or repeated doses of fluconazole will be required. Although much less common than *Candida albicans*, candidiasis caused by non-*albicans Candida* species are less likely to respond to "azole" antifungal therapy. Therapy with vaginal boric acid, 600 mg capsules daily for at least 2 weeks, may be effective.

See Chapters 7 and 8.

Case 3: Adnexal mass

1 In gynecology, adnexal masses are very common, typically presenting both diagnostic and therapeutic dilemmas. As in this patient, most are detected incidentally. In the USA, a woman has a 5–10% lifetime risk of undergoing surgery for a suspected ovarian neoplasm. Although most are benign, the goal of the evaluation is to exclude malignancy.

2 Two factors are important to consider. Is the patient symptomatic? In this case she is not. Next, could this adnexal mass be malignant? Masses with a low likelihood of cancer can often be managed conservatively. Conversely, those that are more likely to be malignant are best managed with prompt surgery by a gynecologic oncologist. Masses that are less clearly benign or malignant usually require surgery. The differential diagnosis is limitless, including both gynecologic and non-gynecologic sources. The most important diagnostic factors are the woman's age and whether she is pre- or postmenopausal. Masses in younger premenopausal women are almost always gynecologic – usually functional cysts. In contrast, adnexal masses in postmenopausal older women are often benign neoplasms (eg, cystadenoma).

The initial evaluation should include a physical examination, including a rectal examination. Palpation of a smooth, mobile mass with cystic (compressible) consistency is reassuring for a benign etiology. Examinations in obese women are of limited value.

Next, the patient should undergo transvaginal ultrasonography (TVU). No alternative imaging modality has comparable accuracy, ease, and availability. However, it is important to recognize that image quality and interpretation vary widely. Each physician should be aware of any limitations in his or her own center and be wary of scans performed elsewhere. The history, pelvic examination, and TVU should provide enough information to develop a plan.

3 Effectively, there are two different types of ovarian cysts – simple and complex. Simple cysts resemble a "water balloon" – they are unilocular, thin-walled sonolucent cysts with smooth regular borders. Overwhelmingly, they are benign. If this patient is found to have a simple cyst, then she could be managed expectantly. Simple cysts <10 cm in size will spontaneously resolve in up to 75% of cases without intervention, regardless of menopausal status. Complex cysts may have any number of findings. Typically, the TVU may indicate the diagnosis of one of a handful of common benign conditions such as a hemorrhagic cyst/endometrioma, dermoid, or hydrosalpinx.

4 The value of the CA-125 measurement is mainly to distinguish between benign and malignant masses in postmenopausal women. CA-125 levels are generally less valuable in premenopausal women due to the numerous benign reasons (fibroids, menses, hepatitis) for non-specific elevation. However, extreme values can be helpful – a markedly elevated CA-125 level would raise a much greater concern for malignancy.

5 No. Aspiration of a malignant mass may induce spillage and seeding of cancer cells in the abdomen, thereby changing the stage and prognosis. The diagnosis is still in question and will require a more definitive procedure.

6 Minimally invasive laparoscopic surgery is the most appropriate and desirable treatment for most women with an adnexal mass due to the shortened length of hospital stay, decreased pain, and quicker recovery time. At a minimum, this patient with several suspicious findings should be counseled about laparoscopic unilateral salpingo-oophorectomy (USO). Intraoperatively, peritoneal washings are collected, the USO is performed, and a frozen section can determine the diagnosis with reasonable certainty. If a benign diagnosis is confirmed, either the operation may be terminated or – depending on preoperative counseling – a contralateral USO may be performed with or without other indicated procedures (eg, hysterectomy).

Malignant features would suggest the need for a more comprehensive staging operation that could be completed laparoscopically by skilled providers. Women with ovarian cancer whose care is managed by a gynecologic oncologist have improved overall survival rates. In this case, it would reflect identification of unexpected occult metastases requiring adjuvant chemotherapy.

Case Table 3.1 Referral guidelines to gynecologic oncology for a newly diagnosed pelvic mass

Premenopausal (<50 years)
(a) CA-125 levels >200 U/mL
(b) Ascites
(c) Evidence of abdominal or distant metastases (by examination or imaging study)
(d) Family history of breast or ovarian cancer (in a first-degree relative)

Postmenopausal (≥50 years)
(a) Elevated CA-125 levels
(b) Ascites
(c) Nodular or fixed pelvic mass
(d) Evidence of abdominal or distant metastases (by examination or imaging study)
(e) Family history of breast or ovarian cancer (in a first-degree relative)

See Chapters 1, 10, 16, and 33.

Case 4: Amenorrhea

1 Primary amenorrhea is the absence of menstruation by age 16. This patient is considered to have *secondary amenorrhea* – defined as cessation of an established menstruation for 3 months in a woman with a history of regular cycles, but now without menses.

2 The initial priority is to make sure that she is not pregnant. Once that has been ruled out, a detailed history of reproductive events leading up to the occurrence of amenorrhea is obtained. General questions about health and lifestyle may identify a history of systemic illness or any pattern of excessive stress (physical, psychological, or nutritional) that could affect hypothalamic function. A history of past and/or present use of medication – particularly oral contraceptives or other types of hormonal contraception (Depo-Provera) – can be very illuminating.

The patient's overall body habitus, height, and weight should be determined. This may reveal very low body weight (decreased percentage of body fat) associated with hypothalamic amenorrhea, or upper body segment obesity (truncal obesity), often associated with insulin resistance and hyperandrogenism. The presence of hirsutism would indicate the possibility of polycystic ovarian syndrome (PCOS), or less likely an adrenal or ovarian androgen-producing tumor if progression is rapid or associated with virilization. A rapid pulse may suggest hyperthyroidism, whereas a slow pulse may indicate the possibility of hypothyroidism. Signs of Graves disease, such as exophthalmos, lid retraction, or tremor would suggest thyroid dysfunction, as would a palpable goiter or other nodule.

Initially, the simplest panel would be FSH (follicle-stimulating hormone), TSH (thyroid-stimulating hormone), and prolactin.

3 This patient does not have evidence for thyroid dysfunction or prolactinoma. She has a normal reproductive tract and either too much unopposed estrogen or not enough. Administration of progestin for a week to induce withdrawal bleeding could be the next step. If she does not have bleeding, then an estrogen/progesterone challenge would be helpful in differentiating between a structural problem (eg, Asherman syndrome) and hypogonadotropic hypogonadism (eg, Sheehan syndrome). A "positive" withdrawal bleed after progestin therapy would suggest PCOS or some type of hypothalamic dysfunction. She appears to have eugonadotropic hypogonadism – most likely to be PCOS. However, to make a more definitive diagnosis, a panel of testosterone, DHEA (dehydroepiandrosterone), and 17-hydroxyprogesterone would be helpful.

4 Oral contraceptives are very effective agents in the long-term management of PCOS. They break the cycle through suppression of pituitary LH (luteinizing hormone) secretion, suppression of ovarian androgen secretion, and increased production of circulating sex hormone-binding globulin (SHBG). Oral contraceptives are also associated with a reduction in the risk of endometrial cancer. Alternatively, cyclic progestin therapy is an option. Metformin and other insulin-sensitizing agents have been explored, but are currently unproven therapeutic options.

5 Yes – obesity contributes substantially to reproductive and metabolic abnormalities in women with PCOS. Weight loss can improve the fundamental aspects of the endocrine syndrome by decreasing circulating androgen levels and causing spontaneous resumption of menses. Other benefits include decreased circulating testosterone levels largely mediated through increases in SHBG. In addition, weight loss can result in significant improvement in the risk of diabetes and cardiovascular disease. Lifestyle modification (diet and exercise) should be promoted as the main primary treatment for all obese women with PCOS.

See Chapters 22 and 23.

Case 5: Endometrial cancer

1 Any episode of postmenopausal bleeding should prompt the physician to consider the diagnosis of endometrial cancer. It is the most common malignancy of the reproductive organs: women have a 2% lifetime risk. Fortunately, most etiologies of postmenopausal bleeding will have a benign etiology. Endometrial polyps are most common, but atrophic vaginitis, trauma, or other lesions of the genital tract (eg, urethral prolapse) may be identified.

2 Initially, a careful history may provide a sense of the duration, amount, and consistency of the bleeding. When "bleeding" consists only of pinkish staining on toilet paper noted on wiping, then it may suggest a benign estrogen-deficient diagnosis. In this patient, having heavier bleeding similar to her "period" is more concerning. A careful pelvic examination is required to rule out a vulvar cancer, vaginal trauma, cervical lesion, or some other obvious cause. An endometrial biopsy (see Chapter 4) should be performed to make the diagnosis. If the results are equivocal, a transvaginal ultrasound may be helpful, but dilation and curettage with diagnostic hysteroscopy may also be required.

3 The vast majority of patients should undergo systematic surgical staging with pelvic washings, hysterectomy, bilateral salpingo-oophorectomy, and bilateral pelvic and para-aortic lymphadenectomy. Increasingly, minimally invasive laparoscopic surgery or robotic-assisted surgery has replaced open laparotomy for treatment of this malignancy.

Rarely, young women with grade 1 endometrioid adenocarcinoma associated with atypical endometrial hyperplasia, who wish to preserve fertility, may be treated with high-dose progestins. Women at increased risk of mortality secondary to comorbidities can be treated primarily by radiation.

Preoperatively, only a physical examination and a chest radiograph are required for the clinical stage I patient with usual (grade 1 endometrioid) histology.

Case Table 5.1 Criteria for referral to gynecologic oncologist

- The ability to completely and adequately surgically stage the patient is not readily available at the time of the initial procedure
- Preoperative histology (grade 3, papillary serous, clear cell, carcinosarcoma) suggests a high risk for extrauterine spread
- The final pathology result reveals an unexpected endometrial cancer after hysterectomy performed for other indications
- There is evidence for cervical or extrauterine disease
- The pelvic washings are positive for malignant cells
- Recurrent disease is diagnosed or suspected
- Non-surgical therapy is contemplated

---

4 This patient would be assigned as a stage IB, grade 13 endometrial cancer. Her surgical–pathologic findings are considered to be "intermediate risk." Most clinicians would refer her for consideration of vaginal brachytherapy to reduce her risk of local relapse.

5 Monitoring for recurrent endometrial cancer depends on the stage and treatment of the original diagnosis. Routine Pap tests have not proven that helpful during follow-up visits, are not cost-effective, and are probably not necessary. For those women who have not received radiation therapy, pelvic examinations every 3–4 months for 2 years, then twice-yearly after surgical treatment of endometrial cancer, are recommended.
See Chapters 4 and 32.

Case 6: Preterm labor

1 Labor is a clinical diagnosis that includes two elements: (1) regular phasic uterine contractions increasing in frequency and intensity, and (2) progressive cervical effacement and dilation. Preterm (premature) labor refers to labor occurring before 37 weeks' gestation. It is not possible to make a diagnosis of preterm labor in this patient, because – although she is experiencing regular uterine contractions – her cervix is long and closed.

2 Of preterm births 20% are iatrogenic, meaning that obstetric care providers recommend delivery for either maternal or fetal indications,

including pre-eclampsia, placenta previa, placental abruption, and diabetes. The remainder are due to preterm labor, which represents a syndrome rather than a diagnosis because the etiologies are varied. The major causes of preterm labor include intra-amniotic infection/inflammation (20–30%) and preterm premature rupture of membranes (PROM; 30%). Of preterm labors 30–50% have no known cause and are regarded as spontaneous (idiopathic) preterm labors.

3 This woman is at high risk of preterm delivery. Screening tests currently available for the prediction of preterm birth fall into four broad categories:

(a) *Home uterine activity monitoring.* Although uterine contractions are a prerequisite for preterm labor, home uterine activity monitoring does not reduce the incidence of preterm birth and, as such, is not recommended.

(b) *Risk factor scoring.* A number of risk factors for preterm labor have been identified (listed below). However, reliance on risk factor scoring alone will fail to identify over 50% of pregnancies that deliver preterm (low sensitivity) and most women designated "at risk" will deliver at term (low positive predictive value [PPV]).

Case Table 6.1 Risk factors for preterm labor

- Prior preterm birth
- African-American race
- Age <18 or >40 years
- Poor nutrition
- Anemia
- Low pre-pregnancy weight
- Low socioeconomic status
- Absent prenatal care
- Bacteriuria/urinary tract infection
- Genital and/or gingival disease
- Cigarette smoking
- Cervical injury or anomaly
- Uterine anomaly or fibroids
- Excessive uterine activity
- Premature cervical dilation (>21 cm) and/or effacement (>80%)
- Overdistended uterus (twins, polyhydramnios)
- ? Vaginal bleeding
- ?? Strenuous work
- ?? High personal stress

(c) *Assessment of cervical maturation.* Transvaginal ultrasound is the "gold standard" for the measurement of cervical length. A strong inverse correlation exists between residual cervical length and preterm birth. The mean cervical length at 22–24 weeks' gestation is 3.5 cm (10th to 90th percentile: 2.5–4.5 cm). A cervical length of ≤1.5 cm at 22–24 weeks occurs in <2% of low-risk women, but is predictive of delivery before 28 and 32 weeks in 60% and 90% of cases, respectively.

(d) *Biochemical/endocrine markers.* A number of biochemical/endocrine markers have been associated with preterm delivery, including, but not limited to, activin, inhibin, follistatin, fibronectin, collagenase, progesterone, and estradiol-17β. To date, only fetal fibronectin (fFN) is established and approved by the US Food and Drug Administration (FDA) as a screening test for preterm birth. Elevated levels of fFN (>50 ng/mL) in cervicovaginal secretions at 22–34 weeks are associated with premature birth, although the PPV of a positive fFN test at 22–24 weeks, for spontaneous preterm birth before 28 weeks and 37 weeks, is only 13% and 36%, respectively. The primary value of this test therefore lies in its negative predictive value (NPV): 99.9% of patients with a negative fFN test will not deliver within 7 days and 98% will still be pregnant in 14 days. Fortunately, 80% of high-risk symptomatic patients will have a negative fFN.

4 In many instances, premature labor represents a necessary escape of the fetus from a hostile intrauterine environment. As such, aggressive intervention to stop labor in such cases may be counterproductive. *Absolute contraindications* to tocolytic therapy include non-reassuring fetal testing (previously referred to as "fetal distress"), chorioamnionitis, intrauterine fetal demise, a lethal fetal structural anomaly or chromosomal defect (such as trisomy 13 or 18), and any maternal condition precluding expectant management (such as severe pre-eclampsia). *Relative contraindications* include unexplained vaginal bleeding, preterm PROM, and a favorable gestational age (commonly defined as >34 weeks).

5 Bed rest is recommended in 20% of all pregnancies with an estimated cost of >US$250 million per year in the USA alone. There is no proven benefit to bed rest in women at risk for preterm labor. Intravenous hydration is also commonly recommended, but without proven benefit.

6 There are two reasons to administer antibiotics to women at imminent risk of preterm birth:

(a) *Antibiotics to prevent preterm birth.* Broad-spectrum antibiotic administration in the setting of preterm PROM <34 weeks' gestation has been shown to prolong latency, delay preterm birth, and improve short-term perinatal outcome. However, there is no consistent evidence of prolonged latency in the setting of preterm labor with intact membranes. As such, antibiotics for this indication are not recommended.

(b) *Chemoprophylaxis against group B β-hemolytic streptococcal (GBS) infection.* Premature neonates are at increased risk of early onset neonatal GBS sepsis. As such, all women at imminent risk of preterm delivery should receive intrapartum GBS chemoprophylaxis. If such a woman has had a negative GBS perineal culture within the previous 5 weeks, GBS prophylaxis can be withheld. In this case, a perineal GBS culture should be sent and GBS chemoprophylaxis initiated immediately (intravenous penicillin 5 mU loading dose followed by 2.5 mU 4-hourly until delivery). If the episode of preterm labor stabilizes and continued expectant management is recommended, then GBS chemoprophylaxis can be stopped and restarted in labor, depending on the result of GBS culture.

7 Pharmacologic tocolytic therapy has been the cornerstone of modern management for preterm labor. However, there are no reliable and consistent data that any tocolytic agent can delay delivery for longer than 24–48 hours. As such, the goal of tocolysis is to delay delivery for 48 hours to allow administration of a full course of antenatal corticosteroids and the patient to be transferred to a tertiary care center. A number of agents are now available for short-term tocolysis (listed below). No single tocolytic agent has a clear therapeutic advantage. As such, the side-effect profile of each of the drugs will often determine which to use in a given clinical setting. Nifedipine (a calcium channel blocker) or magnesium sulfate is commonly used as a first-line agent in the USA, whereas oxytocin receptor antagonists (such as atosiban) are used more commonly in Europe. Magnesium sulfate has the added advantage of being neuroprotective in infants born <32 weeks' gestation. Prostaglandin synthesis inhibitors (such as indomet-

acin), although very effective in delaying preterm birth, have been associated with a number of serious neonatal complications, especially if given shortly before delivery. The only agent that is FDA approved in the USA for the treatment of preterm labor is the β-adrenergic agonist, ritodrine hydrochloride; unfortunately, this drug is no longer marketed in North America because it is too dangerous to administer to pregnant women.

Case Table 6.2 Options for short-term tocolytic therapy

Tocolytic agent	Route of administration (dosage)		Efficacy[a]
Magnesium sulfate	IV (4–6 g bolus, then 2–3 g/h infusion)		Effective
β-Adrenergic agonists			
– Terbutaline sulfate	IV (2 μg/min infusion, maximum 80 μg/min)	SC (0.25 mg every 20 min)	Effective
– Ritodrine hydrochloride		IV (50 μg/min infusion, maximum 350 μg/min)	Effective
		IM (5–10 mg every 2–4 h)	Effective
Prostaglandin inhibitors			
– Indometacin	Oral (25–50 mg every 4–6 h)	Rectal (100 mg every 12 h)	Effective
Calcium channel blockers			
– Nifedipine	Oral (20–30 mg every 4–8 h)		Effective
Oxytocin antagonists			
– Atosiban	IV (1 μmol/L per min infusion, maximum 32 μmol/L per min)		Effective
Others			
– Ethanol	(historical interest only)		
– Nitroglycerin	TD (10–50 mg daily)	IV (100 μg bolus, 1–10 μg/kg per min infusion)	Effective Unproven Unproven

[a]Efficacy is defined as proven benefit in delaying delivery by 24–48 hours compared with placebo or standard control.
IM, intramuscular; IV, intravenous; SC, subcutaneous; TD, three times daily.

8 There is increasing evidence that progesterone supplementation – not treatment – from 16–20 weeks through 34–36 weeks may reduce the rate of preterm birth and improve short-term perinatal outcome in some high-risk women, specifically women with a history of a prior unexplained preterm birth and women with cervical shortening

(<1.5 cm at 22–24 weeks). Recent studies suggest that multiple pregnancies are not likely to benefit from progesterone supplementation. Note that this is progesterone prophylaxis in women at high risk, not treatment with progesterone in women who present in preterm labor. See Chapters 57 and 42.

Case 7: Preterm PROM

1 Premature rupture of membranes (PROM) is defined as rupture of membranes before the onset of labor (uterine contractions) and can occur at any gestational age. Preterm PROM (PPROM) refers to PROM <37 weeks' gestation. Specific risk factors in this case include a history of a connective tissue disease (SLE), use of chronic steroids, and first- and second-trimester bleeding. Other risk factors that should be asked about include prior PPROM (recurrence risk is 20–30% compared with 4% in women with a prior uncomplicated delivery), placental abruption (may account for 10–15% of PPROM), a history of cervical insufficiency, cervicovaginal infection or chorioamnionitis, amniocentesis or chorionic villous sampling, cigarette smoking, multiple gestation, polyhydramnios, *in utero* diethylstilbestrol (DES) exposure, anemia, and demographic factors (such as low socioeconomic class and unmarried status). Factors that are known *not* to be associated with PPROM include coitus, cervical examinations, maternal exercise, and parity.

2 PROM is a *clinical* diagnosis. It is usually suggested by a history of watery vaginal discharge, and confirmed on sterile speculum examination by finding a pool of vaginal fluid that has an alkaline pH (it turns yellow nitrazine paper blue) and demonstrates microscopic ferning on drying. Findings of diminished amniotic fluid volume on ultrasound may further suggest the diagnosis. However, normal amniotic fluid volume on ultrasound does not exclude the diagnosis. If equivocal, transabdominal instillation of dye into the amniotic cavity (indigo carmine rather than methylene blue because of the association of methylene blue dye with methemoglobinemia) and documentation of leakage of dye into the vagina by staining of a tampon within 20–30 min will confirm the diagnosis. However, this amnio/dye test ("tampon test") is rarely performed because of the risks of amniocentesis, which includes PPROM.

3 Your differential diagnosis should include urinary incontinence, vaginal discharge or infection, cervical mucus, and a "show" (early labor).

4 *Neonatal complications* are related primarily to prematurity. PPROM is associated with a fourfold increase in perinatal mortality and a threefold increase in neonatal morbidity, including respiratory distress syndrome (RDS), intra-amniotic infection (occurs in 15–30% of women with PPROM and accounts for 3–20% of neonatal deaths), and intraventricular hemorrhage (IVH). Other neonatal complications include fetal pulmonary hypoplasia (develops in 25% of PPROM <22 weeks), skeletal deformities (complicates 12% of PPROM and is related to the severity and duration of PPROM), cord prolapse (especially if non-vertex presentation), and increased cesarean section delivery (for malpresentation). Placental abruption is associated with PPROM in 10–15% of cases; whether it is a cause or a result of PPROM is unclear.

Maternal complications include chorioamnionitis (occurs in 15–30% of women with PPROM compared with 1% at term) and postpartum endometritis.

5 Yes. She has no evidence of non-reassuring fetal testing ("fetal distress"), unstoppable preterm labor, unexplained bleeding, intra-amniotic infection (chorioamnionitis), and she is not at a favorable gestational age (>34 weeks). However, the likelihood of this woman going into labor within 24–48 hours and 7 days is 50% and 70–90%, respectively. As intra-amniotic infection/inflammation is a major cause of PPROM, amniocentesis should be considered to exclude subclinical infection. Laboratory values consistent with infection include evidence of bacteria on Gram stain or culture, glucose <20 mg/dL, white blood cell count (WBC) >100 cells/mm^3, and lactate dehydrogenase (LDH) ≥400 U/L.

6 Yes. Both the American Congress of Obstetricians and Gynecologists (ACOG) and the National Institutes of Health (NIH) recommend administration of a single course of antenatal steroids in a patient with PPROM <32 weeks' gestation to decrease RDS, necrotizing enterocolitis (NEC), and IVH by approximately 50%.

7 When managing patients with PPROM, obstetric care providers have to weigh the risk of prematurity against the risk of expectant management, primarily ascending infection. As such, the management of PPROM should be individualized. In general, PPROM is a relative contraindication to the use of tocolytic agents. Tocolysis may be able to delay delivery by 1–2 days, but does not appear to improve perinatal morbidity or mortality, and may be associated with increased incidence of maternal and neonatal infectious morbidity. Prophylactic broad-spectrum antibiotics have been shown to prolong latency in the setting of PPROM, but it is unclear whether this translates into an improvement in perinatal outcome or whether antibiotics can prevent intra-amniotic infection. Several broad-spectrum antibiotic regimens have been studied and there is currently no evidence to recommend one regimen over another. Delivery is recommended immediately if there is evidence of intra-amniotic infection (chorioamnionitis), excessive unexplained vaginal bleeding, non-reassuring fetal testing ("fetal distress"), preterm labor, or once a favorable gestational age has been reached (>34 weeks).

See Chapter 59.

Case 8: Post-term pregnancy

1 The mean duration of pregnancy is 40 weeks (280 days) dated from the first day of the last normal menstrual period (LMP). "Term" refers to the period from 37 weeks to 42 weeks of gestation. Post-term (prolonged) pregnancy is defined as a gestational age of ≥42.0 weeks (≥294 days) dated from the LMP. The incidence of post-term pregnancy depends on the population mix (including percentage of primigravid women, women with pregnancy complications, and incidence of preterm birth) and on local practice patterns (such as the rate of elective cesarean section delivery and routine labor induction). Overall, approximately 10% (range 3–14%) of low-risk singleton pregnancies continue beyond 42 weeks' gestation and 4% (2–7%) will continue beyond 43 weeks in the absence of obstetric intervention. A policy of routine dating ultrasound examination at the first prenatal visit (as is commonly done in Europe but not the USA) will substantially decrease the incidence of post-term pregnancy.

2 Risk factors for post-term pregnancy include primiparity and prior post-term pregnancy. In rare instances, post-term pregnancy may be associated with placental sulfatase deficiency or fetal anencephaly (in the absence of polyhydramnios). However, most post-term pregnancies have no known cause.

3 Accurate pregnancy dating is critical to the diagnosis of post-term pregnancy. Gestational age can be regarded as accurate if two or more of the following criteria are present:

Case Table 8.1 Confirmation of gestational age

Clinical criteria
- ≥39.0 weeks have elapsed since the LMP in a woman with a regular menstrual cycle and no immediate antecedent use of oral contraceptives
- Fetal heart tones have been documented for ≥20 weeks by non-electronic fetoscope or for ≥30 weeks by Doppler ultrasound

Laboratory criteria
- ≥36 weeks have elapsed since a positive (serum βhCG) pregnancy test
- Ultrasound estimation of gestational age is considered accurate if it is based on crown–rump measurements obtained at 6–11 weeks' gestation OR it is based on biparietal diameter measurements obtained before 20 weeks' gestation

4 The timely onset of labor and delivery is a critical determinant of perinatal outcome. Post-term pregnancy is associated with a significant increase in perinatal morbidity and mortality. When pregnancies exceed 42 weeks, perinatal mortality (stillbirths plus early neonatal deaths) increases to 4–7 per 1,000 deliveries compared with 2–3 per 1,000 deliveries at 40 weeks. Perinatal mortality at 43 weeks is fourfold higher than that at 40 weeks, and is five- to sevenfold higher at 44 weeks.

Fetal morbidity is also increased after 42 weeks. Post-term infants are on average larger than term infants (around 2.5–10% of fetuses delivered after 42 weeks exceed 4,500 g in weight compared with 0.8–1% at 40 weeks) and, as such, are predisposed to complications associated with fetal macrosomia, including prolonged labor, cephalopelvic disproportion, and shoulder dystocia with resultant neurologic injury. Moreover, 20–40% of post-term fetuses suffer from "fetal dysmaturity (postmaturity) syndrome" with evidence of IUGR (intrauterine growth restriction) secondary to chronic uteroplacental insufficiency. Such pregnancies are at increased risk of umbilical cord compression, non-reassuring fetal testing, meconium aspiration, short-term neonatal complications (including hypoglycemia and seizures), and long-term neurologic sequelae.

At 1 and 2 years of age, the general intelligence quotient (IQ), physical milestones, and frequency of intercurrent illnesses is the same for normal term infants and those from uncomplicated prolonged pregnancies.

5 Although much of the focus of post-term pregnancy has been on the fetus, studies have shown that post-term pregnancy also poses significant risk to the mother (see below).

Case Table 8.2 Maternal risks of post-term pregnancy

Maternal complication	Incidence (%)
Labor dystocia	9–12 (versus 2–7 at term)
Cesarean section delivery	1.5- to 2-fold increase
Severe perineal trauma	3.3 (versus 2.6 at term)
Postpartum hemorrhage	10 (versus 8 at term)

6 In the past, the American Congress of Obstetricians and Gynecologists (ACOG) has recommended induction of labor for well-dated low-risk pregnancy sometime during week 43 of gestation. More recently, however, the ACOG has been unwilling to describe any specific upper limit of gestational age for expectantly managed pregnancies. The decision of whether or not to proceed with induction of labor should be made together with the patient, and should take into account such factors as precise gestational age, fetal wellbeing, amniotic fluid volume, and the degree of dilation and effacement of the cervix. Most practitioners now routinely offer induction of labor at 41 weeks' gestation and few will allow pregnancy to continue beyond 42 weeks.

7 Given that the decision has been made to continue expectant management of this low-risk pregnancy at 41 weeks' gestation, antepartum fetal surveillance should probably be initiated. Despite universal acceptance of antepartum fetal testing in post-term pregnancies (>42 weeks), there is insufficient evidence to show that it significantly improves perinatal outcome or that there is any benefit to routine fetal testing at 40–42 weeks' gestation. Moreover, no single antenatal surveillance protocol for monitoring fetal wellbeing in post-term pregnancy appears to be superior to any other. Most authorities recommend twice-weekly fetal non-stress testing, biophysical profile, and/or ultrasound with amniotic fluid estimation. Delivery should be effected immediately if there is evidence of fetal compromise or oligohydramnios.

See Chapters 52, 60, and 62.

Case 9: Gestational diabetes

1 GDM refers to any form of glucose intolerance with the onset of pregnancy or first recognized during pregnancy, and complicates approximately 5% of all pregnancies. It likely includes some women who have undiagnosed pregestational diabetes.

2 Patients with GDM are typically asymptomatic. There is a small cohort of pregnant women in whom routine screening for GDM is not cost-effective. These are women under age 25 who have normal body mass index (BMI $<25\,kg/m^2$), no first-degree relatives with diabetes, no risk factors (such as a history of GDM, insulin resistance/PCOS [polycystic ovarian syndrome], a prior macrosomic infant, a prior unexplained late fetal demise, and women with persistent glycosuria), and who are not members of ethnic or racial groups with a high prevalence of diabetes (such as Hispanic, Native American, Asian, or African–American). As such patients are rare, most experts and organizations recommend screening for GDM in all pregnant women. The ideal time to screen for GDM is 24–28 weeks of gestation. For women at high risk of developing GDM (listed above), early screening for GDM is recommended at the first prenatal visit. If the early screen is negative, it should be repeated at 24–28 weeks.

3 The most common screening test for GDM is the glucose load test (GLT) – also known as the glucose challenge test (GCT) – which is a non-fasting 50-g oral glucose challenge followed by a venous plasma glucose measurement at 1 hour. Most authorities consider the GLT to be positive if the 1-hour glucose measurement is >140 mg/dL. Use of a lower cut-off (such as >130 mg/dL) will increase the detection rate of women with GDM, but will result in a substantial increase in the false-positive rate.

There is no GLT cut-off that should be regarded as diagnostic of GDM. A definitive diagnosis of GDM requires a 3-hour glucose tolerance test (GTT). In pregnancy, the GTT involves 3 days of carbohydrate loading followed by a 100-g oral glucose challenge after an overnight fast. Venous plasma glucose is measured fasting and at 1 hour, 2 hours, and 3 hours. Although there is agreement that two or more abnormal values are required to confirm the diagnosis, there is little consensus about the glucose values that define the upper range of normal in pregnancy (see below). Most institutions use the National Diabetes Data Group (NDDG) or Carpenter and Coustan cut-offs. Measurement of glycated hemoglobin (HbA1c) levels is not useful in making the diagnosis of GDM, although it may be useful in the diagnosis of pregestational diabetes.

Case Table 9.1 Diagnostic threshold for GDM during 100-g GTT

| | Plasma glucose values (mg/dL) (mmol/L)[a] | | |
	NDDG	Sacks et al.	Carpenter and Coustan
Fasting	105 (5.8)	96 (5.3)	95 (5.2)
1-hour	190 (10.6)	172 (9.4)	180 (9.9)
2-hour	165 (9.2)	152 (8.3)	155 (8.6)
3-hour	145 (8.1)	131 (7.2)	140 (7.7)

[a]Values in parentheses are mmol/L.

4 GDM poses little risk to the mother. Such women are not at risk of diabetic ketoacidosis (DKA), which is primarily a disease of absolute insulin deficiency. However, GDM has been associated with an increase in infant birth trauma and perinatal morbidity and mortality. The risk to the fetus/infant is directly related to its size. Fetal macrosomia is defined as an estimated fetal weight (not birthweight) of ≥4,500 g. It is a single cut-off that is unrelated to gestational age, the sex of the baby, or the presence or absence of diabetes, or to the actual birthweight.

The goal of antepartum treatment of GDM is to prevent fetal macrosomia and its resultant complications by maintaining maternal blood glucose at desirable levels throughout gestation, defined as a fasting glucose level <95 mg/dL and 1-hour postprandial level <140 mg/dL. Initial recommendations should include a diabetic diet (36 kcal/kg or 15 kcal/lb of ideal body weight plus 100 kcal per trimester given as 40–50% carbohydrate, 20% protein, and 30–40% fat to avoid protein catabolism), moderate exercise, daily home glucose monitoring, and weekly antepartum visits to monitor glycemic control. If diet alone does not maintain blood glucose at desirable levels, hypoglycemic therapy may be required. If initial fasting glucose levels are >95 mg/dL, treatment can be started immediately because "you can't diet more than fasting."

Insulin (which has to be given several times a day by injection) remains the "gold standard" for the medical management of GDM. The use of oral hypoglycemic agents has traditionally been avoided in pregnancy because of concerns over fetal teratogenesis and prolonged neonatal hypoglycemia. However, recent studies suggest that second-generation hypoglycemic agents (glyburide, glipizide) do not cross the placenta, are safe in pregnancy, and can achieve adequate glycemic control in 85% of pregnancies complicated by GDM.

5 As noted above, the complications of GDM are related primarily to fetal macrosomia, including an increased risk of cesarean section delivery, operative vaginal delivery, and birth injury to both the mother (vaginal, perineal, and rectal trauma) and fetus (including orthopedic and neurologic injury). Shoulder dystocia with resultant brachial plexus injury (Erb's palsy) is a serious consequence of fetal macrosomia, and further increased in the setting of GDM because the macrosomia of diabetes is associated with increased diameters in the upper thorax of the fetus.

The use of elective cesarean section delivery to reduce the risk of maternal and fetal birth injury in the setting of fetal macrosomia remains controversial. According to current ACOG guidelines, an elective cesarean section delivery at or after 39 weeks' gestation should be recommended for all non-diabetic women who have a fetus with an estimated fetal weight (EFW) ≥5,000 g (or ≥4,500 g in a diabetic individual) to minimize the risk of birth trauma. Furthermore, it is recommended that a discussion be held about the safest route of delivery with non-diabetic women who have a fetus with an EFW ≥4,500 g (or ≥4,000 g in a diabetic individual) and that this discussion be documented in the medical record.

6 If the patient declines elective cesarean section delivery, spontaneous labor should be awaited. Induction of labor for so-called "impending macrosomia" does not decrease the risk of cesarean section delivery or intrapartum complications, and is therefore not routinely recommended. If she is still undelivered at 41 weeks' gestation, she should be counseled again about induction of labor and/or elective cesarean section.

During labor, maternal glucose levels should be maintained at 100–120 mg/dL to minimize the risk of intrapartum fetal hypoxic–ischemic injury. Continuous fetal monitoring is recommended throughout labor and the progress of labor should be carefully charted. Internal monitors such as an intrauterine pressure catheter (IUPC) and/or fetal scalp electrode can be used, if indicated. Neonatal blood glucose levels should be measured within 1 hour of birth and early feeding encouraged.

Delivery of the fetus and placenta effectively removes the source of the anti-insulin (counter-regulatory) hormones that cause GDM. As such, no further management is required in the immediate postpartum period. A 2-hour non-pregnant GTT should be performed at 6–8 weeks postpartum in all women with GDM to exclude pre-gestational diabetes.
See Chapter 45.

Case 10: Pre-eclampsia

1 Pre-eclampsia (gestational proteinuric hypertension) is defined as new-onset significant hypertension and proteinuria after 20 weeks' gestation. The correct technique to measure blood pressure (BP) in pregnancy is in the sitting position at rest for at least 5 minutes using an appropriate size BP cuff placed on the upper arm at the level of the heart and using the fifth Korotkoff sound (disappearance) to designate the diastolic BP. Significant hypertension refers to a sustained elevation in BP of ≥140 mmHg systolic and/or ≥90 mmHg diastolic in a previously normotensive parturient. Of note, an increase over the pregnancy in systolic BP of ≥30 mmHg and/or diastolic BP of ≥30 mmHg and ≥15 mmHg, respectively, is no longer sufficient to make the diagnosis. Significant proteinuria refers to a new finding of ≥1+ protein on urine dipstick or, more objectively, ≥300 mg protein in a 24-hour urine collection.

The original definition of pre-eclampsia included non-dependent edema (ie, swelling of the hands and face), but this is no longer a prerequisite for the diagnosis.

The diagnosis of pre-eclampsia should be made only after 20 weeks' gestation. Evidence of gestational proteinuric hypertension before 20 weeks' gestation should raise the possibility of an underlying molar pregnancy, drug withdrawal, antiphospholipid antibody syndrome, or (rarely) a chromosomal abnormality in the fetus.

2 Once a diagnosis of pre-eclampsia has been made, the patient should be allocated to one of two categories: "mild" or "severe" pre-eclampsia. There is no category of "moderate" pre-eclampsia. *Mild pre-eclampsia* includes all women with a diagnosis of pre-eclampsia, but without features of severe disease. *Severe pre-eclampsia* refers to women who meet the diagnostic criteria for pre-eclampsia and have one or more of the criteria listed below. Note that only one of the listed criteria is required for the patient to be assigned to the severe category.

Case Table 10.1 Features of "severe" pre-eclampsia

Symptoms
- Symptoms of central nervous system dysfunction (blurred vision, scotomas, altered mental status, and/or severe headache)
- Symptoms of liver capsule distention (right upper quadrant and/or epigastric pain)

Signs
- Severe BP elevation (defined as BP ≥160/110 mmHg on two occasions at least 6 hours apart)
- Pulmonary edema
- Eclampsia (generalized seizures and/or unexplained coma)
- Cerebrovascular accident (stroke)
- Fetal intrauterine growth restriction (IUGR)

Laboratory findings
- Proteinuria (>5 g/24 h)
- Renal failure or oliguria (<500 mL/24 h)
- Hepatocellular injury (serum transaminase levels two or more times normal)
- Thrombocytopenia (<100,000 platelets/mm^3)
- Coagulopathy
- HELLP (**h**emolysis, **e**levated **l**iver enzymes, **l**ow **p**latelets) syndrome

3 Pre-eclampsia is a multisystem disorder specific to human pregnancy and the puerperium. It does not occur naturally in any other animal species. More precisely, it is a disease of the placenta because it has also been described in pregnancies where there is trophoblast but no fetal tissue (complete molar pregnancies). It complicates 5–7% of all pregnancies.

The pathophysiology of pre-eclampsia remains unclear. At least six hypotheses have been proposed, including: (1) genetic imprinting; (2) immune maladaptation; (3) placental ischemia; (4) generalized endothelial dysfunction; (5) defective free fatty acid, lipoprotein, and/or lipid peroxidase metabolism; and (6) an imbalance in pro- and antiangiogenic factor expression. The primary defect appears to be a complete or partial failure of the second wave of trophoblast invasion, which is responsible for remodeling of the maternal spiral arterioles and establishment of the definitive uteroplacental circulation. This process is typically complete by 16–18 weeks' gestation. If this process is deficient (so-called "shallow endovascular invasion" of the placenta), the spiral arterioles are unable to dilate adequately to meet the demands of the growing fetoplacental unit. This leads, in turn, to placental ischemia with the release of a "toxemic factor" that damages the vasculature throughout the maternal circulation, resulting in widespread vasospasm and endothelial injury, which manifests clinically as pre-eclampsia. The blueprint for the development of pre-eclampsia

is therefore laid down early in gestation, although the clinical manifestations appear only in the latter half of pregnancy.

4 A number of risk factors for pre-eclampsia have been described (listed below). That said, it is not possible to accurately predict whether or not an individual will develop pre-eclampsia in a given pregnancy. Moreover, pre-eclampsia cannot be effectively prevented. Despite promising early studies, low-dose aspirin, dietary supplementation with elemental calcium, bed rest, sodium restriction, and/or vitamin C and E supplementation does not appear to prevent pre-eclampsia in either high- or low-risk populations.

Case Table 10.2 Risk factors for pre-eclampsia

Risk factor	Relative risk
Nulliparity	3
African–American origin	15
Extremes of age (<18 or >40 years)	3
Multiple gestation	4
Family history of pre-eclampsia (first-degree relative on the maternal or paternal side)	5
Prior history of pre-eclampsia	10–14
Chronic hypertension	10
Chronic renal disease	20
Antiphospholipid antibody syndrome	10
Diabetes mellitus	2
Collagen vascular disease (such as systemic lupus erythematosus)	2–3
Obesity	2
Angiotensinogen gene *T235*	
– homozygous	20
– heterozygous	4

5 Delivery is the only effective treatment for pre-eclampsia. It should be considered in all women with mild pre-eclampsia once a favorable gestational age has been reached (usually regarded as 36–37 weeks). Delivery is also recommended for all women with severe pre-eclampsia regardless of gestational age, with three possible exceptions:
- Severe pre-eclampsia by proteinuria alone (because the amount of protein in the urine does not correlate with maternal or perinatal outcome)
- Severe pre-eclampsia by IUGR alone remote from term with good fetal testing (although such women should be kept in hospital with daily fetal testing)
- Severe pre-eclampsia by BP criteria alone <32 weeks' gestation (a number of studies have suggested that it may be both reasonable and safe to continue the pregnancy in this setting with careful BP control and delivery at 34 weeks).

The magnitude of BP elevation is not predictive of eclampsia (defined as the occurrence of one or more generalized convulsions and/or coma in the setting of pre-eclampsia and in the absence of other neurologic conditions). Although routine use of antihypertensive medications does not change the course of pre-eclampsia for either the mother or the fetus, BP control is important to prevent maternal cerebrovascular accident (stroke), which is usually associated with a BP ≥170/120 mmHg. For this reason, antihypertensive medications can be used while affecting delivery to maintain BP <160/110 mmHg.

Once the decision has been made to proceed with delivery, the patient should be given magnesium sulfate seizure prophylaxis during labor and for 24–48 hours postpartum. If circumstances permit, antenatal corticosteroids should be administered and delivery delayed for 24–48 hours to allow them to exert their protective effect on the fetus. **6** Once the decision has been made to proceed with delivery, there is generally no proven benefit to a cesarean section, and attempted vaginal delivery is a reasonable option. That said, however, the chance of affecting a successful vaginal delivery in a woman with severe pre-eclampsia, remote from term with an unfavorable cervical examina-tion, is only 14–20%. Every effort should be made to avoid prolonged induction of labor. If there is no response to cervical ripening after 12 hours, cesarean section delivery should be considered.

Pre-eclampsia and its complications typically resolve within a few days of delivery (with the noted exception of stroke). Diuresis (>4 L/day) is the most accurate clinical indicator of resolution. Fetal prognosis depends largely on gestational age at delivery and the presence or absence of complications of prematurity (such as respiratory distress syndrome, necrotizing enterocolitis, intraventricular hemorrhage, and chronic lung disease).

See Chapter 44.

Further reading

Belfort MA, Saade GR, Foley MR, Phelan JP, Dildy GA, eds (2010) *Critical Care Obstetrics*, 5th edn. Hoboken, NJ: Wiley-Blackwell.

Cunningham FG, Leveno KJ, Bloom SL, Hauth JC, Rouse D, Sprong CY, eds (2009) *Williams Obstetrics*, 23rd edn. New York: McGraw-Hill.

Fritz MA, Speroff L, eds (2010) *Clinical Gynecologic Endocrinology and Infertility*, 8th edn. Philadelphia, PA: Lippincott-Raven.

Gabbe SG, Niebyl JR, Simpson JL, eds (2004). *Obstetrics: Normal and abnormal pregnancies*, 4th edn. New York: Churchill Livingstone.

Hoffman BL, Schorge JO, Schaffer JI, Halvorson LM, Bradshaw KD, Cunningham FG, eds (2012) *Williams Gynecology*, 2nd edn. New York: McGraw-Hill.

Karlan BY, Bristow RE, Li AJ, eds (2012) *Gynecologic Oncology: Clinical practice & surgical atlas*. New York: McGraw-Hill.

Queenan JT, Spong CY, Lockwood CJ, eds (2012) *Queenan's Management of High-Risk Pregnancy: An evidence-based approach*, 6th edn. Malden, MA: Wiley-Blackwell Publishing.

Strauss J III, Barbieri RL, eds (2009) *Yen and Jaffe's Reproductive Endocrinology: Physiology, pathophysiology, and clinical management*, 6th edn. Philadelphia, PA: Saunders-Elsevier.

Walters MD, Karram MM, eds (2006). *Urogynecology and Reconstructive Pelvic Surgery*, 3rd edn. St Louis, MO: Mosby.

Weiner CP, Buhimschi CS (2004) *Drugs for Pregnant and Lactating Women*. New York: Churchill Livingstone.

Obstetrics and Gynecology at a Glance, Fourth Edition. Errol R. Norwitz and John O. Schorge.

162 © 2013 John Wiley & Sons, Ltd. Published 2013 by John Wiley & Sons, Ltd.

Index

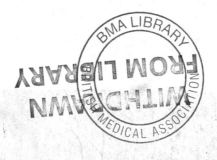